Phlebotomy

Worktext and Procedures Manual

ELSEVIER

evolve

To access your Student Resources, visit:

http://evolve.elsevier.com/Warekois/phlebotomy

Evolve® Student Resources for *Warekois: Phlebotomy: Worktext and Procedures Manual,* offer the following features:

Student Resources

- **Weblinks**
  Links to places of interest on the web specifically for phlebotomy.

- **Content Updates**
  Find out the latest information on relevant issues in the field.

Phlebotomy

Worktext and Procedures Manual

Robin S. Warekois, MT(ASCP)

VCU Health Systems/MCV
Department of Pathology
Sales Support for Outreach/Client Services
Richmond, Virginia

Richard Robinson, NASW

Sherborn, Massachusetts

Second Edition

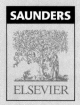

SAUNDERS

ELSEVIER

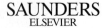

11830 Westline Industrial Drive
St. Louis, MO 63146

PHLEBOTOMY: WORKTEXT AND
PROCEDURES MANUAL

ISBN 13: 978-1-4160-0035-8
ISBN 10: 1-4160-0035-6

Notice

Knowledge and best practice in this field are constantly changing. As new research and experience broaden our knowledge, changes in practice, treatment and drug therapy may become necessary or appropriate. Readers are advised to check the most current information provided (i) on procedures featured or (ii) by the manufacturer of each product to be administered, to verify the recommended dose or formula, the method and duration of administration, and contraindications. It is the responsibility of the practitioner, relying on their own experience and knowledge of the patient, to make diagnoses, to determine dosages and the best treatment for each individual patient, and to take all appropriate safety precautions. To the fullest extent of the law, neither the Publisher nor the Authors assume any liability for any injury and/or damage to persons or property arising out of or related to any use of the material contained in this book.

Library of Congress Control Number: 2007920191

Publishing Director: Andrew Allen
Executive Editor: Loren Wilson
Developmental Editor: Ellen Wurm
Publishing Services Manager: Pat Joiner
Project Manager: Gena Magouirk
Design Direction: Julia Dummitt
Text Designer: Julia Dummitt

Printed in China

Last digit is the print number: 9 8 7 6 5 4 3 2

Acknowledgments

Many people have helped bring this new edition of *Phlebotomy: Worktext and Procedures Manual* into being, and we are in their debt. In particular, we appreciate the efforts of Dennis Tremblay and Susan Marino of Brigham and Women's Hospital, whose suggestions on safety and infection control helped improve this edition significantly. This book would not have been possible without the dedication of our two editors at Elsevier: Mindy Hutchinson, who began the project, and Ellen Wurm, who labored long to complete it. We are grateful for their patience, hard work, and devotion to this new edition. They have our deepest thanks.

Robin Warekois
Richard Robinson

Preface

The successful practice of phlebotomy requires a combination of highly skilled technique; wide knowledge of the current health care environment; and a sympathetic approach to patients of all ages, backgrounds, and medical conditions. We have designed *Phlebotomy: Worktext and Procedures Manual, Second Edition* to provide a complete introduction to the practice of phlebotomy in all its aspects. We believe its emphasis on procedures, its up-to-date and thorough professional information, and its comprehensive approach to the many situations encountered by the modern phlebotomist make it a unique and valuable offering in the field of phlebotomy training.

Who Will Benefit From This Book?

Phlebotomy: Worktext and Procedures Manual, Second Edition is suitable for phlebotomy certification programs, medical technologist and medical laboratory technician programs, medical assisting programs, and nurse training. No prior training in phlebotomy is assumed. The text may also be used by experienced phlebotomists, allied health professionals, or nurses seeking to expand or update their training in phlebotomy.

Why is This Book Important to the Profession?

Students, above all, learn by doing. Teaching phlebotomy technique is at the heart of this book, and we have therefore designed it as a worktext for both the classroom and the laboratory. Each major skill in phlebotomy, from handwashing to venipuncture to preparing a blood smear, is shown and described in step-by-step, fully illustrated procedures. We believe these will provide the student with an invaluable visual tool for understanding the essentials of the techniques before, during, and after their practical lab experience.

In addition to thorough training in the skills of phlebotomy, this text provides an introduction to development of skills beyond blood collection with a chapter on point-of-care testing. In this way, phlebotomy students can begin their training as multiskilled health professionals ready for the challenges of the modern health care workplace.

Organization

The text is divided into 5 units. Unit 1 provides an introduction and general information needed for working in a health care facility. Unit 2 covers the basics needed to study phlebotomy, from medical terminology to anatomy and physiology. Unit 3 features the various methods of specimen collection, including venipuncture, dermal puncture, arterial blood collection, and special procedures. Unit 4 presents specimen handling and processing, and Unit 5 concludes the text with a section on professional issues.

Distinctive Features and Learning Aids

Phlebotomy courses are offered in a variety of settings. *Phlebotomy: Worktext and Procedures Manual, Second Edition* provides the essential learning tools students need to succeed in each of them. Because we believe that students learn best when they know the "why" as well as the "how," we explain the reasoning behind the clinical information they must learn to become successful phlebotomists.

This approach is strengthened by key features of each chapter, including *boxes*, *tables*, and *figures*, which summarize key information and illustrate difficult concepts. Features also include those illustrated on the next three pages.

In addition to these chapter features, a comprehensive *Glossary* is found at the end of the book, along with appendices of *Spanish phrases* important in phlebotomy. Finally, a *Mock Certification Exam* provides students the opportunity to test themselves at the end of the course as they prepare for certification.

New to This Edition

A new edition offers the opportunity to both update and improve. We have taken advantage of this opportunity in *Phlebotomy: Worktext and Procedures Manual, Second Edition*. Every chapter has been reviewed and updated as needed while maintaining the approach and features that made the first edition a success.

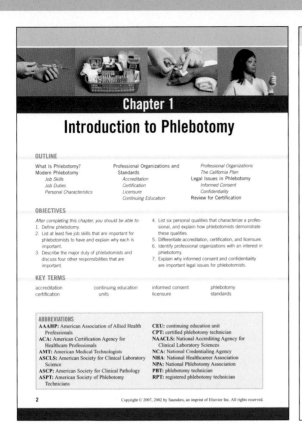

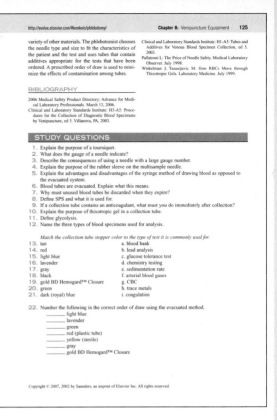

• Detailed *Objectives*, *Key Terms*, *Abbreviations*, and *Study Questions*, which serve as a study guide for the student and provide the instructor with the framework for regular assignments.

• Each major skill in phlebotomy is shown and described in step-by-step, fully illustrated *Procedures*.

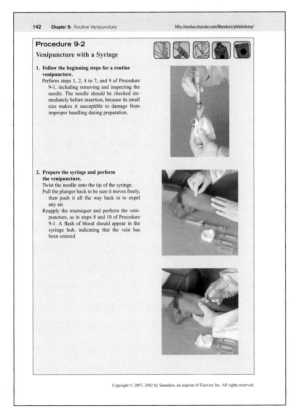

Additives: K_2 EDTA
Specimen: Plasma, whole blood

ORDER OF DRAW

Patients often need to have more than one test performed and therefore more than one tube filled. Because the same multisample needle is used to fill all the tubes, material from an earlier tube could be transferred into a later tube if it contacts the needle. Good technique can reduce this risk somewhat (discussed in more detail in the next chapter); however, it cannot eliminate it entirely. For this reason, the Clinical and Laboratory Standards Institute (CLSI) has developed a set of standards dictating the proper **order of draw** for a multitube draw. The order is the same for syringe samples as for direct filling from a multisample needle. The order-of-draw standards have undergone several revisions within the past decade, and not all institutions have adopted the most recent set of standards (termed H3-A5). It is important for you to follow the order of draw used at your institution, even if it differs from the order below.

1. Blood culture tubes (which are sterile) are drawn first. This prevents the transfer of unsterilized material from other tubes into the sterile tube.
2. Light blue-topped tubes (for coagulation tests) are next. These tubes are always drawn before tubes containing other kinds of anticoagulants, because other additives could contaminate this tube and interfere with coagulation testing.
3. Red/gray (gold BD Hemogard™) tubes and plastic red-top tubes are next. These contain clot activators, which would interfere with many other samples if passed into other tubes. Glass red-top tubes, which do not contain additives, may also be drawn now.
4. Green tubes are drawn next. The heparin from the green tube is less likely to interfere with EDTA-containing tubes than vice versa.
5. Lavender tubes are next. EDTA binds many metals in addition to calcium, so it can cause problems with many test results, including giving falsely low calcium and falsely high potassium readings. For this reason, lavender tubes are drawn near the end.
6. The gray-topped tube is last. This tube contains potassium oxalate. The potassium would elevate the potassium levels measured in electrolyte analysis, and oxalate can damage cell membranes. Also, another additive, sodium

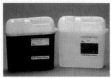

Figure 8-11
Needle disposal systems reduce the risk of accidental injury while removing the needle. (From Bonewit-West K: Clinical Procedures for Medical Assistants, ed 6. Philadelphia, Saunders, 2004.)

fluoride, elevates sodium levels and inhibits many enzymes.

Other color tubes are typically drawn after these six, but you should check the instructions on the manufacturer's package insert, and your lab procedures manual, for specific information. The glass red-top tube (but not the plastic red-top tube) may be drawn after the sterile tube, if your institution allows it.

NEEDLE DISPOSAL CONTAINERS

Once you have withdrawn the needle from the patient's arm, it must be handled with extreme care to avoid an accidental needle stick. A used needle is considered biohazardous waste and must be treated as such. Dispose of the needle and needle adapter immediately after activating the needle safety device. Needles must be placed in a clearly marked, puncture-resistant biohazard disposal container (Figure 8-11). Containers must be closable or sealable, puncture resistant, leakproof, and labeled with the correct biohazard symbol.

You must become familiar with the system in use at your workplace. Practice with a new system *before* you draw your first sample.

REVIEW FOR CERTIFICATION

The phlebotomist's tray includes tourniquets for locating veins; antiseptics and disinfectants for cleaning the puncture site; a variety of needles in different sizes, including multisample needles, syringe needles, and butterflies; needle adapters or tube holders; evacuated collection tubes; bandages; and a

• *Review for Certification* and *Certification Exam Preparation*, allowing the student to assess his or her progress toward preparedness for the certification exam.

CERTIFICATION EXAM PREPARATION

1. Which of the following is not an anticoagulant?
   a. thixotropic gel
   b. sodium heparin
   c. sodium citrate
   d. EDTA

2. The most common antiseptic used in routine venipuncture is:
   a. povidone-iodine solution
   b. bleach
   c. isopropyl alcohol
   d. chlorhexidine gluconate

3. How many times may a needle be used before discarding it?
   a. 1
   b. 2
   c. 3
   d. no limit

4. Which of the following indicates the largest-sized needle?
   a. 20 gauge
   b. 23 gauge
   c. 16 gauge
   d. 21 gauge

5. Complete blood clotting takes _____ minutes.
   a. 10 to 20
   b. 25 to 45
   c. 30 to 60
   d. 30 to 40

6. Serum contains:
   a. fibrinogen
   b. clotting factors
   c. plasma
   d. none of the above

7. Which color-coded tube does not contain any additives?
   a. red (plastic tube)
   b. red (glass tube)
   c. gold BD Hemogard™
   d. dark blue

8. EDTA prevents coagulation in the blood tubes by:
   a. inactivating thrombin
   b. binding calcium
   c. inactivating thromboplastin
   d. inhibiting glycolysis

9. Tubes with gray stoppers are used for:
   a. sedimentation rate tests
   b. glucose tolerance tests
   c. coagulation studies
   d. CBC

10. Tubes with green stoppers may contain:
    a. sodium citrate
    b. sodium heparin
    c. sodium oxalate
    d. sodium phosphate

11. The smaller the gauge number, the:
    a. larger the lumen diameter
    b. longer the needle
    c. shorter the needle
    d. smaller the lumen diameter

12. The syringe method of draw is useful for patients:
    a. who are very young
    b. who are obese
    c. who have large veins
    d. who have fragile or small veins

13. The additive sodium citrate is used in blood collection to test for:
    a. blood alcohol
    b. sedimentation rate
    c. lactic acid
    d. lead

14. The most common gauge used for a *routine* venipuncture is:
    a. 16
    b. 20
    c. 25
    d. 23

• *Flashbacks* and *Flash Forwards*, which directly link students to material they have encountered before or will cover in more depth in the future.

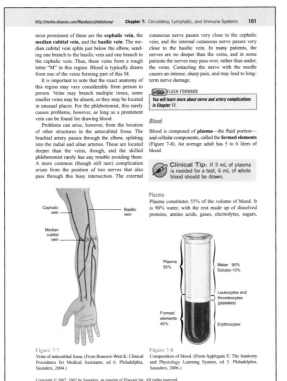

Routine venipuncture is the most common procedure a phlebotomist performs. The single most important step in venipuncture is positive identification of the patient. This is done by matching the information on the requisition with, for inpatients, the information on the patient's identification band or, for outpatients, the information provided by the patient. Although most patients are suitable candidates for drawing blood with evacuated tubes, patients with fragile veins may be better candidates for syringe collection, with the blood being transferred to evacuated tubes after the draw.

REQUISITIONS

All blood collection procedures begin with a request for a test from the treating physician. The laboratory processes this request and generates a **requisition**. The requisition is the form the phlebotomist uses to determine what type of sample to collect from the patient (Figure 9-1).

Requisitions may be computer generated or handwritten. At a minimum, the requisition has the following information:

• Patient demographics—full name, date of birth (DOB), sex, and race.

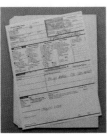

Figure 9-1
The phlebotomist uses the requisition form to determine what type of sample to collect from the patient. The requisition may be computer-generated or written by hand.

• If an inpatient, hospital identification (ID) number and room number and bed.
• Name or code of the physician making the request.
• Tests requested with the accompanying ICD-9 code.
• Test status (e.g., stat, timed, fasting).

The requisition may also contain information about the patient's status, such as potential bleeding complications or puncture sites to avoid. The number and type of tubes to collect may also be indicated. Test names may be abbreviated, so it is important to know the meaning of test abbreviations.

FLASHBACK
Most common lab tests and their abbreviations were covered in Chapters 2, 6, and 7.

The information on the requisition serves several purposes. First, it allows you to identify the patient correctly and may provide some helpful information about the patient. Second, it tells you what specimen should be collected. And third, it allows you to gather the necessary equipment for the collection before you encounter the patient. Computer-generated requisitions may also have a set of labels used for the collection tubes. The requisition may not indicate any special handling procedures, and you may be required to consult the laboratory resources to ensure both correct collection and handling of samples. For instance, a sample for a bilirubin test must always be shielded from light after collection, even though the requisition does not state this.

FLASH FORWARD
Special collection procedures are covered in Chapter 14.

The requisition may arrive in one of several ways. Requisitions for inpatients are usually picked up at either the lab or the nursing station. Outpatients typically carry their own requisitions with them. Emergency requisitions may be telephoned in to the lab; in this case, the phlebotomist picks up the form at the unit where the patient is located.

There are several steps you should perform when you receive requisitions:

• Examine them to make sure that each has all the necessary information: Full name, DOB, ordering physician, and test ICD-9 codes.
• Check for duplicates. If there are several requisitions for one patient, group them together so

• *Clinical Tips*, which offer students pearls of wisdom they can use in the clinical setting.

most prominent of these are the **cephalic vein**, the **median cubital vein**, and the **basilic vein**. The median cubital vein splits just below the elbow, sending one branch to the basilic vein and one branch to the cephalic vein. Thus, these veins form a rough letter "M" in this region. Blood is typically drawn from one of the veins forming part of this M.

It is important to note that the exact anatomy of this region may vary considerably from person to person. Veins may branch multiple times, some smaller veins may be absent, or they may be located in unusual places. For the phlebotomist, this rarely causes problems, however, as long as a prominent vein can be found for drawing blood.

Problems can arise, however, from the location of other structures in the antecubital fossa. The brachial artery passes through the elbow, splitting into the radial and ulnar arteries. These are located deeper than the veins, though, and the skilled phlebotomist rarely has any trouble avoiding them. A more common (though still rare) complication arises from the position of two nerves that also pass through this busy intersection. The external

cutaneous nerve passes very close to the cephalic vein, and the internal cutaneous nerve passes very close to the basilic vein. In many patients, the nerves are no deeper than the veins, and in some patients the nerves may pass over, rather than under, the veins. Contacting the nerve with the needle causes an intense, sharp pain, and may lead to long-term nerve damage.

FLASH FORWARD
You will learn more about nerve and artery complications in Chapter 11.

Blood

Blood is composed of **plasma**—the fluid portion—and cellular components, called the **formed elements** (Figure 7-8). An average adult has 5 to 6 liters of blood.

⟢ **Clinical Tip:** If 3 mL of plasma is needed for a test, 6 mL of whole blood should be drawn.

Plasma
Plasma constitutes 55% of the volume of blood. It is 90% water, with the rest made up of dissolved proteins, amino acids, gases, electrolytes, sugars,

Cephalic vein

Basilic vein

Median cubital vein

Plasma 55%

Water 90%
Solutes 10%

Leukocytes and thrombocytes (platelets)

Formed elements 45%

Erythrocytes

Figure 7-7
Veins of antecubital fossa. (From Bonewit-West K: Clinical Procedures for Medical Assistants, ed 6. Philadelphia, Saunders, 2004.)

Figure 7-8
Composition of blood. (From Applegate E: The Anatomy and Physiology Learning System, ed 3. Philadelphia, Saunders, 2006.)

- Most importantly, **safety protocols and equipment** have undergone significant changes since the first edition of this textbook appeared. For this edition, we have entirely revised procedures, discussions, illustrations, and guidelines throughout the book to reflect the most current guidelines from OSHA, CLSI, and other governmental and professional organizations.
- **New photography** of procedures and equipment show the latest equipment and safety practices so students receive the most current information in the field.
- **Legal issues** have also changed dramatically in the past several years, and in this new edition, we discuss patient confidentiality in light of the many changes HIPAA has brought to the health care setting. Important changes in these two areas are reflected not only throughout the text, but also in our popular *Mock Certification Exam* at the end of the book.
- The text has been updated throughout to reflect the most recent changes in the CLSI Approved Standard—Sixth Edition (H3-A6, November, 2007)

Ancillaries

For the Instructor

With the second edition, we are offering several assets.

TEACH

- **TEACH Lesson Plan Manual,** available via Evolve. The TEACH Lesson Plan Manual provides instructors with customizable lesson plans and lecture outlines based on learning objectives. With these valuable resources, instructors will save valuable preparation time and create a learning environment that fully engages students in classroom preparation. The lesson plans are keyed chapter-by-chapter and are divided into 50-minute units in a 3-column format. In addition to the lesson plans, instructors will have unique lecture outlines in PowerPoint with lecture notes, thought-provoking questions, and unique ideas for lectures.

CD

- Test bank: an ExamView test bank of approximately 600 multiple-choice questions that feature rationales, cognitive levels, and page number references to the text. The test bank can be used for class reviews, quizzes, or exams.
- Image Collection: all of the images from the book are available as .JPGs and can be downloaded into PowerPoint presentations. These can be also used during lecture to illustrate important concepts.

Evolve Website

- Test bank: an ExamView test bank of approximately 600 multiple-choice questions that feature rationales, cognitive levels, and page number references to the text. The test bank can be used for class reviews, quizzes, or exams.
- Image Collection: all of the images from the book are available as .JPGs and can be downloaded into PowerPoint presentations. These can also be used during lecture to illustrate important concepts.
- TEACH assets containing all TEACH resources.

For the Student

The following assets are available via the **Evolve Website**:

- Weblinks: links to places of interest on the web specifically for phlebotomy.
- Content Updates: the latest information on relevant issues in the field.

Procedure Photo Credits

Procedure 4-1

Steps 1, 3, 4, 5, 6 (From Kinn ME, Woods MA: The Medical Assistant: Administrative and Clinical, ed 8. Philadelphia, WB Saunders, 1999.)

Step 2 (From Chester GA: Modern Medical Assisting. Philadelphia, WB Saunders, 1999.)

Procedure 9-1

Steps 11, 12, 13, 14 (Courtesy of Zack Bent. From Garrels M, Oatis CS: Laboratory Testing for Ambulatory Settings. Philadelphia, Saunders, 2000.)

Procedure 9-2

Steps 1, 2, 3, 4, 5 (Courtesy of Zack Bent. From Garrels M, Oatis CS: Laboratory Testing for Ambulatory Settings. Philadelphia, Saunders, 2006.)

Procedure 10-1

Steps 2, 3, 5, 6, 7, 8 (Courtesy of Zack Bent. From Garrels M, Oatis CS: Laboratory Testing for Ambulatory Settings. Philadelphia, Saunders, 2006.)

Step 5 (From Bonewit-West K: Clinical Procedures for Medical Assistants, ed 6. Philadelphia, Saunders, 2004.)

Procedure 10-2

Step 1 (From Stepp CA, Woods MA: Laboratory Procedures for Medical Office Personnel. Philadelphia, WB Saunders, 1998.)

Procedure 10-3

Step 1 (Courtesy of Zack Bent. From Garrels M, Oatis CS: Laboratory Testing for Ambulatory Settings. Philadelphia, Saunders, 2006.)

Step 2 (From Chester GA: Modern Medical Assisting. Philadelphia, WB Saunders, 1998.)

Procedure 11-1

Steps 1, 4 (Courtesy of Zack Bent. From Garrels M, Oatis CS: Laboratory Testing for Ambulatory Settings. Philadelphia, Saunders, 2006.)

Steps 2, 7 (From Bonewit-West K: Clinical Procedures for Medical Assistants, ed 6. Philadelphia, Saunders, 2004.)

Procedure 13-2

Steps 3, 4 (From Potter P, Perry A: Fundamentals of Nursing, ed 6. St. Louis, Mosby, 2005.)

Step 6 (From Stepp CA, Woods MA: Laboratory Procedures for Medical Office Personnel. Philadelphia, WB Saunders, 1998.)

Procedure 14-1

Steps 1, 2, 3 (From Leahy JM, Kizilay PE: Foundations of Nursing Practice: A Nursing Process Approach. Philadelphia, WB Saunders, 1998.)

Procedure 15-1

Steps 1, 2, 3 (From Stepp CA, Woods MA: Laboratory Procedures for Medical Office Personnel. Philadelphia, WB Saunders, 1998.)

Procedure 15-2

Step 1 (From Bonewit-West K: Clinical Procedures for Medical Assistants, ed 6. Philadelphia, Saunders, 2004.)

Icons Used in This Book

The OSHA Standards must be followed when performing most of the procedures presented in this text. Icons have been incorporated into the procedures to assist in following these standards. An illustration of each icon along with its description is outlined below.

 HANDWASHING is an important medical aseptic practice and is crucial in preventing the transmission of pathogens in the medical office. The phlebotomist should wash the hands frequently, using the proper handwashing technique. When performing venipuncture procedures, the hands should always be washed before and after patient contact, before applying gloves and after removing gloves, and after contact with blood or other potentially infectious materials. An alchol-based agent may be used as a handwashing alternative and may be preferable unless the hands are visibly soiled.

 Clean disposable GLOVES should be worn when it is anticipated that you will have hand contact with blood and other potentially infectious materials, mucous membranes, and contaminated articles or surfaces.

 Appropriate PROTECTIVE CLOTHING such as gowns, aprons, and laboratory coats should be worn when gross contamination can reasonably be anticipated during performance of a task or procedure.

 FACE SHIELDS or MASKS in combination with EYE PROTECTION DEVICES must be worn whenever splashes, spray, spatter, or droplets of blood or other potentially infectious materials may be generated, posing a hazard through contact with your eyes, nose, or mouth.

 Place infectious waste in BIOHAZARD CONTAINERS that are closeable, leak-proof, and suitably constructed to contain the contents during handling, storage, transport, or shipping. The containers must be labeled or color-coded and closed before removal to prevent the contents from spilling.

 Place used disposable syringes, needles, lancets, and other sharp items in puncture-resistant SHARPS CONTAINERS located as close as practical to the area in which the items are used.

Contents

UNIT 3   Specimen Collection

UNIT 4 Specimen Handling

UNIT 5 Professional Issues

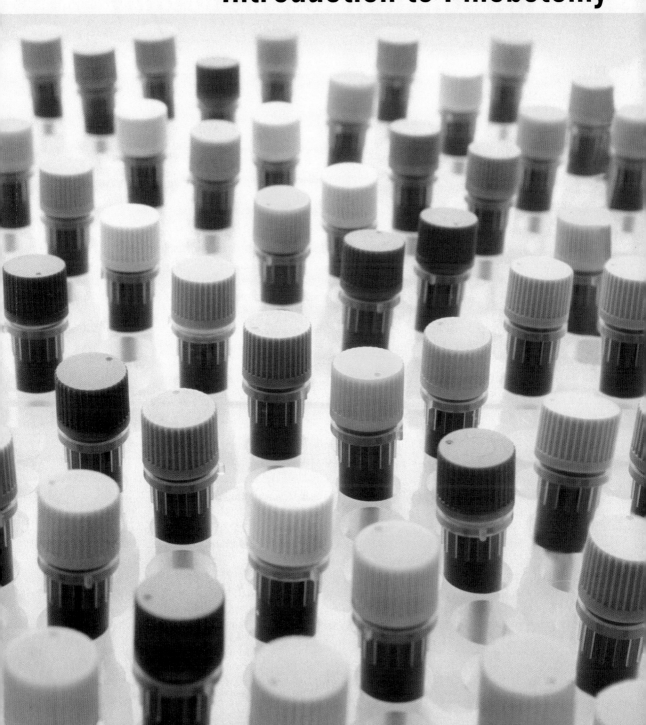

UNIT 1

Introduction to Phlebotomy

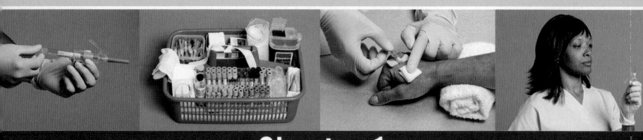

Chapter 1

Introduction to Phlebotomy

OUTLINE

What Is Phlebotomy?
Modern Phlebotomy
   Job Skills
   Job Duties
   Personal Characteristics

Professional Organizations and
   Standards
   Accreditation
   Certification
   Licensure
   Continuing Education

Professional Organizations
The California Plan
Legal Issues in Phlebotomy
   Informed Consent
   Confidentiality
Review for Certification

OBJECTIVES

After completing this chapter, you should be able to:
1. Define phlebotomy.
2. List at least five job skills that are important for phlebotomists to have and explain why each is important.
3. Describe the major duty of phlebotomists and discuss four other responsibilities that are important.
4. List six personal qualities that characterize a professional, and explain how phlebotomists demonstrate these qualities.
5. Differentiate accreditation, certification, and licensure.
6. Identify professional organizations with an interest in phlebotomy.
7. Explain why informed consent and confidentiality are important legal issues for phlebotomists.

KEY TERMS

accreditation
certification

continuing education
   units

informed consent
licensure

phlebotomy
standards

ABBREVIATIONS

AAAHP: American Association of Allied Health Professionals
ACA: American Certification Agency for Healthcare Professionals
AMT: American Medical Technologists
ASCLS: American Society for Clinical Laboratory Science
ASCP: American Society for Clinical Pathology
ASPT: American Society of Phlebotomy Technicians

CEU: continuing education unit
CPT: certified phlebotomy technician
NAACLS: National Accrediting Agency for Clinical Laboratory Sciences
NCA: National Credentialing Agency
NHA: National Healthcareer Association
NPA: National Phlebotomy Association
PBT: phlebotomy technician
RPT: registered phlebotomy technician

Phlebotomy is the practice of drawing blood. The modern phlebotomist is a trained professional with a wide variety of job skills and personal characteristics, including communication skills, organizational skills, and compassion. After initial training, the phlebotomist may become certified by one or more professional organizations. Continuing education courses keep the phlebotomist up-to-date on the latest changes in techniques and regulations in the field. The phlebotomist must also be aware of important legal issues, including patient confidentiality and informed consent.

WHAT IS PHLEBOTOMY?

Phlebotomy is the practice of drawing blood. The word phlebotomy is derived from Greek: phlebo- means vein, and -tomy means to make an incision. Phlebotomy is an ancient profession, dating back at least 3500 years to the time of the Egyptians. The earliest phlebotomists drew blood in an attempt to cure disease. In Europe during the Middle Ages,

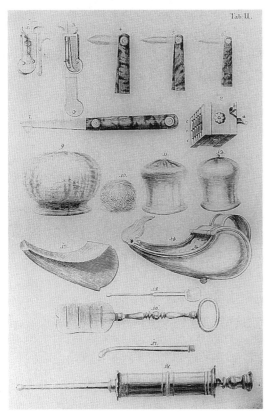

Figure 1-1
Tools of the earliest phlebotomists. (From Brambilla GA: Instrumentarium chirurgicum. Vienna, Matthias Andreas Schmidt, 1781. Courtesy U.S. National Library of Medicine, History of Medicine Division, Bethesda, MD.)

barber-surgeons performed bloodletting to balance the four humors, or bodily fluids, because an imbalance of the humors was thought to underlie disease. The familiar stripes on the barber's pole date from this period, with red symbolizing blood and white symbolizing bandages. Early phlebotomists' tools included lancets (called fleams) and suction cups (Figure 1-1), and they used ornate ceramic bowls to collect the blood. Phlebotomists also applied leeches to patients' skin for hours at a time to remove blood.

MODERN PHLEBOTOMY

Modern phlebotomy shares little more than a name with these ancient practices. Today, phlebotomy is performed primarily for diagnosis and monitoring of a patient's condition, and it involves highly developed and rigorously tested procedures and equipment to ensure the safety and comfort of the patient and the integrity of the sample collected.

Job Skills

Today's phlebotomist is highly trained and uses a wide variety of skills in the workplace. Technical skills are required to collect specimens for analysis, and developing these skills will constitute a large part of your training. A phlebotomist also needs to be highly organized and detail oriented in order to deal with the large number of samples that may be collected in a short time, while ensuring that each sample is properly labeled and correctly handled. Equally important are interpersonal skills. As a phlebotomist, you will spend a large part of your working day interacting with people, both patients and medical personnel (Figure 1-2). Another important job skill is being able to handle stress. A phlebotomist must occasionally deal with difficult patients, malfunctioning equipment, or demands for immediate action. As your technical skills increase, these situations will become less stressful, but the job will always carry some stress. Being able to cope with this in a calm, professional manner is vital to being a successful phlebotomist.

Job Duties

The principal purpose of phlebotomy is to obtain blood samples, at the request of a physician, for analysis in the laboratory. Performing these duties correctly ensures that patients receive prompt and complete medical care. Failure to perform these duties correctly can lead to significant adverse consequences for the

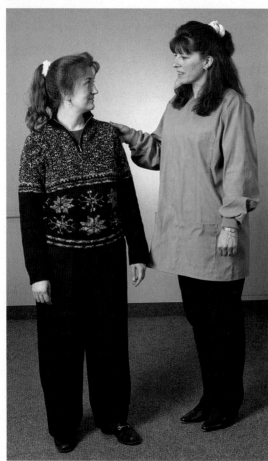

Figure 1-2
Phlebotomists spend much of the day interacting with people, and interpersonal skills are a vital part of the job.

patient, including improper care and even death. Later chapters cover the details of how to perform each step of each procedure you will be required to perform. In brief, the steps in a routine collection are:

1. Correctly and positively identify the patient.
2. Choose the appropriate equipment for obtaining the sample.
3. Select and prepare the site for collection.
4. Collect the sample, ensuring patient comfort and safety.
5. Correctly label the sample and transport it to the lab in a timely manner, using appropriate handling procedures.

Beyond these responsibilities, phlebotomists must also:

1. Adhere to all safety regulations.
2. Effectively interact with both patients and health care professionals.

3. Keep accurate records and be knowledgeable about the computer operations of the lab.
4. Develop other health care skills, such as taking blood pressure, collecting nonblood specimens, processing specimens, instructing patients on collecting nonblood specimens (such as urine), performing point-of-care testing and quality-control procedures and maintenance on point-of-care instruments, and performing some basic laboratory tests.

Personal Characteristics

As a phlebotomist, you will often be the first medical professional a patient meets. You therefore represent not just yourself or the lab but the entire health care facility. This public relations aspect of your work is important, because it sets the tone for the patient's stay in the health care facility. How you present yourself has an effect on everyone you interact with.

The phlebotomist is a member of the health care profession and must display professional behavior at all times. Professionalism is both an attitude toward your work and a set of specific characteristics. A professional displays the following characteristics.

Dependability

The phlebotomist plays a crucial role in the health care institution and is depended on to perform that role skillfully, efficiently, and without constant supervision. The phlebotomist must report to work on time and avoid all unnecessary absences or tardiness. Failure to do so can affect patient care both indirectly, by decreasing the overall functioning of the laboratory, and directly, by preventing a patient from having a sample collected in a timely manner for monitoring of medication, for example.

Honesty and Integrity

Because the phlebotomist often works without supervision, it is crucial that he or she be a person of unquestioned integrity. Everyone makes errors, and you will be no exception. It is vital for the health of your patients that you admit errors when they are made.

Positive Attitude

Your attitude affects everyone you interact with, and having a positive attitude toward your job makes others around you more positive as well. This is especially important in your interactions with patients.

Empathy and Compassion

The phlebotomist is often called on to interact with patients experiencing health crises or undergoing painful or unpleasant treatments. Patients may be worried about the procedure you are performing, the condition for which they are being treated, or the cost of their care. By being sensitive to patients' concerns and taking the time to reassure anxious patients, you can help make their stay less stressful.

Professional Detachment

Conversely, it is important to remain emotionally detached from patients. You will encounter many distressing situations in your career. Becoming emotionally involved on a personal level does not help your patients and can lead to stress and burnout. Your approach to patients in distress must be sympathetic and understanding, but you must retain enough professional distance to allow you to do your job efficiently. Developing this balanced approach is a significant step in your professional growth.

Professional Appearance

Appearance has a significant impact on how the phlebotomist is thought of by patients and treated by coworkers, including superiors. First impressions are often lasting ones. Cleanliness is critical, and conservative clothing and grooming is the general rule. Avoid long, brightly painted fingernails or long, dangling earrings; exposed piercings other than pierced ears; strong perfume; and gaudy makeup. Specific standards are usually set by the employer.

Interpersonal Skills

The phlebotomist must be able to communicate effectively with patients and coworkers. Patients may be fearful, uncooperative, or excessively talkative. In all cases, the phlebotomist must be able to communicate clearly to the patient what is to be done and to obtain consent for the procedure. By speaking slowly and clearly in a courteous tone, you will usually be able to gain the patient's trust, which is necessary to perform the procedure effectively. Nonverbal communication is important as well. By making eye contact, smiling, and appearing relaxed, calm, and prepared, you communicate confidence and professionalism to the patient. Finally, take the time to reassure anxious patients by listening to their needs. Take the time to answer questions. Patients need some attention—they are people, not just names on requisition forms.

Telephone Skills

The phlebotomist is often required to answer calls and take messages in the laboratory. The information that comes in over the phone may be critical for patient care or for the operation of the lab. It is essential that you display the same high level of professionalism in answering the phone as in dealing directly with patients or coworkers. If you are staffing the desk:

- Answer the phone promptly.
- Identify the department and yourself, and ask how you can help.
- Write everything down, including the name of the person calling and the date and time of the call. Be prepared to take a message by having writing materials at hand.
- Speak slowly and clearly.
- Do not put the caller on hold before determining whether this is an emergency call.
- Make every attempt to help, but give only accurate information. If you do not know the answer to a question, find out and call back, if necessary.

An example of these steps is illustrated in Box 1-1.

BOX 1-1 Answering the Phone

Here is an example of the correct way to answer the phone in the clinical lab:

[Phone rings]

Phlebotomist: Good afternoon, this is the clinical lab at Mercy Hospital, Sandy speaking. How may I help you?

Caller: This is Dr. Tom Watson from Fairview Clinic. Can you tell me if the results from the fecal test on a patient on Three West are ready yet?

Phlebotomist: I will try to find out. Can you tell me the patient identification number on the test request?

Caller: Yes, it was 243576-1.

Phlebotomist: Thank you. Can you hold while I check?

Caller: Yes.

Phlebotomist: Thank you. Please hold [places call on hold]. Dr. Watson? I'm sorry, the results are not back yet—we've had a slight delay here. May I take your number and call you when they are ready? It should be about 2 hours.

Caller: Yes. I'm at 555-5555.

Phlebotomist: [Writes down number.] I will call you as soon as the results are ready.

Caller: Thank you.

Phlebotomist: Thank you. Good-bye.

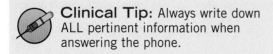
Clinical Tip: Always write down ALL pertinent information when answering the phone.

PROFESSIONAL ORGANIZATIONS AND STANDARDS

The high standards necessary for the proper practice of modern phlebotomy have led to the creation of several different organizations that develop standards and monitor training in the field. There are four aspects of this type of professional monitoring: accreditation, certification, licensure, and continuing medical education. Accreditation is for institutions that train phlebotomists, while the other three are for phlebotomists themselves. Some of the organizations and the services they provide are shown in Table 1-1.

Accreditation

Programs that train phlebotomists receive **accreditation** or **approval** from a professional organization by meeting and documenting established requirements, called **standards**. An accredited education program exposes students to both classroom and clinical experiences and fully prepares them to become professional phlebotomists. As shown in Table 1-1, the organizations that provide accreditation or approval are American Allied Health, Inc., American Association of Allied Health Professionals (AAAHP), the American Medical Technologists (AMT), the American Society of Phlebotomy Technicians (ASPT), the National Accrediting Agency for Clinical Laboratory Sciences (NAACLS), and the National Phlebotomy Association (NPA). The program you are enrolled in may be accredited by one or more of these organizations. As discussed later, California accredits training programs within that state.

Certification

After completing an accredited or approved program, you are eligible to take a certifying exam. **Certification** is evidence that an individual has demonstrated proficiency in a particular area of practice. As shown in Table 1-1, the organizations that offer certification are the AAAHP, the American Certification Agency for Healthcare Professionals (ACA), the AMT, the American Society for Clinical Pathology (ASCP), the ASPT, the National Credentialing Agency (NCA), the National Healthcareer Association (NHA), and the NPA. Once you pass the exam, you may use the title shown in Table 1-1 as part of your professional name.

Licensure

Licensure is a documented permit issued by a government agency, either municipal or state, that grants the bearer permission to perform a particular service or procedure. This permit is issued after a person has met the educational and experience requirements set by the agency and has passed an exam demonstrating competency. Sometimes an agency recognizes successful passage of a national certification exam in place of the state licensure exam. This process is called *reciprocity*. The individual must petition the state licensing agency to grant reciprocity. As of late 2005, only California required licensure of phlebotomists (see below). The state of Louisiana requires phlebotomists to apply for certification through the State Board of Medical Examiners, after receiving certification from one of the private national organizations.

Continuing Education

Certification programs usually require phlebotomists to participate in continuing education programs and earn a certain number of **continuing education units** (CEUs) to remain certified. These programs provide updates on new information, regulations, and techniques and help you refresh the skills you use less frequently. Larger health care institutions often sponsor such programs on-site. As shown in Table 1-1, the organizations that provide continuing education are the AAAHP, the AMT, the American Society for Clinical Laboratory Science (ASCLS), the ASCP, the ASPT, and the NPA.

Professional Organizations

Membership in a professional organization for phlebotomists offers an additional way to follow changes in the field and to learn important new information. Some of the organizations listed in Table 1-1 publish journals with useful articles or sponsor workshops or seminars.

The California Plan

Phlebotomists in California fall under a set of state regulations governing their education, training, and certification. Those who wish to become phlebotomists must show proof of having met several

TABLE 1-1 Organizations That Provide Accreditation, Certification, or Continuing Education

Name	Accredits or Approves Training Programs	Certifies Phlebotomists (Title Awarded)	Offers Continuing Education Units
American Allied Health, Inc Testing and Certification P.O. Box 6474 Springdale, Arkansas 72766-6474 (479) 248-4646 Americanalliedhealth@yahoo.com	Yes	Yes	Yes
American Association of Allied Health Professionals (AAAHP) 803 E. Main St. Havelock, SC 28532 (252) 447-9609 www.aaahp.com	Yes	Yes	Yes
American Certification Agency for Healthcare Professionals (ACA) PO Box 58 Osceola, IN 46561 (574) 277-4538 http://www.acacert.com	No	Yes	No
American Medical Technologists (AMT) 710 Higgins Rd. Park Ridge, IL 60068-5765 (847) 823-5169 http://www.amt1.com	Yes	Yes Registered phlebotomy technician—RPT (AMT)	Yes
American Society for Clinical Laboratory Science (ASCLS) 6701 Democracy Boulevard, Suite 300 Bethesda, MD 20817 (301) 657-2768 http://www.ascls.org	No	No	Yes
American Society for Clinical Pathology (ASCP) 2100 West Harrison St. Chicago, IL 60612 (312) 738-1336 http://www.ascp.org	No	Yes Phlebotomy technician— PBT (ASCP)	Yes
American Society of Phlebotomy Technicians (ASPT) PO Box 1831 Hickory, NC 28603 (828) 299-0078 http://www.aspt.org	Yes	Yes Certified phlebotomy technician—CPT (ASPT)	Yes
National Accrediting Agency for Clinical Laboratory Sciences (NAACLS) 8410 W. Bryn Mawr Ave. Suite 670 Chicago, IL 60631-3415 (773) 714-8880 http://www.naacls.org	Yes	No	No
National Credentialing Agency (NCA) PO Box 15945-289 Lenexa, KS 66285 (913) 438-5110 http://www.nca-info.org	No	Yes Clinical laboratory phlebotomist—CLP1b (NCA)	No

Continued

TABLE 1-1 Organizations That Provide Accreditation, Certification, or Continuing Education—cont'd

Name	Accredits or Approves Training Programs	Certifies Phlebotomists (Title Awarded)	Offers Continuing Education Units
National Phlebotomy Association (NPA) 1901 Brightseat Rd. Landover, MD 20785 (301) 386-4200 www.nationalphlebotomy.org/	Yes	Yes Certified phlebotomy technician—CPT (NPA)	Yes
National Healthcareer Association 134 Evergreen Place 9th Floor East Orange, NJ 07018 (800) 499-9092 http://www.nhanow.com	Yes	Yes Certified phlebotomy technologist—CPT (NHA)	Yes

educational requirements, including:

- High school diploma or equivalent.
- Forty hours of classroom instruction in phlebotomy in a state-accredited program.
- Forty hours of practical training in phlebotomy in a state-accredited program, including at least 50 venipunctures and 10 skin punctures.
- Certification from a national phlebotomy organization that is itself approved by the state to administer exams and issue certification.

Once you have met all these requirements, you are eligible to apply to the state for certification to practice phlebotomy. State certification is for 2 years, with renewal based on meeting continuing education requirements.

The initial certification granted is as a certified phlebotomy technician level I (CPT-I), which enables phlebotomists to perform dermal punctures and venipunctures without supervision and arterial punctures with the supervision of a physician, registered nurse, or certified respiratory therapist. After a CPT-I has performed 20 successful supervised arterial punctures, he or she can apply to become a CPT-II, with the ability to perform unsupervised punctures.

Practicing phlebotomists may need to show proof of classroom instruction to obtain state certification, even if they are already certified by a national organization.

California has led the way in many areas of governmental regulation, and these changes in the regulation of phlebotomists may signal the beginning of similar movements in other states. Regardless of whether you plan to practice in California, it is wise to get the maximum amount of training before you start your career as a phlebotomist.

LEGAL ISSUES IN PHLEBOTOMY

Like every other profession, phlebotomy is bound by laws and regulations governing the workplace, relations with customers (patients), and the privacy of privileged information, such as medical records. Failure to observe these laws and regulations may be cause for dismissal, and may lead to a law suit against you or your institution. These issues are covered in more detail in Chapter 18. Here, we stress the two most important legal aspects of the phlebotomist's profession: informed consent and confidentiality.

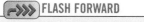

FLASH FORWARD

Legal issues are discussed in more detail in Chapter 18.

Informed Consent

Informed consent means that a patient must be informed of intended treatments and their risks before they are performed. For the phlebotomist, this means that the patient must understand that his or her blood is to be drawn and must consent to that procedure before the phlebotomist may proceed. The patient has the right to refuse any and all medical treatments, including phlebotomy procedures requested by the physician. When a patient refuses, follow your institution's policy to ensure that the patient's doctor is notified promptly.

Confidentiality

All information regarding a patient's condition, including the types of tests ordered or the results of those tests, is confidential medical information. For the phlebotomist, this means that information regarding a patient should never be discussed with a coworker who is not involved in that patient's treatment. Discussions should never occur in common rooms or public areas such as elevators, hallways, waiting rooms, or cafeterias.

These and other issues are summarized in the Patient's Bill of Rights, created by the American Hospital Association, and presented in Chapter 18, Box 18-1.

The privacy of medical information is covered by the Health Insurance Portability and Accountability Act (HIPAA), a law that went into effect in 1996. Under HIPAA, medical institutions must have procedures in place to actively protect the confidentiality of medical information.

REVIEW FOR CERTIFICATION

The modern professional phlebotomist must display technical, organizational, and interpersonal skills. The ability to communicate effectively with patients, the public, and coworkers is critical. Phlebotomy can be a stressful profession, and it is important to remain professionally detached even while showing compassion and care for all patients.

Phlebotomy training occurs at institutions that have received accreditation from one or more national agencies. After completing course work and practical training, the phlebotomist is eligible to take a national exam and receive certification from a national phlebotomy organization. Continuing education is often required to maintain certification. California and Louisiana are the first states to create state certification requirements.

Significant legal issues in phlebotomy include confidentiality and informed consent. The phlebotomist should never disclose information about a patient to third parties who are not involved in the patient's care. Every patient has the right to refuse treatment, including the withdrawal of blood.

BIBLIOGRAPHY

Clutterbuck H: On the Proper Administration of Blood-Letting, for the Prevention and Cure of Disease. London, 1840.

Ernst DJ: Is the Phlebotomist Obsolete? Medical Laboratory Observer. October 1997.

Fidler JR: The Role of the Phlebotomy Technician: Skills and Knowledge Required for Successful Clinical Performance. Evaluation & the Health Professions. September 1997.

Henry JB: Clinical Diagnosis and Management by Laboratory Methods, ed 21. Philadelphia, WB Saunders, 2006.

Mahon C, Smith LA, Burns C: An Introduction to Clinical Laboratory Science. Philadelphia, WB Saunders, 1998.

Murdock SS, Murdock JR: From Leeches to Luers: The History of Phlebotomy. Journal of Medical Technology. September/October 1987.

Narlock VR, Reyes CN, Nyberg D: Developing a Phlebotomy Curriculum: Didactic and Practical Aspects. Journal of Medical Technology. September/October 1987.

STUDY QUESTIONS

1. What is phlebotomy?
2. List five personal characteristics of a professional phlebotomist.
3. Besides drawing blood samples, what other skills may a phlebotomist be trained to perform?
4. What is licensure?
5. Explain the purpose of continuing education units.
6. List three organizations that provide accreditation for phlebotomy programs.
7. List three organizations that provide certification for phlebotomists.
8. Why would a phlebotomist wish to become a member of a professional organization?
9. What is informed consent?
10. What is confidentiality?
11. Describe some of the ancient phlebotomy practices and their uses.
12. Describe modern-day phlebotomy practices, their use in modern health care, and their similarities to ancient phlebotomy practices.
13. List and explain at least four steps and responsibilities in the phlebotomist's job-related duties.
14. List at least four of the required personal characteristics of the phlebotomist.
15. Explain which one of these four personal characteristics you feel is the most important characteristic to possess.
16. List the two most important legal aspects of the phlebotomist's profession.

CERTIFICATION EXAM PREPARATION

1. Phlebotomy skills would not include:
   a. organization
   b. handling patient correspondence
   c. interpersonal skills
   d. being able to handle stress

2. The monitoring system for institutions that train phlebotomists is known as:
   a. certification
   b. accreditation
   c. licensure
   d. continuing education units

3. Once phlebotomists are certified, continuing education programs allow them to earn:
   a. CEUs
   b. licensing points
   c. accreditation
   d. a degree

4. Informed consent means:
   a. Patients must ask their doctors if they can have blood drawn.
   b. Patients waive their rights.
   c. Patients must be informed of intended treatments and their risks before they are performed.
   d. The phlebotomist may draw a patient's blood without the patient's permission.

5. Which is not a required personal characteristic of a professional phlebotomist?
   a. dependability
   b. honesty
   c. compassion
   d. sense of humor

6. When a patient refuses to have blood drawn, the phlebotomist should:
   a. persuade the patient to comply
   b. perform the phlebotomy
   c. notify a family member
   d. ensure that the patient's doctor is notified promptly

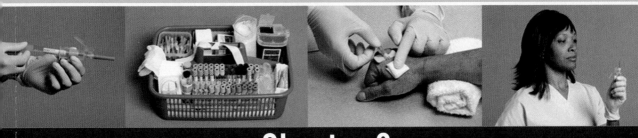

Chapter 2

Health Care Structure

OUTLINE

OBJECTIVES

After completing this chapter, you should be able to:

1. Describe the overall structure of a typical hospital.
2. Explain the roles of each of the following hospital branches and list the kinds of jobs included:
   a. fiscal services
   b. support services
   c. nursing services
3. Describe the departments and functions of the professional services branch of the hospital.
4. List the kinds of personnel who may work in the laboratory.
5. Describe the functions of the anatomic and surgical pathology laboratory.
6. List the major departments of the clinical laboratory.
7. Describe the kinds of samples typically analyzed and the kinds of tests that may be performed in

each of the following clinical laboratory sections:
   a. hematology
   b. coagulation
   c. chemistry
   d. microbiology
   e. urinalysis
   f. serology and immunology
   g. blood bank and immunohematology
8. Explain the role of molecular diagnostics and flow cytometry in laboratory testing.
9. Explain how laboratory quality is monitored and list at least four organizations that are involved in ensuring quality laboratory testing.
10. Describe other health care settings where a phlebotomist may work.

KEY TERMS

anatomic and surgical
  pathology area
autologous donation
blood bank

blood type
chemistry panel

Clinical and Laboratory
  Standards Institute
Continued

KEY TERMS—cont'd

Clinical Lab Improve-
  ment Act of 1988
clinical laboratory
clinical pathology area
coagulation
College of American
  Pathologists
complete blood count
culture and sensitivity

flow cytometry
forensic
health maintenance
  organization
hemolyzed
hemostasis
icteric
immunohematology
Joint Commission on

Accreditation of
Healthcare
Organizations
lipemic
molecular diagnostics
nursing home
physician office lab
preferred provider
  organization

professional services
reagent
reference laboratory
serum separator tube
stat
urgent care center

ABBREVIATIONS

AIDS: acquired immunodeficiency syndrome
ALP: alkaline phosphatase
ALT: alanine aminotransferase
APTT: activated partial thromboplastin time
AST: aspartate aminotransferase
BUN: blood urea nitrogen
C&S: culture and sensitivity
CAP: College of American Pathologists
CBC: complete blood count
CCU: cardiac care unit
CK: creatine kinase
CLIA '88: Clinical Lab Improvement Act of 1988
CLS: clinical laboratory scientist
CLSI: Clinical Laboratory Standards Institute
CLT: clinical laboratory technician
CNA: certified nursing assistant
CT: computed tomography
diff: differential
EIA: enzyme immunoassay
ER: emergency room
ESR: erythrocyte sedimentation rate
FBS: fasting blood sugar
GGT: γ-glutamyltransferase
GTT: glucose tolerance test
HCT: hematocrit
HDL: high-density lipoprotein
Hgb: hemoglobin
HIV: human immunodeficiency virus
HMO: health maintenance organization
ICU: intensive care unit

INR: international normalized ratio
JCAHO: Joint Commission on Accreditation of
  Healthcare Organizations
LD: lactate dehydrogenase
LDL: low-density lipoprotein
LIS: laboratory information services
LPN: licensed practical nurse
MCH: mean corpuscular hemoglobin
MCHC: mean corpuscular hemoglobin
  concentration
MCV: mean corpuscular volume
MIS: manager of information services
MLT: medical laboratory technician
MRI: magnetic resonance imaging
MT: medical technologist
NCCLS: National Committee for Clinical
  Laboratory Standards
OR: operating room
PCA: patient care assistant
PCT: patient care technician
PET: positron emission tomography
POL: physician office lab
PPO: preferred provider organization
PT: prothrombin time
RBC: red blood cell (or count)
RDW: red cell distribution width
RIA: radioimmunoassay
RN: registered nurse
SST: serum separator tube
WBC: white blood cell (or count)

Although phlebotomists may be employed in a variety of health care settings, including health maintenance organizations, clinics, urgent care centers, nursing homes, or physician office laboratories, most phlebotomists work in hospitals, in the clinical laboratory. The various departments within the clinical laboratory are all involved in the analysis of patient samples, whether they are blood, urine, or other body fluids or tissues. All clinical labs must meet standards set by a variety of national organizations in order to be certified. In this chapter, you will learn about the organizational structures found in hospitals, how the phlebotomist fits into the larger health care environment, and how each department in the laboratory works with others to provide the many services offered.

HOSPITAL ORGANIZATION

The hospital laboratory in which a phlebotomist works is one part of a large organization. The medical staff is overseen by the chief of staff, and the central administration of the hospital is the responsibility of the hospital administrator. The hospital administrator also oversees the four branches of support personnel: fiscal services, support services, nursing services, and professional services. Each branch is headed by an assistant administrator. Professional services includes the clinical laboratory in which the phlebotomist works and is discussed in detail later.

Fiscal Services

This branch is responsible for admissions and medical records, as well as for billing, accounting, and other financial aspects of the hospital.

Support Services

This branch includes all aspects of the physical plant of the hospital, such as cleaning, maintenance, and security, as well as food service, purchasing, and human resources.

Nursing Services

Nursing services personnel provide direct care to patients. Phlebotomists have a great deal of direct contact with nursing personnel. Some nursing services departments have their own phlebotomy team. Nursing services includes a wide range of people with various levels of education and training, including the registered nurse (RN), licensed practical nurse (LPN), certified nursing assistant (CNA), patient care technician (PCT) or patient care assistant (PCA), and ward clerk or unit secretary. Nursing staff is divided among a number of units within the hospital, depending on the size of the institution. The most common divisions are the emergency room (ER), operating room (OR), intensive care unit (ICU), cardiac care unit (CCU), nursery, and labor and delivery, as well as inpatient floors for medical, surgical, and psychiatric patients.

Professional Services

Professional services personnel provide services at the request of physicians who aid in the diagnosis and treatment of patients. Each department provides specialized services.

Pharmacy

The pharmacy prepares and dispenses drugs that have been prescribed by physicians.

Physical Therapy

Physical therapists assess patients both before and after treatment and devise plans of physical treatment. Physical therapists design exercises, stretching programs, and other physical treatments to aid in a patient's rehabilitation after injury or illness.

Occupational Therapy

Occupational therapists assess patients and design adaptive aids or compensatory strategies to help people with physical or mental impairments perform tasks of daily living and reach their maximum potential.

Respiratory Therapy

Respiratory therapists provide treatment for respiratory disorders. They often perform arterial punctures for the determination of arterial blood gases.

>>> FLASH FORWARD

You will learn about arterial blood collection in Chapter 13.

Radiology

The radiologist interprets a wide range of diagnostic and therapeutic procedures using various forms of radiant energy. The radiological technologist performs radiographs, computed tomography (CT) scans, magnetic resonance imaging (MRI) scans, positron emission tomography (PET) scans, and fluoroscopy.

Nuclear Medicine

This department uses radioisotopes to perform tests and treat diseases. Radioisotopes are unstable forms of certain elements that can be detected as they break down. They are often used as tracers; when injected into a patient's bloodstream, they can be tracked to reveal the structure and function of internal organs. In large doses, radioisotopes can be used to destroy cancerous tissue.

Radiation Therapy

This department also treats cancer, using x-rays or other high-energy radiation sources to destroy the tumor.

Clinical Laboratory

The **clinical laboratory** analyzes samples from patients at the request of physicians or other health care personnel. The samples may be blood, urine, or other body fluids, or they may be cells from aspiration procedures or pieces of tissue from biopsies. Results of these tests are used for making a diagnosis, monitoring treatment, or determining a patient's prognosis. The lab is divided into two main areas: the **anatomic and surgical pathology area**, which analyzes the characteristics of cells and tissues, and the **clinical pathology area**, which analyzes blood and other body fluids. The phlebotomist works in the clinical pathology area of the clinical laboratory.

INTRODUCTION TO THE CLINICAL LABORATORY

Personnel

The clinical laboratory is usually under the supervision of a pathologist, who is a physician with special training in laboratory analysis of tissues and fluids. A laboratory manager directs the administrative functions of the laboratory, including hiring personnel. Management staff may include a manager of information services (MIS) and a laboratory information services (LIS) coordinator. Section supervisors supervise personnel, monitor equipment maintenance, and monitor test results. Clinical laboratory scientists (CLSs) or medical technologists (MTs) and clinical laboratory technicians (CLTs) or medical laboratory technicians (MLTs) run routine tests, perform equipment maintenance, and collect specimens. MTs and CLSs have bachelor of science degrees in clinical laboratory science–medical technology, whereas CLTs and MLTs have associate's degrees. Phlebotomists collect blood specimens for analysis in the lab. Phlebotomists obtain certification from a nationally recognized certifying agency.

Departments of the Anatomic and Surgical Pathology Area

This area is usually divided into three sections, or departments.

Cytology

The cytology department processes and stains cells that are shed into body fluids or removed from tissue with a needle (aspiration) and examines them for the presence of cancer or other diseases. The cytotechnologist assists in this work. One of the most common tests performed in cytology is the Pap smear.

Histology

The histology department prepares tissues from autopsy, surgery, or biopsy for microscopic examination by a pathologist. Special stains are used to highlight particular cell morphology. The histotechnologist helps prepare samples for the pathologist to examine.

Cytogenetics

The cytogenetics department examines chromosomes for evidence of genetic disease, such as Down syndrome.

Departments of the Clinical Pathology Area

Blood and other body fluids can be analyzed in a number of different ways, and the divisions within the clinical pathology area reflect these differences. The number of sections in this area depends on the size of the hospital. In some labs, some functions may be combined. The clinical departments in a typical lab are:

- Hematology and coagulation
- Chemistry
- Blood transfusion medicine
- Serology or immunology
- Microbiology
- Urinalysis and microscopy
- Molecular diagnostics
- Referrals
- Phlebotomy

FUNCTIONS OF THE CLINICAL PATHOLOGY LABORATORY DEPARTMENTS

Hematology

The hematology department analyzes blood for evidence of diseases affecting the blood-forming tissues and the cells produced by those tissues—namely, the red blood cells (RBCs), white blood cells (WBCs), and platelets. This department also analyzes the clotting ability of the blood

FLASH FORWARD

You will learn about the composition and function of blood in Chapter 7.

Hematology tests are most often performed on whole blood, which is blood that has not coagulated (clotted). To prevent the blood from clotting after it is collected from the patient, the blood is drawn into a tube containing an anticoagulant (usually a chemical called EDTA). Thus, the blood cells remain freely suspended in the liquid component of the blood, just as they are inside the body.

TABLE 2-1 Complete Blood Count

Test	Purpose
White blood count (WBC)	Counts the number of WBCs in a sample of known volume
Differential (diff)	Classifies and counts the different types of WBCs; morphological (shape) abnormalities in RBCs or platelets detected by the analyzer can be checked by manual examination of a blood smear under a microscope
Platelet count	Counts the number of platelets in a sample of known volume
Mean platelet volume (MPV)	Assesses platelet volume and size
Red blood count (RBC)	Counts the number of RBCs in a sample of known volume
Hematocrit (HCT)	Determines the percentage of blood volume attributable to RBCs
Hemoglobin (Hgb)	Determines the level of Hgb in the blood as a whole; this determines the oxygen-carrying capacity
Red Cell Indices	
Mean corpuscular Hgb (MCH)	Determines the average amount of Hgb in an RBC
Mean corpuscular Hgb concentration (MCHC)	Determines the ratio of Hgb in a cell to the size of the cell
Mean corpuscular volume (MCV)	Determines the volume of the average RBC, which can be used to assess morphological abnormalities
Red cell distribution width (RDW)	Determines the range of sizes of RBCs

⌐≫≫ FLASH FORWARD

You will learn about anticoagulants and other tube additives in Chapter 8.

In the hematology lab, blood is analyzed in a computer-controlled instrument that counts and identifies the various types of cells. The most common hematology test is the **complete blood count (CBC).** This automated test, performed by a machine, includes a white blood count, red blood count, and platelet count. It may also include a white cell differential, which determines the different kinds of white cells present. Among other applications, the CBC is used to diagnose types of anemia, leukemia, infectious diseases, and other conditions that affect the number and types of blood cells. The complete range of tests included in the CBC is given in Table 2-1. Other common hematology tests are listed in Table 2-2.

⌐≫≫ FLASH FORWARD

You will learn about the types of blood cells in Chapter 7.

Flow cytometry is a special analytical technique that is used in hematology, immunology, or anatomic pathology. Flow cytometry identifies cellular markers on the surface of WBCs. This is done to determine lymphocyte subclasses in patients with acquired immunodeficiency syndrome (AIDS), as a measure of the disease process, and to determine CD4/CD8 ratios of helper to suppressor cells, as a means of tracking the health of patients infected with human immunodeficiency virus (HIV). It is also used to classify malignancies, aiding in the development of treatment plans.

TABLE 2-2 Other Hematology Tests

Test	Purpose
Body fluid analysis	Determines the number and types of cells in body fluids
Bone marrow	Determines the number and types of cells in bone marrow
Osmotic fragility	Determines the response of RBCs to changes in water concentrations, which correlate with certain blood disorders
Plasma hemoglobin	Determines whether the plasma contains significant Hgb, indicating hemolysis within the circulation
Reticulocyte count	Evaluates bone marrow delivery of RBCs into the peripheral circulation
Sickle cell (solubility test)	Determines whether RBCs containing hemoglobin S are present; used to diagnose sickle cell anemia; most often performed on children

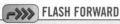

FLASH FORWARD

You will learn about special patient populations, including patients with HIV, in Chapter 12.

Coagulation and Hemostasis

This department is usually part of the hematology department, but it may be separate in larger hospitals.

Coagulation depends on the presence of clotting factors and platelets. **Hemostasis** refers to the process by which the body stops blood from leaking out of a wound; as you will learn in Chapter 7, hemostasis involves both coagulation and other processes.

Coagulation tests are performed on plasma (Box 2-1). Coagulation studies (samples) are collected in a tube containing the anticoagulant citrate, which preserves the coagulation factors better than other anticoagulants do. Coagulation tests are most often performed to monitor anticoagulant therapy, for instance, in a patient who has had a thrombotic stroke, heart attack, or thrombophlebitis. Drugs to prevent the formation of clots help avoid the recurrence of stroke, but the dose must be adjusted to allow a minimal level of clotting. The activated partial thromboplastin time (APTT) is used to monitor intravenous heparin therapy, and the prothrombin time (PT) and international normalized ratio (INR) are used to monitor oral warfarin (Coumadin) therapy. These tests are also used to diagnose a variety of clotting disorders, including hemophilia.

Chemistry

The chemistry department performs a wide range of tests on the chemical components of blood. Most tests are automated, and advances in the instruments used to perform these tests now allow them to be run using very small samples. In many cases, this means that less blood is needed from the patient, which can decrease patient discomfort

significantly. For patients who require frequent blood monitoring, it can also reduce the chance of developing anemia. The clinical pathology laboratory must keep records of the amount of blood drawn from each patient.

Clinical Tip: Always draw the smallest amount of blood consistent with the tests ordered.

Chemistry Department Sections

Sections within the chemistry department include the following.

Electrophoresis

This section separates chemical components of blood based on differences in electrical charge. Electrophoresis is most often used to analyze hemoglobin, enzymes, and other proteins.

Toxicology

This section analyzes plasma for levels of drugs and poisons, performing therapeutic drug monitoring, identifying illegal drugs, and detecting lead and other toxic substances.

Immunochemistry

This section uses antibodies in the testing reagent to detect a wide range of substances in the blood. Antibodies are immune system proteins that can be tailored to bind specifically to substances such as hormones, enzymes, or certain drugs, thereby allowing their detection. In a radioimmunoassay (RIA), the antibody is linked to a radioactive molecule; in an enzyme immunoassay (EIA), the antibody is linked to an enzyme, which causes a color change in solution when the substance of interest is present.

Specimen Collection for Chemistry

Chemistry tests are performed on either serum or plasma. Serum is collected in a tube without anticoagulants (a plain red-top tube) or in a **serum separator tube** (SST), and the blood is allowed to clot for at least 30 minutes before the serum is separated. When results are needed very quickly (a **stat requisition**), blood can be collected in a tube with clot activators. After clotting, serum is separated out by centrifugation. A centrifuge spins the sample at high speeds to separate components based on density. Plasma, which is also used for stat results, is collected with either heparin or fluoride.

BOX 2-1 Coagulation Tests

Activated clotting time
Activated partial thromboplastin time
Bleeding time
Factor activity assays
Fibrinogen and fibrin degradation tests
International Normalized Ratio
Prothrombin time
Thrombin time

> →》》 **FLASH FORWARD**
>
> *You will learn more about serum and plasma in Chapter 7.*

Serum is normally a clear, pale yellow fluid. The quality of the serum sample can be degraded by both the patient's condition and the collection technique. Liver disease can increase the amount of bilirubin in the serum, making it appear a darker yellow (called **icteric** serum). Recent ingestion of fats or other lipids can make the sample cloudy (**lipemic** serum). Hemolysis, or breakage of RBCs, can give the serum a pink tinge (**hemolyzed** serum). Many lab tests measure the substance of interest by photometry, in which the substance is reacted to form a colored solution whose intensity is detected by passing light through the sample. If the original sample is degraded by hemolysis or other contamination, however, the results of photometry tests can be erroneous.

Serum quality can also be affected by post-collection handling procedures. Some samples must be chilled during transport, whereas others must be protected from light. Some tests must be performed within 1 hour of collection.

> →》》 **FLASH FORWARD**
>
> *You will learn more about special specimen handling procedures in Chapters 14 and 16.*

Chemistry tests are also performed on other body fluids, such as urine, cerebrospinal fluid, or synovial fluid (from joints).

Chemistry Tests

Chemistry tests may be performed as either single tests or as groups, called **chemistry panels**. The most common tests and panels are shown in Table 2-3.

TABLE 2-3 Common Chemistry Tests and Panels

Test or Panel	Purpose	Test or Panel	Purpose

Glucose
Fasting blood sugar (FBS)
2-Hour postprandial
   glucose (2 h PPBS)
Glucose tolerance test (GTT)
	Elevated levels indicate
	   diabetes mellitus
		Protein/total protein
		Albumin	

Glycolated hemoglobin
   (Hgb Alc)
	Elevated levels indicate
	   diabetes mellitus
		Coronary Risk
		Cholesterol
		Triglycerides
		High-density lipoprotein
		   (HDL)
		Low-density lipoprotein
		   (LDL)
			Assesses risk for heart disease

Electrolytes Potassium (K) Chloride (Cl) Sodium (Na) Bicarbonate	A group of tests that evaluates levels of ions in the blood		

Chem 7	Used as a general metabolic
	   screen; includes glucose,
	   electrolytes, and blood urea
	   nitrogen
		Myocardial Infarction
		AST
		Creatine kinase (CK)
		CK isoenzymes
		Lactate dehydrogenase (LD)
		Troponin
			Determines the occurrence and
			   timing of a myocardial
			   infarction

Liver Function Panel
Enzymes and bilirubin
Alkaline phosphatase (ALP)
Alanine aminotransferase
   (ALT)
Aspartate aminotransferase
   (AST)
γ-Glutamyl transferase
   (GGT)
	Assesses liver function	**General Health**
		Chem 7
		ALP
		AST
		LD
		Cholesterol
		Triglycerides
		Uric acid
		Total protein/albumin
		Bilirubin
		Calcium
			Assess overall health standard
			   of patient

Renal Disease Blood urea nitrogen (BUN) Creatinine Creatinine clearance Phosphorus and calcium	Assesses kidney function	**Lipid Panel** Triglyceride Cholesterol LDL & HDL	Assesses risk for cardiac/ stroke

Microbiology

The microbiology department isolates and identifies pathogenic microorganisms in patient samples and is responsible for infection control in the health care institution. Microbiology comprises bacteriology (the study of bacteria), mycology (the study of fungi), parasitology (the study of parasites), and virology (the study of viruses). Specimens to be tested include blood, urine, throat swabs, sputum, feces, pus, and other body fluids.

> **⤳》》 FLASH FORWARD**
>
> *Collection of blood cultures is discussed in Chapter 14, and nonblood samples in Chapter 15.*

The most common microbiology tests are **culture and sensitivity** (C&S) tests, which detect and identify microorganisms and determine the most effective antibiotic therapy. Bacteria are identified by their nutritional requirements, and by the staining characteristics (shape and color) detected with Gram's stain. Results are usually available in 24 to 48 hours. Identification of fungi usually takes much longer, because they take longer to grow in culture.

Urinalysis and Clinical Microscopy

Urine is examined to assess kidney disease and metabolic disorders that alter the levels of substances in the urine. Diabetes, for instance, causes elevated glucose, and damage to the kidneys themselves may lead to protein in the urine. Many urinalysis tests are performed with paper test strips, which are dipped into the sample. The **reagents** (test chemicals) embedded in the paper change color, indicating the results of the test. The range of tests performed on urine is shown in Table 2-4.

Feces may be examined for blood—called occult blood—as a screen for colorectal cancer. They are also examined for parasites and their ova (eggs). Other body fluids (e.g., spinal fluid, joint fluid) may also be analyzed in this section.

Serology or Immunology

The serology or immunology department evaluates the patient's immune response through the detection of antibodies. Antibodies are proteins that help fight infection by binding to surface molecules of the infective agent, called *antigens* (Table 2-5).

TABLE 2-4 Complete Urinalysis

Test	Purpose
Color	Detects blood, bilirubin, and other pigments
Clarity	Detects crystalline and cellular elements
Specific gravity	Measures urine concentration
Chemical Exam	
pH	Determines the acidity of the urine
Protein	Elevated levels indicate kidney disease
Glucose	Elevated levels indicate diabetes mellitus
Ketones	Elevated levels indicate diabetes mellitus or starvation
Bilirubin	Elevated levels indicate liver disease
Urobilinogen	Elevated levels indicate liver disease or hemolytic disorder
Nitrite	Detects bacterial infection
Leukocyte esterase	Detects WBCs
Blood	Detects RBCs or hemoglobin
Microscopic Exam	
Cells and other structures	Detects WBCs, RBCs, epithelial cells, bacteria, yeast, parasites; detects crystals and casts (structures sloughed off renal tubules)

TABLE 2-5 A Sample of Common Immunology Tests

Test	Purpose
ANA (antinuclear antibodies)	Detects autoimmune disease
Anti-diphtheria toxin antibody	Detects exposure to diphtheria
Anti-Haemophilus influenza B antibody	Detects exposure to Haemophilus influenza B
Anti-Lyme antibodies	Detects exposure to Lyme disease
C-reactive protein	Elevated levels indicate inflammatory disease
Cryoglobulins	Detects abnormal proteins in the blood
Rheumatoid factor	Detects rheumatoid arthritis
T and B cell markers	Used to quantify types of white blood cells

Antibodies are found in the serum; thus, samples for serology testing are serum samples, collected in either a plain red-top tube or an SST. Antibodies may be formed in response to infection by microorganisms such as bacteria, fungi, parasites, or viruses. For example, the presence of antibodies against HIV is a sign of exposure to that virus. Similarly, antibodies are used to diagnose syphilis, hepatitis, infectious mononucleosis, and other communicable diseases. Antibodies may also form against antigens in the body's own tissues, in a process called *autoimmunity*. Detection of such autoantibodies is part of the diagnostic process for systemic lupus erythematosus, for instance.

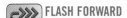 **FLASH FORWARD**

The immune system is discussed in Chapter 7.

Blood Bank or Immunohematology

The **blood bank** or **immunohematology** department deals with blood used for transfusions. Blood is tested there to identify the blood type of both patient and donor blood to determine their compatibility. Compatibility testing is performed to ensure that the patient's immune system does not reject the donor blood.

Specimens for this department are drawn in a plain red-top tube and a special pink-top tube containing EDTA. The strictest attention must be paid to patient identification and sample labeling. A fatal transfusion reaction can occur if identification and labeling are incorrect.

Blood type is due to the presence and type of particular antigens on the surface of RBCs. In routine blood typing, two major antigen groups are tested for: the ABO group and the Rh group. In addition, there are dozens of other antigens that can be determined to improve the match. This is important for patients receiving multiple transfusions over a lifetime, such as for sickle cell disease or kidney disease.

In compatibility testing, patient serum is mixed with donor red cells to look for clumping of cells, caused by a reaction between the patient's antibodies and antigens on the donor RBCs. If clumping is seen, the donor blood cannot be used. Patients can also donate their own blood for use at a later time, called **autologous donation**. This is often done several weeks before a patient is scheduled for surgery.

The blood bank also performs direct antiglobulin testing (Coombs' test) on newborn infants to assess the risk of hemolytic anemia. This test determines the presence of maternal antibodies in the child's circulation that act against the child's antigens. During pregnancy, the mother may be tested to determine whether and how much antibody is present.

The blood bank department may also process donated blood to obtain blood components. Blood is donated and handled by the unit, which is equivalent to a pint. Using a centrifuge, blood can be separated in several different ways to obtain the following components:

- Packed cells, consisting of RBCs, WBCs, and platelets, without plasma.
- Fresh frozen plasma, collected from a unit of blood and immediately frozen.
- Platelets, harvested from several units of blood and combined in a single packet.
- Cryoprecipitate, the component of fresh plasma that has clotting factors.
- Each of these has specific uses. For instance, cryoprecipitate may be used for patients with clotting disorders.

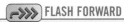 **FLASH FORWARD**

You will learn about blood bank collections in Chapter 14.

Molecular Diagnostics

Molecular diagnostics refers to genetic and biochemical techniques used to diagnose genetic disorders, analyze forensic evidence, track disease, or identify microbiologic pathogens. At the heart of these techniques is the analysis of the DNA in the sample. In the clinical lab, molecular diagnostic techniques are used most commonly to identify infectious agents such as HIV and genetic diseases such as cystic fibrosis; to test for parentage; and to perform **forensic** studies on criminal evidence. Specimens analyzed include blood, body fluids, skin cells, hair, and other body tissues that contain DNA. Special tubes and handling procedures are required for these specimens. The most important aspect of this type of test is to keep the sample free from contamination with DNA from other sources. Keeping the lab clean is very important, and usually only authorized personnel are allowed entrance.

Referrals

The referrals department handles and ships specimens for any tests not done by the laboratory. These are most often newer tests, and may require special equipment or training not available in the lab. Some of these tests are approved diagnostic tests, while others are used for research only. Often, physicians will call the referral department requesting information about a new and uncommon test. Referral personnel will do research to find a laboratory that performs the test so the specimen can be sent to that lab. Frequently a hospital lab will contract with a single large national commercial lab to handle all of the tests not done in-house.

STANDARDS AND ACCREDITATION FOR THE CLINICAL LABORATORY

The clinical laboratory must meet rigorous performance standards to ensure the quality of its procedures and results. Congress passed the **Clinical Lab Improvement Act of 1988** (CLIA '88), which mandated the regulation of all facilities that perform patient testing. Standards and guidelines are set by the **Clinical and Laboratory Standards Institute** (CLSI), a nonprofit organization formerly known as the National Committee for Clinical Laboratory Standards (NCCLS). Laboratories that meet these standards are eligible to receive accreditation from one or more agencies. Accreditation is required for the health care facility to receive Medicare or Medicaid reimbursement. Agencies involved in the accreditation of clinical laboratories are the following:

- **Joint Commission on Accreditation of Healthcare Organizations** (JCAHO). Laboratories must be inspected and accredited every 2 years.
- **College of American Pathologists** (CAP). Inspection and accreditation occur every 2 years. Beginning in 2006, unannounced inspections will occur within 6 months of the accreditation renewal date.
- State agencies. In states with their own licensure requirements, these agencies require labs to participate in proficiency testing and inspections.

OTHER HEALTH CARE SETTINGS

In addition to hospitals, phlebotomists may be employed in other health care settings, including:

- **Health maintenance organizations** (HMOs). HMOs have become major providers of health care in the last two decades. HMOs typically function as full-service outpatient clinics, providing all or almost all medical specialties under one roof.

- **Preferred provider organizations** (PPO). A PPO is a group of doctors and hospitals who offer their services to large employers to provide health care to employees.
- **Urgent care centers**. An urgent care center is an outpatient clinic that provides walk-in services to patients who cannot wait for scheduled appointments with their primary health care providers, or who do not have a primary health care provider.
- **Physician office lab** (POL). Physicians in a group practice may employ a phlebotomist to collect patient samples, which are then usually analyzed by a separate reference laboratory or, if the facility is large enough, in an on-site lab.
- **Reference laboratory**. A reference laboratory is an independent laboratory that analyzes samples from other health care facilities. The phlebotomist may travel to other facilities to obtain samples or collect samples on-site from outpatients referred there by their health care providers.
- **Nursing home**. Phlebotomists may be employed by a nursing home to obtain samples from clients for analysis by a reference laboratory.

REVIEW FOR CERTIFICATION

Most phlebotomists work in hospitals, in the clinical laboratory. The clinical lab is divided into two major sections: the anatomic and surgical pathology area, and the clinical pathology area. Clinical pathology is further divided into a number of departments, each responsible for the analysis of one or more types of samples. Hematology analyzes the cells of the blood, coagulation and hemostasis is concerned with the coagulation process, and chemistry measures the chemical composition of the fluid portion. Microbiology tests for bacterial and other infections, and urinalysis and clinical microscopy is responsible for urine and feces analysis. Serology or immunology is concerned with elements of the immune response, and blood bank or immunohematology focuses on compatibility testing and blood storage. Finally, molecular diagnostics analyzes DNA in a variety of tissues.

All clinical labs are monitored and accredited by one or more national organizations. Other health care settings in which the phlebotomist may work include HMOs, reference labs, urgent care centers, and nursing homes.

BIBLIOGRAPHY

Berger D: A Brief History of Medical Diagnosis and the Birth of the Clinical Laboratory, Parts 1 & 2. Medical Laboratory Observer. July 1999.

Butch S: Professional Organizations: Part of the Package. Advance for Medical Laboratory Professionals. February 28, 2000.

Doig K, Beck SJ, Kolenc K: CLT and CLS Job Responsibilities: Current Distinctions and Updates. Clinical Laboratory Science. Summer 2001.

Henry JB: Clinical Diagnosis and Management by Laboratory Methods, ed 21. Philadelphia, WB Saunders, 2006.

Mahon C, Smith LA, Burns C: An Introduction to Clinical Laboratory Science. Philadelphia, WB Saunders, 1998.

STUDY QUESTIONS

1. Name the four branches of support personnel in the hospital organizational system.
2. Name the two main areas of the laboratory and identify which area the phlebotomist works in.
3. Name the specialty of the physician who oversees the lab.
4. Name two common lab tests performed in the coagulation department and which therapy each test monitors.
5. Describe the tests the immunology department performs.
6. Define molecular diagnostics.
7. Name five liver function tests.
8. Culture and sensitivity testing is performed in which department?
9. Describe the importance of CLIA '88.
10. Hospitals are accredited by JCAHO, which stands for what?
11. What organization sets laboratory standards and guidelines?
12. Name four health care settings, besides the hospital, in which a phlebotomist may be employed.
13. Name the laboratory that has a special specimen/patient identification system. What might be the outcome of mislabeling or mishandling specimens within this lab?
14. Describe the details the technologist looks for in compatibility testing to determine test results.
15. Define what professional services are and give at least two examples.

CERTIFICATION EXAM PREPARATION

1. Fiscal services is responsible for:
   a. cleaning and maintenance
   b. performing tests
   c. diagnosis and treatment of the patient
   d. admitting, medical records, and billing

2. Other than the laboratory, the _____ department may also draw arterial blood gases.
   a. physical therapy
   b. occupational therapy
   c. respiratory therapy
   d. radiology

3. The _____ department uses radio-isotopes to perform tests.
   a. respiratory therapy
   b. cytogenetics
   c. nuclear medicine
   d. hematology

4. The laboratory is under the direction of a:
   a. pathologist
   b. phlebotomist
   c. pharmacist
   d. medical assistant

5. The coagulation department tests samples for:
   a. complete blood counts
   b. prothrombin times
   c. electrolytes
   d. bacterial growth

6. A CBC is performed in the _____ department.
   a. chemistry
   b. urinalysis
   c. serology
   d. hematology

7. APTT testing monitors:
   a. chemotherapy
   b. physical therapy
   c. heparin therapy
   d. warfarin therapy

8. The chemistry department section associated with drug analysis is known as:
   a. immunology
   b. cardiology
   c. toxicology
   d. electrophoresis

9. The _____ department identifies pathogenic microorganisms in patient samples.
   a. virology
   b. microbiology
   c. mycology
   d. parasitology

10. A culture and sensitivity test is analyzed in which department?
    a. urinalysis
    b. hematology
    c. microbiology
    d. chemistry

11. Occult blood testing is performed on:
    a. plasma
    b. feces
    c. serum
    d. cerebrospinal fluid

12. When patients donate their blood for use during their own surgery, this is known as:
    a. autologous donation
    b. platelet donation
    c. cryoprecipitate donation
    d. fresh frozen plasma donation

13. Independent labs that analyze samples from other health care facilities are known as:
    a. physician office labs
    b. urgent care centers
    c. reference labs
    d. waived labs

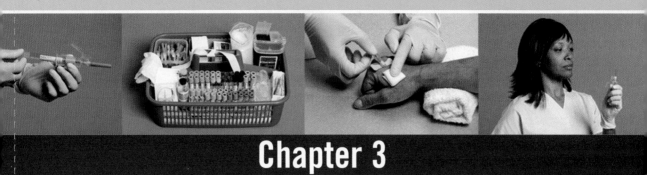

Chapter 3

Safety

OBJECTIVES

After completing this chapter, you should be able to:

1. Define OSHA and explain its role in workplace safety.
2. List eight types of safety hazards.
3. Describe six general precautions that can reduce the risk of injury.
4. Explain steps to be taken to lessen the risk of physical or sharps hazards.
5. List the items that must be included on a hazardous chemical label according to the OSHA Hazardous Communication Standard.
6. Explain the purpose of the materials safety data sheet.
7. List two other kinds of labels used to identify hazardous materials.
8. Describe the components of a chemical hygiene plan.
9. Discuss safety precautions to be used when handling hazardous chemicals.
10. Identify the radioactive hazard symbol.
11. Describe precautions to be taken to reduce the risk of electrical hazards.
12. Describe the four classes of fire, and identify the type(s) of fire extinguisher to be used to combat each.
13. Explain what to do in case of:
  a. bleeding wound
  b. no sign of breathing
  c. shock
  d. latex sensitivity

KEY TERMS

allergic contact dermatitis
anaphylaxis
cardiopulmonary resuscitation
chemical hygiene plan
Department of Transportation label

irritant contact dermatitis
latex sensitivity
materials safety data sheet
National Fire Protection
  Association label

Occupational Safety
  and Health Administration
radioactive hazard symbol
sharps

Like any workplace, a hospital or other health care facility contains certain hazards that must be treated with caution and respect in order to prevent injury. These hazards include biological, physical, chemical, fire, electrical, and radioactive factors, as well as the most significant hazard involved in phlebotomy—sharps in the form of needles, lancets, and glass. Latex sensitivity is also a growing concern in the workplace. Here, we discuss the variety of potential hazards you may encounter and outline the proper precautions to take to prevent accidents or injuries. The Occupational Safety and Health Administration (OSHA) is the governmental agency responsible for workplace safety.

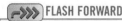 **FLASH FORWARD**

The special precautions needed for infection control are covered in Chapter 4.

OCCUPATIONAL SAFETY AND HEALTH ADMINISTRATION

Workplace safety is regulated by the **Occupational Safety and Health Administration** (OSHA). OSHA regulations are designed both to inform workers about hazards in the workplace (e.g., by requiring that workers know the health effects of the chemicals they use) and protect workers from harm (e.g., by requiring that there be an emergency shower nearby in case of chemical spills). OSHA regulations are revised as needed to increase workplace safety in light of new information or new hazards. Therefore you should keep up-to-date on all relevant information as it changes throughout your career.

TYPES OF SAFETY HAZARDS

Despite their goal of promoting health, health care facilities can be dangerous places for people who are not aware of the potential risks. Types of hazards include:

- Biological: infectious agents, including airborne or blood-borne organisms such as bacteria and viruses.

- Physical: wet floors, heavy lifting (e.g., boxes, patient transfers).
- Sharps: needles, lancets, broken glass.
- Chemical: preservatives and reagents (laboratory-grade chemicals).
- Radioactive or x-ray: equipment and reagents.
- Electrical: dangerous high-voltage equipment.
- Fire or explosive: open flames, oxygen, and chemicals (e.g., nitrous oxide).
- Latex sensitivity: allergic reaction to latex in gloves or other equipment.

In addition to specific safety precautions for phlebotomy procedures, there are a number of general precautions that can reduce your risk of injury:

1. *Avoid putting anything in your mouth in the work area.* This means no eating, drinking, smoking, or chewing gum while in the laboratory area. Never put pens or pencils in your mouth.
2. *Avoid hand-eye contact in the work area.* Do not rub your eyes, handle contact lenses, or apply cosmetics.
3. *Never store food or beverages in the same refrigerator with reagents or specimens.*
4. *Do not let anything hang loose that might get contaminated or caught in equipment.* Tie back shoulder-length hair, and never wear long chains, large or dangling earrings, or loose bracelets.
5. *Protect your feet from spills, slips, and falling objects.* Never wear open-toe or open-back shoes. Shoes should be sturdy and made of nonabsorbent material, with nonskid soles.
6. *Always wear the appropriate personal protective equipment when handling specimens.*

Physical Hazards

Avoiding physical hazards in the workplace is mostly a matter of common sense, plus learning some important habits:

- Avoid running. This is not only a safety rule but also a consideration for patients, who may become concerned or agitated.
- Watch for wet floors.

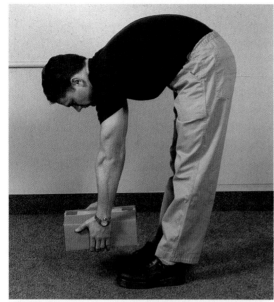

A

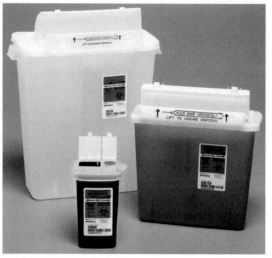

Figure 3-2
Sharps containers.

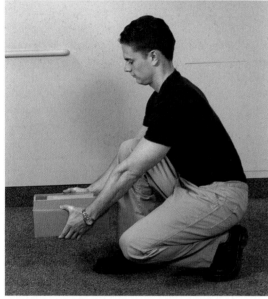

B

Figure 3-1
A, Improper lifting technique. **B**, Proper lifting technique. The knees should be bent while lifting; this allows the legs to bear the weight, instead of the back.

- Bend your knees when lifting heavy objects or transferring a patient (Figure 3-1).
- Maintain a clean, organized work area.

Sharps Hazards

Sharps, especially needles and lancets, are the most common hazards you will encounter as a phlebotomist. To prevent contact, never manually recap a needle. As you will learn in Chapter 8, needle recapping devices or special removal devices are available,

so you should never have to place the cap on an exposed needle by hand before disposing of it. Also, used needles should never be removed from a syringe by hand, and you should never bend or break a needle. Always dispose of sharps immediately after use in a puncture-resistant container (Figure 3-2). It is best to keep the needle disposal device within arm's reach during the procedure.

Safety engineering for sharps includes shielded or self-blunting needles for both vacuum tubes and butterflies, as well as syringe needles with cylindrical sheaths, used when injecting blood into vacuum tubes. The needle stick Safety and Prevention Act of 2001 require that all employers switch to safety needle devices to minimize the risk of accidental sticks, and solicit employee input in choosing safer devices. Failure to comply with the 2001 regulation can result in high fines for the institution and the individual who violates the act.

If you are stuck by a used needle or other sharp object that has been in contact with blood, or you get blood in your eyes, nose, mouth, or broken skin:

1. *Immediately* flood the exposed area with water and clean any wound with soap and water or a skin disinfectant.
2. Report this immediately to your employer. Your employer is required to keep a log of such incidents.
3. Seek immediate medical attention.

Some phlebotomists may be tempted to cut some safety corners, especially as they gain more confidence in their handling of needles and other sharps. But there is never a good enough reason to take such risks. The risk of infection is always present, and there can be months of psychological trauma while waiting to learn the results of serologic testing after an accidental needle stick. In many institutions, not following safety procedures is grounds for dismissal.

Clinical Tip: Remember, never manually recap a needle.

Chemical Hazards

You will encounter many different chemicals in your work as a phlebotomist, including several that can be quite harmful if handled improperly. Hydrochloric acid, which burns mucosal tissue and skin, is used as a preservative for urine. Bleach, which causes irritation of mucosal tissue and skin, is used as a disinfectant.

Identification of Chemicals

The safe handling of chemicals begins with proper labeling. All chemicals should have labels that identify the chemical by name, and you should read the label carefully before using any chemical. *Do not use a chemical that is not labeled.*

The OSHA Hazardous Communication Standard requires that all manufacturers label hazardous material (Figure 3-3). The label must have:

- A warning to alert you to the hazard.
- An explanation of the hazard.
- A list of precautions to reduce the risk.
- First-aid measures to be used in case of exposure.

OSHA also requires that each chemical come with a Materials Safety Data Sheet (MSDS), which provides information about the chemical, its hazards, and procedures for cleanup and first aid. These data sheets must be kept on file in the workplace, and you have a right to review them.

Clinical Tip: "Right-to-know" laws allow you to review information on chemical hazards in the workplace.

Two other types of labels are used to identify hazardous materials. The **Department of Transportation** (DOT) **label** (Figure 3-4) displays the type of hazard, the United Nations hazard class number, and an identifying number. **The National Fire Protection Association** (NFPA) label (Figure 3-5) is a design recognized by firefighters that warns of the location of hazardous materials in the event of a fire. It uses a diamond-shaped symbol whose four quadrants indicate the relative danger level in four different areas: health, fire, chemical stability, and specific hazard types. Primarily designed for fixed installations, this symbol has been widely used to indicate hazards at the entrances to laboratory facilities within buildings.

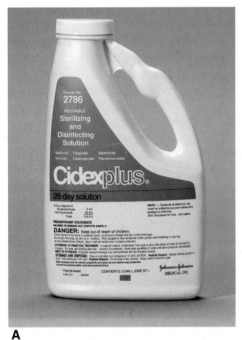

PRECAUTIONARY STATEMENTS
HAZARDS TO HUMANS AND DOMESTIC ANIMALS
DANGER: Keep out of reach of children.
Direct contact is corrosive to exposed tissue, causing eye damage and skin irritation/damage. Do not get into eyes, on skin or on clothing. Wear goggles or face shield and rubber gloves when handling or pouring. Avoid contamination of food. Use in well ventilated area in closed containers.
STATEMENT OF PRACTICAL TREATMENT: In case of contact, immediately flush eyes or skin with plenty of water for at least 15 minutes. For eyes, get medical attention. Harmful if swallowed. Drink large quantities of water and call a physician immediately.
NOTE TO PHYSICIAN: Probable mucosal damage may contraindicate the use of gastric lavage.
STORAGE AND DISPOSAL: Store at controlled room temperature 15°-30°C (59°-86°F).
Pesticide disposal: Discard residual solution in drain. Flush thoroughly with water.
Container disposal: Do not reuse empty container. Wrap container and put in trash.
Refer to package insert for material compatibility information and more detailed usage/product data.
Use with polycarbonate plastic could cause equipment failure.

*TRADEMARK   CONTENTS: 0.946 L (ONE QT.)
2786 C2-1   830006

A   **B**

Figure 3-3
Examples of OSHA-mandated labeling. **A,** Hazardous chemical container label. **B,** The label must indicate the possible hazards of the chemical. (From Bonewit-West K: Clinical Procedures for Medical Assistants, ed 6. Philadelphia, WB Saunders, 2004.)

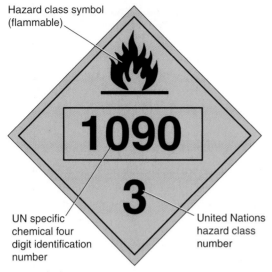

Hazard class symbol (flammable)

1090

3

UN specific chemical four digit identification number

United Nations hazard class number

Figure 3-4
DOT label displaying the type of hazard, the United Nations hazard class number, and an identifying number.

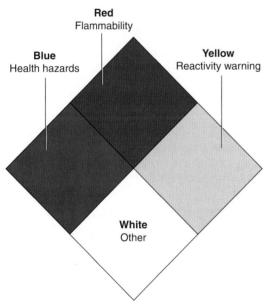

Red
Flammability

Blue
Health hazards

Yellow
Reactivity warning

White
Other

Figure 3-5
NFPA label.

Reducing Risk
OSHA further requires that every workplace develop and train its employees in a **chemical hygiene plan**. The plan describes all safety procedures, special precautions, and emergency procedures used when working with chemicals. Each employee must receive training in the details of the plan.

Although some chemicals are more dangerous than others, you should treat every chemical as if it were hazardous. This means that you should always use proper protective equipment when working with chemicals, including eye protection, a lab coat, and gloves.

Follow protocols and instructions carefully. For instance, if a protocol says to add an acid to water, do not add the water to the acid instead. Combining acid and water releases heat. By adding acid to water, you allow the large amount of water to heat up slowly. By adding water to concentrated acid, the small amount of water may boil on contact (Figure 3-6).

> **Clinical Tip:** Never add water to acid. Always add acid to water.

Other important precautions include:

- Follow the written chemical hygiene plan.
- Never mix chemicals together unless you are following an approved protocol.
- Never store chemicals above eye level.
- Know the location of safety showers and eyewash stations in the lab.

When Accidents Happen
Despite precautions, chemical accidents do occasionally occur. In such cases, you must be prepared to act quickly to prevent or minimize a serious injury.

If a chemical spills on you, proceed immediately to the safety shower or eyewash station. Flush the affected area with water for a minimum of 15 minutes,

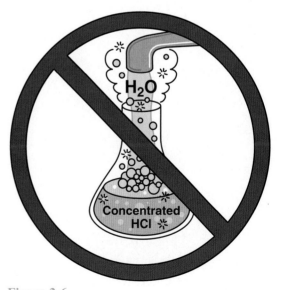

Figure 3-6
Adding water to concentrated acid is very dangerous.

and then proceed to the emergency room to be evaluated for further treatment.

If a chemical spills on the floor or a work surface, alert nearby personnel of the danger, and then follow lab protocol for cleanup. Cleanup kits should be available, with different types of equipment and neutralizing chemicals used for different types of spills.

Radioactive Hazards

Radioactive materials are used in health care facilities to perform diagnostic tests and deliver treatment. In areas in which radioactivity is used, the **radioactive hazard symbol** is displayed (Figure 3-7). Although the duties of a phlebotomist do not involve direct handling of radioactive materials, you may be exposed to small amounts of such materials when drawing blood from a patient in the radiology department, for instance, or when drawing blood from a patient receiving radioactive treatments. You may be exposed to x-rays in the emergency room.

The effects of radiation exposure increase with both the length of exposure and the dose of radiation. Pregnant women need to be especially careful to minimize their exposure because of the risk to the fetus. There are several important guidelines to follow to minimize your risk:

- Recognize the radioactive hazard symbol.
- Exercise extra caution in areas where radioactive materials are in use.

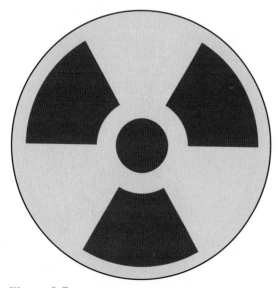

Figure 3-7
Radioactive hazard symbol.

- Learn your institution's procedures for minimizing exposure and responding to accidents.

Pregnant women in the first trimester should not enter a patient's room or a laboratory facility if there is a radiation alert posted at the door, to prevent possible adverse effect on the fetus.

Electrical Hazards

Electrical hazards in the lab may result in shock or fire. General rules of electrical safety apply in health care institutions as well, including:

- Avoid using extension cords.
- Report frayed cords, overloaded circuits, and ungrounded equipment.
- Unplug a piece of equipment before servicing it.
- If a piece of equipment is marked with an electrical caution warning, do not attempt to open it, even for inspection. It may contain batteries or electrical capacitors that store electricity even when unplugged.
- Know the location of the circuit breaker box for the equipment you are using.
- Avoid contact with any electrical equipment while drawing blood. Electricity may pass through you and the needle and shock the patient.

Emergency Response to Electrical Shock

If someone receives an electrical shock in the workplace, turn off the equipment, either by unplugging it or by switching off the circuit breaker. In the event you cannot turn off the electricity, break contact between the source and the victim using a *nonconductive* material, such as a wooden broom handle. Do not touch the victim until the risk of further shock is removed. Call for medical assistance (call 911), start **cardiopulmonary resuscitation** (CPR) if indicated, and keep the victim warm.

Fire and Explosive Hazards

Fires or explosions in the lab may occur due to chemical or electrical accidents, as well as carelessness with flames or other fire sources. In addition to preventive measures, the most important steps to take to minimize the risk of injury are:

- Pull the fire alarm immediately if smoke or flames are present.
- Know the location of fire extinguishers and fire blankets.

- Know how to use a fire extinguisher.
- Know the location of emergency exits.

Classes of Fire

There are five classes of fire, as identified by the NFPA, based on the fire's fuel source. These correspond to the type of extinguisher that should be used to combat the fire, as shown in Table 3-1. Type A fire extinguishers may contain water or dry chemicals. Type B extinguishers may contain dry chemicals, carbon dioxide, or environmentally safe fluorocarbons. Type C extinguishers are safe for electrical fires. Type D extinguishing agents are dry powders that may be contained in a pressurized extinguisher or in sealed cans for careful application. The newest class of extinguisher is the type K unit, which is used for kitchens or grease fires.

Emergency Action in Case of Fire

If a fire occurs in the workplace:

- Pull the nearest alarm.
- Call the fire department.
- Remove patients from danger.
- Close windows and doors to prevent fire spread.
- If the fire is small and isolated from other fuel sources, use an extinguisher to combat it.
- If the fire is not isolated or threatens to block exits, evacuate immediately. Leave through the nearest exit, using the stairs, not the elevator.

MRI Hazards

A magnetic resonance imaging (MRI) machine uses an extremely powerful magnet to create images of the body. The strength of the magnet poses significant safety risks when proper precautions are not taken. The magnet is strong enough to pull metal objects toward it from across the room at great speed. Warning signs are posted outside the MRI examination room. Anyone entering the MRI examination room must remove all metallic objects, including jewelry, belt buckles, and even zippers. People with implanted metallic devices may be barred from entering. The instructions of the MRI staff must be followed to prevent serious injury or death.

EMERGENCY FIRST-AID PROCEDURES

A full review of first-aid techniques is beyond the scope of this chapter. Here we review the most common types of emergencies and the major steps that should be taken to deal with them. Health care workers should be trained in the techniques of CPR and should refresh their skills biannually.

Bleeding Aid

1. Apply direct pressure to a bleeding wound, placing a clean cloth against the wound first, if available.
2. Elevate the limb, unless you suspect a fracture.
3. Maintain pressure until medical assistance is available.

Breathing Aid

1. Determine whether the victim is conscious by asking loudly, "Are you OK?" If there is no response and breathing has stopped, alert emergency medical personnel (either within the hospital or by calling 911) and begin rescue breathing.
2. With the victim on a firm, flat surface, position the victim's head by placing one hand on the forehead and one hand under the chin. Exert slight pressure on the forehead and pull up gently on the chin.
3. Check for breathing by placing your ear over the victim's nose and mouth. Also observe the chest for any breathing action.
4. If there are no signs of spontaneous breathing, pinch the nose shut, place your mouth over the victim's mouth, and exhale. Give two slow breaths. (Many authorities recommend using a device such as a face shield with a one-way valve as a barrier between your mouth and the victim's mouth rather than direct mouth-to-mouth contact. Your institution will probably provide training in the use of these devices.)
5. If the victim's chest does not rise, the airway is blocked and must be cleared before proceeding.
6. If the airway is clear, continue the rescue breathing cycle of one slow breath every five seconds, pausing so you can take a breath between each rescue breath. Continue until spontaneous breathing occurs or until professional assistance arrives.

Table 3-1 Classes of Fire

Class	Fuel	Extinguisher
A	Wood, paper, cloth	A, ABC
B	Grease, oil, flammable liquids	ABC, BC, halogenated agents
C	Safe for use on energized electrical equipment	
D	Flammable metals	Special equipment
K	Cooking oils and grease	Special equipment

Shock Prevention

1. Recognize the early signs of shock: pale, cold, or clammy skin; rapid pulse; shallow breathing; weakness; possible nausea or vomiting.
2. Keep the victim lying down.
3. Elevate the legs, unless you suspect a fracture.
4. In case of vomiting, keep the airway open by turning the victim's head to the side and sweeping out his or her mouth with your finger.
5. Keep the victim warm.
6. Call for professional assistance.

DISASTER EMERGENCY PLAN

Most institutions have disaster emergency plans that describe procedures in the event of large-scale disasters such as flood, fire, earthquake, and the like. Learn your institution's procedures so that you are prepared to respond in an emergency.

LATEX SENSITIVITY

Latex sensitivity is an emerging and important problem in the health care field. Following the development of OSHA's Universal Precautions Standards in the 1980s, the use of natural rubber latex gloves for infection control skyrocketed. Since then, the incidence of latex sensitivity has grown from a trickle to a flood. It is an issue that every health care worker must be concerned about.

Regulations by the Food and Drug Administration (FDA) require the labeling of medical gloves that contain natural rubber latex or powder. Glove boxes are required to bear caution statements whose wording depends on the actual content of the gloves.

The reaction to latex products can take one of three forms. **Irritant contact dermatitis** occurs as a result of direct skin contact with materials left on the latex surface during manufacturing, such as processing chemicals. Redness, swelling, and itching may occur within minutes to hours of exposure. Removing the glove and washing the exposed area are enough to reduce the reaction within several hours. The skin may become highly sensitized with repeat exposure.

Allergic contact dermatitis is a true allergic response, in which the body's immune system reacts to the proteins or other components of the latex that are absorbed through the skin. Perspiration increases absorption. Absorption may also occur through inhalation of glove powder. Symptoms may not be localized to the exposed area.

Anaphylaxis is a rapid, severe immune reaction that can be life-threatening if not treated. During anaphylaxis, the airway may swell shut, the heart rate may increase, and the blood pressure drops. Epinephrine injection and emergency room management are needed for anaphylaxis.

Preventing Latex Reactions

Individuals with known sensitivity to latex should wear a medical alert bracelet. Patients should be asked about allergies or other reactions to previous latex exposure. The substances causing latex allergy are similar to ones found in chestnuts and some tropical fruits such as kiwi, avocado, and banana. Patients should be asked about allergies or reactions to any of these fruits. There are a variety of alternatives to latex-containing gloves, and these should be available for use.

REVIEW FOR CERTIFICATION

Safety is a paramount concern in the health care workplace. OSHA is responsible for workplace safety and has created rules and regulations to improve safety. These regulations govern the handling of sharps, chemicals, and other occupational hazards. The phlebotomist must pay close attention to workplace safety and learn the most effective ways to avoid hazards such as physical, chemical, biological, electrical, fire, and radioactive dangers. Most important of all is the danger of accidental contamination with blood or other body fluids. Latex sensitivity is a growing problem. Nonlatex gloves may be useful.

BIBLIOGRAPHY

Carroll P, Celia F: What You Need to Know about Latex Allergy. Medical Laboratory Observer. July 2000.

Francis AL: Glove Me Tender. The Scientist. May 15, 2000.

Henry JB: Clinical Diagnosis and Management by Laboratory Methods, ed 21. Philadelphia, WB Saunders, 2006.

Muller BA: Minimizing Latex Exposure and Allergy. Postgraduate Medicine. April 2003.

NCCLS: National Committee for Clinical Laboratory Standards. Villanova, PA, NCCLS.

NIOSH Alert: Preventing allergic reactions to natural rubber latex in the workplace. DHHS Publication No. 97-135. August 1997.

Toraason M, Sussman G, Biagini R, et al: Latex Allergy in the Workplace. Toxicological Sciences. November 2000.

STUDY QUESTIONS

1. Name six types of safety hazards in the workplace and give an example of each.
2. List five safety precautions that can reduce the risk of injury in the workplace.
3. Because needle sticks are a major concern, what should you never do after performing a venipuncture?
4. List the four identifying features that all hazardous material labels must display.
5. Describe the purpose of a materials safety data sheet.
6. Explain the purpose of a chemical hygiene plan.
7. In the event a chemical spills on your arm, what steps should be taken?
8. Describe the steps in the emergency response to electrical shock.
9. List the different types of fire extinguishers and what each contains.
10. Describe the protocol for assistive breathing.
11. Describe three types of reaction associated with latex usage.
12. Name the organization that regulates workplace safety and define its purpose.
13. Explain the process that should be followed in controlling a bleeding emergency.
14. List the signs of shock and what steps to take to prevent further complications.
15. What are the recommendations to follow regarding disaster emergency plans?

CERTIFICATION EXAM PREPARATION

1. OSHA stands for:
   a. Occupational Standards in Health Associations
   b. Outline of Safety Hazards and Accidents
   c. Occupational Safety and Health Administration
   d. Occupational Standards and Health Administration

2. When mixing acids and water, one should:
   a. add acid to water
   b. add water to acid
   c. never mix acids and water together
   d. add equal amounts in an empty container

3. Chemicals should:
   a. be stored above eye level
   b. be labeled properly
   c. be cleaned up using soap and water
   d. be disposed of in the sink

4. The first action to take in the event of fire is:
   a. Call the fire department.
   b. Close windows and doors.
   c. Remove patients from danger.
   d. Pull the fire alarm.

5. In the event of electrical shock, the first thing one should do is:
   a. Call 911.
   b. Attempt to turn off the electrical equipment.
   c. Break contact between the source and the victim.
   d. Start CPR.

6. Class C fires involve:
   a. wood
   b. grease or oil
   c. flammable materials
   d. electrical equipment

7. Which of the following does the NFPA symbol not warn about?
   a. protective equipment
   b. fire
   c. chemical stability
   d. health

8. The first thing to do when giving breathing aid to a victim is:
   a. Clear the airway.
   b. Place the victim on a firm, flat surface.
   c. Begin mouth-to-mouth ventilations.
   d. Determine whether the victim is conscious.

9. Safety equipment in the lab may include:
   a. personal protective equipment
   b. emergency shower
   c. eyewash station
   d. all of the above

10. An MSDS provides information on:
    a. sharps
    b. patients
    c. chemicals
    d. office procedures

11. Reaction to latex products may include:
    a. irritant contact dermatitis
    b. allergic contact dermatitis
    c. anaphylaxis
    d. all of the above

12. The yellow diamond in the NFPA label indicates:
    a. health hazards
    b. flammability
    c. reactivity warning
    d. other

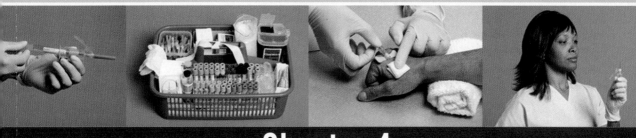

Chapter 4

Infection Control

OUTLINE

Infection
Chain of Infection
   Means of Transmission
Breaking the Chain of Infection
   Hand Hygiene
   Personal Protective Equipment
   Standard Precautions

Occupational Safety and Health
   Administration Bloodborne
   Pathogens Standard
Isolation Control Measures
   Airborne Precautions
   Droplet Precautions
   Contact Precautions

Blood-Borne Pathogens
   Contact with Blood-Borne
   Pathogens
   Viral Survival
Cleaning Up a Spill
Review for Certification

OBJECTIVES

After completing this chapter, you should be able to:

1. Define infection and differentiate between community-acquired and health care–associated infections.
2. Explain how organisms found in a hospital are different from those found in the community.
3. Explain four ways that infectious agents may be transmitted and give examples of each.
4. Discuss the importance of proper hand hygiene in breaking the chain of infection.
5. Describe proper hand-hygiene technique, including the sequence of steps.
6. Define personal protective equipment and describe at least four types.

7. Describe the order and procedure for putting on and removing personal protective equipment.
8. Define OSHA and explain its role in infection control.
9. Define blood-borne pathogen and give examples.
10. Explain how blood-borne pathogens may be transmitted.
11. Explain the components of standard precautions.
12. Define expanded precautions and describe the different types.
13. Given an isolation classification, select the appropriate personal protective equipment.
14. Explain general procedures for cleaning up a blood spill.

KEY TERMS

airborne infection
  isolation precautions
airborne transmission
blood-borne pathogens
chain of infection
common vehicle
  transmission

contact precautions
contact transmission
droplet nuclei
droplet precautions
droplet transmission
expanded precautions
exposure control plan

fomite
health care–associated
  infections
HEPA
infection
isolation
pathogens

personal protective
  equipment
protective environment
reservoir
standard precautions
vectors

The goal of infection control is to develop and maintain an environment that minimizes the risk of acquiring or transmitting infectious agents to hospital personnel, patients and visitors. It is not always possible for you to know if a patient is infectious or is incubating an infection. Therefore, it is important that you understand how infections occur, and that you follow infection control practices and policies to protect yourself and your patients from infectious agents. Infection control requires recognizing potential sources of transmission and breaking the chain of infection. Techniques for preventing transmission include hand hygiene, use of personal protective equipment, and use of both standard and expanded precautions. In Chapter 3, you learned how to recognize and prevent physical safety hazards on the job. In this chapter, we examine in detail the biological hazards with which you may come in contact. By taking appropriate precautions against potentially infectious organisms, you can make the workplace safe for you, your patients, and your coworkers.

INFECTION

The human body is host to a variety of microorganisms that normally do not cause illness. Such organisms are said to colonize the body. For example, the skin has several common types of bacteria that live harmlessly on its surface. Although these microorganisms can live and multiply on and within the body without causing disease, the correct conditions, such as a break in the skin, can allow these organisms to enter the body and cause an **infection**. An infection is an invasion and growth of a microorganism in the human body that causes disease. Infectious organisms, also called **pathogens**, can be viruses, bacteria, fungi, protists, helminths, or prions. Some common infectious organisms are listed in Table 4-1. The number of potential pathogens is large, however, and the list is not comprehensive.

The infectious agents found in a hospital are often more virulent and more resistant to treatment than are most organisms found at large in the community. This is true for three reasons. First, a more virulent organism is more likely to cause a more serious disease, meaning that an infected person is more likely to be admitted for treatment. Second, hospitalized patients usually have a lowered resistance to infection by potential pathogens and opportunistic organisms. Third, treatment with antibiotics may leave the most resistant organisms alive through the process of natural selection. These organisms then cause even more serious disease, requiring more aggressive treatment, usually in a hospital.

Infections contracted by patients during a hospital stay are termed **health care–associated infections**. Health care–associated infections may be due to direct contact with other patients, but are most often caused by failure of hospital personnel to follow infection control practices, such as hand hygiene.

CHAIN OF INFECTION

The **chain of infection** requires a continuous link among three primary elements: the source, the means of transmission, and the susceptible host (Figure 4-1). In addition, other links in this chain include a "portal of exit" (the means by which the infectious agent leaves the source) and a "portal of entry" (the means by which the infectious agent enters the host, resulting in infection or colonization). The source can be an infected person, who may be either symptomatic or asymptomatic. The source may also be a contaminated object (called a **fomite**), such as equipment or supplies, or it may be food or water contaminated with the infectious agent. The susceptible host may be a patient, a health care professional, or a visitor. Microorganisms can be transmitted by contact (either direct or indirect), droplet or airborne routes. The means of transmission of

Table 4-1   Common Infectious Organisms and Diseases They Cause

Organism	Disease
Viruses	
Adenovirus	Upper respiratory infections
Herpes simplex	Oral and genital herpes
Varicella-zoster	Chickenpox, shingles
Poliovirus	Polio
Influenza virus	Influenza, or "flu"
HIV	AIDS
Hepatitis virus (A, B, C, D, E, and G)	Hepatitis
Bacteria	
Staphylococcus aureus	Skin and wound infections, food poisoning
Escherichia coli	Food poisoning; some types are normal residents of the colon
Haemophilus influenzae	Meningitis, pinkeye, and upper respiratory infections
Corynebacterium diphtheriae	Diphtheria
Bordetella pertussis	Pertussis, or whooping cough
Mycobacterium tuberculosis	Tuberculosis
Streptococcus	"Strep throat," rheumatic fever, other types of infections
Neisseria meningitidis	Meningococcal meningitis
Salmonella	Food poisoning
Treponema pallidum	Syphilis
Neisseria gonorrhoeae	Gonorrhea
Fungi	
Cryptococcus neoformans	Cryptococcosis
Candida albicans	Candidiasis
Protists	
Entamoeba histolytica	Amebiasis, dysentery
Giardia lamblia	Giardiasis
Trichomonas vaginalis	Trichomoniasis
Plasmodium	Malaria

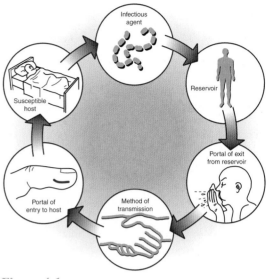

Figure 4-1

The chain of infection. The disease cycle continues to repeat unless measures are taken to stop the cycle, such as practicing meticulous hand hygiene and isolating the patient. (Modified from Polaski A, Warner J: Saunders Fundamentals for Nursing Assistants. Philadelphia, WB Saunders, 1994.)

Means of Transmission

Infectious agents can spread by five different means:

1. Contact, both direct and indirect.
2. Droplet.
3. Airborne.
4. Common vehicle.
5. Vector.

Contact Transmission

Contact transmission is the most frequent and important transmission route for health care–associated infections. Direct contact involves the transfer of microorganisms from an infected or colonized person directly to a susceptible host by physical contact between the source and susceptible host. Indirect contact involves contact between a susceptible host and a fomite, such as a medical instrument, needle, dressing, or bed rail. Phones, pencils, computer keyboards, gloves, and other objects can also act as sources of indirect contact transmission.

Droplet Transmission

Droplets are particles that are generated from the source by coughing, sneezing, or talking. Transmission of infectious agents by this route can also occur from liquid splashes, or aerosols formed by uncapping a blood collection tube or transferring

infectious agents can be as obvious as a puncture with a contaminated needle or as inconspicuous as exposure to airborne droplets from a person with tuberculosis. In some cases, a person may carry and transmit the agent without being sick; this person is considered a **reservoir**. Breaking the chain of infection requires understanding the continuous links in the chain and applying appropriate interventions to interrupt the link between them.

blood from a syringe to a tube. Because droplet particles are bigger than 5 micrometers in size, they are propelled only a short distance before falling and coming to rest. Therefore, **droplet transmission** is likely for only a brief time and within a short distance (approximately 3 feet) of the source, meaning that specialized ventilation or air filtering equipment is not needed to prevent the transmission of infectious agents via droplets.

Airborne Transmission

Airborne transmission involves either airborne **droplet nuclei** or dust particles that contain the infectious microorganism. Droplet nuclei are particles smaller than 5 micrometers that can remain suspended in the air for long periods of time. These droplet nuclei can be transported long distances by air currents and cause disease when inhaled. Droplet nuclei can be formed by sneezing or coughing, or simply by singing or talking. They may also form during aerosol-producing procedures such as suctioning or bronchoscopy. Examples of microbes spread in this manner are *Mycobacterium tuberculosis*, rubeola virus (measles), and varicella-zoster virus (chickenpox). Special ventilation and air handling equipment designed to prevent airborne transmission include **HEPA** (high efficiency particulate air) filters.

Infectious agents found in the environment that can cause disease via the airborne route include *Aspergillus* and anthrax. *Aspergillus* species can be aerosolized from construction dust. Patients who are immunocompromised or immunosuppressed are at risk for *Aspergillus* infection. Anthrax in a finely milled powder can also be transmitted via the airborne route. These agents are not generally thought to be transmitted from person to person.

Common Vehicle Transmission

Common vehicle transmission involves a common source that causes multiple cases of disease. This type of transmission is caused by contaminated items such as food, water, medications, devices, and equipment. Examples of this are food-borne illnesses, such as Salmonellosis and Listeriosis, which can occur by ingesting food (e.g., chicken or hot dogs) contaminated with these bacteria. Although some infectious agents are inactivated in the gastrointestinal tract, many others are not.

Vector Transmission

Some infectious agents are carried by agents such as arthropods (e.g., insects, ticks) that are not harmed by their presence. Such organisms are called **vectors**.

Mosquitoes, for instance, may carry malaria and yellow fever, and ticks may carry Lyme disease and Rocky Mountain spotted fever.

BREAKING THE CHAIN OF INFECTION

The chain of infection is broken by disrupting the continuous chain from source to host, thus preventing transmission of infectious microorganisms. Transmission is prevented by practicing appropriate hand hygiene, using personal protective equipment (PPE), isolating patients at risk of spreading or contracting infections, and using the set of practices known as "standard precautions." Your facility should have an **exposure control plan** that describes all these elements for preventing spread of infection.

Hand Hygiene

Hand hygiene is the single most important and effective means of preventing the spread of infection and antibiotic-resistant microorganisms. Hand hygiene includes washing your hands with plain or antimicrobial soap and water, or disinfecting your hands with an alcohol-based hand agent. An alcohol-based hand agent is the preferred hand hygiene agent because it has greater ability to kill microbes, is less drying than plain or antimicrobial soap and water, and is more convenient. Soap and water should be used when hands are visibly soiled.

While performing your duties, your hands continually come in contact with patients and with potentially infected material and microorganisms. Wearing gloves reduces but does not eliminate the chance of your hands carrying infectious agents. Performing appropriate hand hygiene significantly reduces the likelihood of passing potentially infectious agents on to yourself or other people.

You should perform hand hygiene:

before and after patient contact;
before donning gloves and after removing gloves;
before performing procedures;
after removing personal protective equipment;
after touching contaminated equipment;
before going to break; and
before leaving the lab at the end of your shift.

You may want to routinely disinfect your hands when you enter a patient's room, even if you just disinfected them in the last patient's room, as it gives the patient confidence that you are doing all you can to prevent health care–associated infection.

Clinical Tip: Perform hand hygiene upon entering and before exiting a patient's room and before donning gloves and after removing gloves.

Procedure 4-1 illustrates proper hand-washing technique. To disinfect your hands with waterless alcohol-based antiseptic hand rub, apply the product to the palm of one hand, being sure to pump enough of the product to cover all the surfaces of your hands and fingers. Rub your hands together, covering *all surfaces* of your hands and fingers, until your hands are dry.

Personal Protective Equipment

Personal protective equipment (PPE) are barriers and respirators used alone or in combination to protect skin, mucous membranes, and clothing from contact with infectious agents. PPE includes fluid-resistant gowns, aprons, masks and respirators, face shields, goggles, shoe covers, and gloves. The types of PPE you use depend on the tasks or procedures being performed, the amount of fluids you are working with, and the potential for exposure to these fluids.

Fluid-resistant gowns provide full body coverage and prevent body fluids or spills from passing through and contacting the skin or clothing. The cuffs are designed to close tightly around the wrists and are covered by the gloves as well, for further protection. Alternatively, a cloth gown may be worn to prevent contamination of skin and clothing with transmissible infectious microorganisms when protection from fluid penetration is not necessary.

Face protection is worn to protect mucous membranes of the eyes, mouth, and nose from splashes or sprays of blood, bodily fluids (including excretions and secretions). Face protection includes goggles and mask or a chin-length face shield.

Face shields can prevent droplets or spatters from contacting non-intact skin of the face (Figure 4-2). In some models, the shield can be flipped up out of the way, if necessary. Masks cover the mouth and nose to protect mucous membranes from large droplets of respiratory secretions from a coughing patient and from splashes of blood or body fluids generated during certain procedures (Figure 4-3).

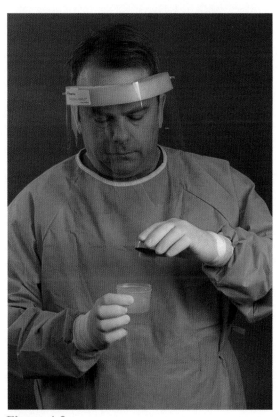

Figure 4-2
A phlebotomist wearing a face shield.

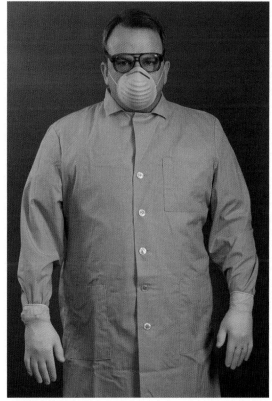

Figure 4-3
A phlebotomist wearing a mask.

Procedure 4-1

Hand-Washing Technique

1. Wet your hands.
   Remove any rings you are wearing, and wet your hands with warm water.

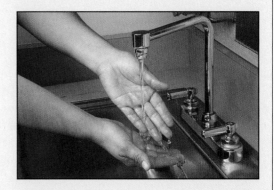

2. Apply soap.
   Antimicrobial soap should be applied from an easily accessible container.

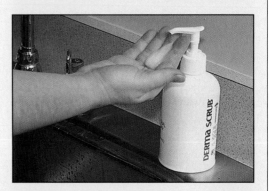

3. Scrub vigorously.
   The friction of rubbing hands together loosens debris and creates a lather to wash away surface material. Rub palms, backs of hands, between fingers, and under nails for at least 15 seconds.

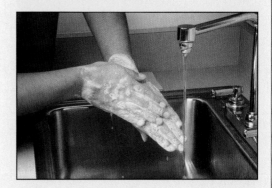

Procedure 4-1—cont'd

Hand-Washing Technique

4. Rinse your hands.

While rinsing the hands, be sure to hold them in a downward position. This allows water and lather to run into the sink instead of back on clean hands.

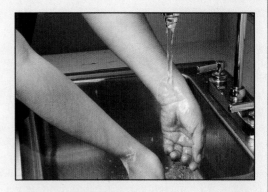

5. Dry your hands.

Use a paper towel, being careful not to touch the paper towel dispenser as you are obtaining the towel. Dry the hands thoroughly.

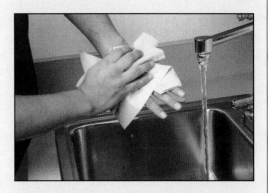

6. Turn off the faucet, using a new dry paper towel

Use a new, dry paper towel to turn off the faucet. (The faucet is considered contaminated, whereas the hands are now considered clean.) When finished, throw the paper towel in the waste container.

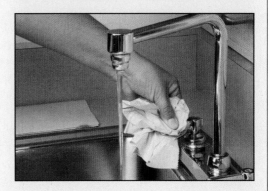

Goggles and mask or face shield must be worn during procedures that may generate splashes of blood, or bodily fluid excretions or secretions. Masks can also worn by health care workers to prevent transmission of infectious microorganisms to the patient (e.g., lung transplant/bone marrow transplant patients). Masks are secured to the head either with elastic loops or two cloth straps for tying behind the head. They also have a metal band at the nose to seal the mask over the bridge of the nose.

Respirators are designed to prevent inhalation of airborne microorganisms. These masks are tight fitting and have filters whose filtration efficiency capability is set by the Occupational Safety and Health Administration (OSHA), and must be certified by the National Institute for Occupational Safety and Health (NIOSH). Such masks are known as N95 masks or N95 respirators, meaning they filter out a minimum of 95% of airborne particles, *if they are worn correctly*. Before you wear a respirator, you must receive medical clearance and be fit-tested to the specific respirator. You must check the fit each time you wear the respirator, by checking for leaks on both inhalation and exhalation.

Gloves are designed to fit tightly over the hand and fingers to allow precision work. Gloves are made of a variety of materials (e.g., latex, vinyl, nitrile) and come in several sizes. They can have cornstarch powder inside as a lubricant. Individuals who are allergic to natural latex proteins or other components of latex gloves may need to wear hypoallergenic gloves or gloves made from synthetic materials. Gloves provide a protective barrier against blood and other body fluids and from contamination of hands with microorganisms.

 Clinical Tip: Gloves are not a fail-safe barrier to contamination. Always perform hand hygiene before donning and after removing gloves.

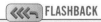 **FLASHBACK**

You learned about latex allergy in Chapter 3.

Shoe covers can protect your shoes and feet from spills of biohazardous materials or chemicals. Shoes that are not protected by shoe covers and that cannot be appropriately disinfected may need to be disposed of after a spill.

Putting on and Removing Personal Protective Equipment

The order in which you don and remove your PPE is chosen to ensure that you do not contaminate your skin or clothing with infectious agents. Procedures for putting on and removing PPE are illustrated in Procedures 4-2 and 4-3.

Standard Precautions

Standard precautions refer to infection control measures that use barrier protection and work practice controls to prevent contact between skin or mucous membranes and blood, other body fluids, and tissues from all persons. Standard precautions are based on the difficulty of identifying all individuals who are infected or harboring infectious agents with whom the health care worker may come in contact. Standard precautions should be the minimum level of precautions applied when coming in contact with all patients. New guidelines for standard precautions were published by the Centers for Disease Control and Prevention (CDC) in 1996.

Standard precautions include:

Hand hygiene: Disinfect hands whether or not gloves are worn. Use an alcohol-based hand agent unless hands are visibly contaminated, then use soap and water.

Gloves: Wear gloves when collecting or handling blood, body fluids, tissue samples, secretions, excretions, and items contaminated with blood or body fluids. Remove gloves promptly after use, and disinfect your hands.

Gowns: Wear fluid-resistant gowns when there is a likelihood of contamination of your clothing or skin with blood or body fluids.

Face protection: Wear appropriate protection (mask and goggles or chin-length face shield) when there is a danger of spray, spatter, or aerosol formation.

Sharps disposal: Dispose of all needles and other sharps in a puncture-proof container, after engaging the safety device. Do not recap the needle.

Respiratory hygiene and cough etiquette: This is a new component of standard precautions that was added in 2003 in response to the SARS (severe acute respiratory syndrome) outbreak in 2003. These infection control measures are aimed at preventing transmission of respiratory infections. These measures apply to patients, their families and friends, and any person with signs of a cold and respiratory infection. These precautions include

Procedure 4-2

Putting on Personal Protective Equipment

Perform hand hygiene before donning PPE.

1. **Put on the gown.**
   Tie the gown behind your back.

2. **Put on the mask, respirator and goggles or face shield.**
   Tie the top strap of the mask, then the bottom. Crimp the metal band down across the bridge of your nose. If you are donning a respirator (not shown), secure the elastic band at the middle of your head and neck. Crimp the metal band down across the bridge of your nose. Perform a fit-check. Don goggles or face shield. Adjust the face shield headband for a firm, comfortable fit.

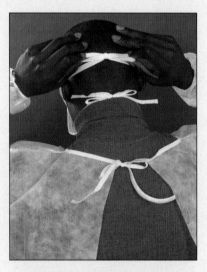

3. **Put on the gloves.**
   Pull the gloves on tightly, and stretch the ends of the gloves over the cuffs of the gown. The gloves should fit snugly over the cuff.

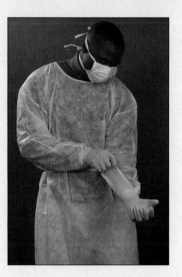

Procedure 4-3

Removing Personal Protective Equipment

The order of removal is important to prevent contamination of your skin and clothing. Except for the respirator, your PPE should be removed at the doorway, before leaving the patient's room or in the anteroom. Remove the respirator outside the room, after the door has been closed, to avoid airborne transmission.

1. **Remove the gloves.**
   The outside of the gloves are contaminated. Pull the gloves off from the open end, turning each inside out as it is removed. To remove the first glove, grasp the *outer* surface near the wrist. To remove the second glove, slide a finger inside and grasp the *inner* surface. This avoids contact between your ungloved finger and the outer, contaminated glove surface. Follow hospital infection control policy for proper disposal.

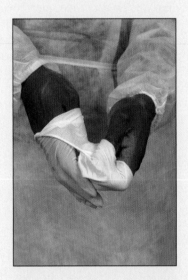

2. **Remove the face shield or goggles.**
   The outside of the goggles or face shield is contaminated. To remove, handle by the clean head band or ear pieces. Follow hospital infection control policy for proper disposal.

3. **Remove the gown.**
   The front and sleeves of the gown are contaminated. Fold the gown with the contaminated side inward. Follow hospital infection control policy for proper disposal.

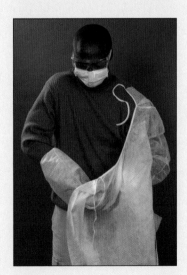

Procedure 4-3—cont'd

Removing Personal Protective Equipment

4. **Remove the mask or respirator.**

   The front of the mask or respirator is contaminated. Grasp the bottom ties or elastics, then the top ones, and remove. Follow hospital infection control policy for proper disposal.

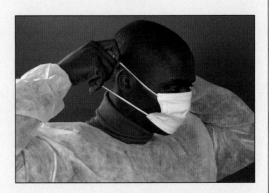

5. **Perform hand hygiene after removing your PPE.**

posting signs to instruct persons who are coughing to cover their mouth and nose with tissues, dispose of used tissues in the trash, and perform hand hygiene after contact with respiratory secretions. There should also be a supply of tissues and alcohol-based hand agents available for these patients, and persons who are coughing should be asked to wear a surgical mask and separate themselves from other patients in the waiting room if possible.

 Clinical Tip: Activate the safety device before disposing of the sharp in the needle box. Never recap a used needle.

OCCUPATIONAL SAFETY AND HEALTH ADMINISTRATION BLOODBORNE PATHOGENS STANDARD

The Occupational Safety and Health Administration (OSHA) is a regulatory enforcement agency for employee health and safety that has authority over all industries, including hospitals and health care facilities. In 1992, OSHA gave the standard precautions the force of law by making them part of a larger set of standards designed to protect health care workers from infection. The blood-borne pathogen rule was revised in 2001 to clarify issues related to sharps safety. The Bloodborne Pathogens Standard set by OSHA includes the following:

- Employers must have a written blood-borne pathogen exposure control plan in the workplace, and it must be readily accessible to employees.
- Employers must provide the proper PPE to employees at no charge, train employees in the use of PPE, and require employees to wear PPE.
- Employers must mandate that all blood and body fluids and other potentially infectious materials are treated as if they are infectious, and must implement work practice and engineering controls to minimize or prevent occupational exposure.
- Employers must provide immunization against hepatitis B virus to employees free of charge. If the employee declines the vaccine, the employer must document that the vaccine was offered by having the employee sign a waiver.
- Employers must provide free medical follow-ups to employees in the event of accidental exposure.
- Employers must provide education and safety training for employees at the time of hire and annually thereafter.

- Employers must provide additional training, education, and containment policies for HIV and HBV research laboratories.
- All biohazardous materials must be appropriately identified with a biohazard label or a color-coded system and contained to prevent leakage. Regulated medical waste must be disposed of into appropriate containers (e.g., sharps and needles into puncture-resistant leakproof containers).
- Employers must provide a written schedule for cleaning, including a procedure for how to clean blood and other potentially infectious materials and the type of disinfectant to use. Employees must carry out a daily and as-needed disinfection protocol on countertops and workspaces (e.g., bleach disinfection).
- Employers must maintain records on occupational exposure and employee training sessions.

Following these mandated standards significantly reduces the likelihood of infection.

ISOLATION CONTROL MEASURES

Isolation means the separation of an infection source from susceptible hosts, thereby breaking the chain of infection. Isolation control measures can be used to protect the patient from infectious agents in the environment or carried by staff or visitors, or can be used to protect staff, visitors, and other patients from patients with certain infectious diseases and conditions. Such patients may be in private rooms with specific isolation precautions (e.g., droplet, contact, airborne) posted outside the door. In some cases, a separate floor of a hospital may be reserved for patients with infections that are transmitted via the airborne route, and therefore require special ventilation and air handling. An example of this is tuberculosis, which requires negative pressure air (so that air flows in, not out, of the unit). Air is exhausted directly to the outside or recirculated through HEPA filtration.

Immunocompromised patients may have their own isolation unit. This is termed a **protective environment** (PE). These units are designed to minimize risk of acquiring environmental fungal infections (e.g., Aspergillosis). Such patients may include chemotherapy patients and transplant patients. PE rooms have HEPA-filtered air and positive air pressure (air flows out, not in) with respect to adjacent areas. In addition, there may be special requirements for wearing gloves, mask, and gowns when providing care for these patients. Be sure to check with the infection control practice policies at your facility.

Isolation precautions are based on a two-tiered system. Tier 1 includes precautions used for all patients in the hospital, without regard to their diagnosis or infection status. Standard precautions are used for tier 1 isolation. Standard precautions are meant to protect against transmission of infectious agents by means of blood, body fluids, secretions, and excretions; through exposure to mucous membranes, nonintact skin surfaces; and through punctures. The purpose of these precautions is to prevent transmission of pathogens regardless of a patient's diagnosis or infection status.

Tier 2 isolation uses **expanded precautions** (EP). This tier is targeted at patients known or suspected to be infected with a highly transmissible pathogen. It also applies to pathogens that are considered epidemiologically important, such as MRSA (methicillin-resistant *Staphylococcus aureus*) and VRE (vancomycin-resistant *Enterococcus*). EPs begin with standard precautions and add additional precautions based on the potential means of transmission of the suspected or identified disease or condition. There are three types of EPs: airborne, droplet, and contact. Some diseases may require a combination of precautions. An example of this is varicella (chickenpox), which requires that a nonimmunized person use both airborne and contact precautions. Immunized persons only need to use contact precautions when caring for a patient with varicella.

Airborne Precautions

In addition to standard precautions, **airborne precautions** are used for patients known or suspected to have a disease transmitted by airborne droplet nuclei. Examples of such illnesses are measles, varicella (including disseminated zoster), and tuberculosis. Airborne precautions include having the patient in a room with special air handling and ventilation. Persons entering the room must perform hand hygiene and wear an N95 respirator. A fit check must be done each time the respirator is put on.

Droplet Precautions

In addition to standard precautions, **droplet precautions** are used for patients known or suspected to have a disease transmitted by large infectious droplets that can be deposited on the conjunctivae or mucous membranes of a susceptible host. Examples

---

BOX 4-1   Diseases for Which Droplet Precautions Should Be Used

Bacterial Diseases
Invasive *Haemophilus influenzae* type b disease, including meningitis, pneumonia, epiglottitis, and sepsis
Invasive *Neisseria meningitidis* disease, including meningitis, pneumonia, and sepsis
Diphtheria (pharyngeal)
Mycoplasma pneumonia
Pertussis
Pneumonic plague
Streptococcal (group A) pharyngitis, pneumonia, or scarlet fever in infants and young children

Viral Diseases
Adenovirus*
Influenza
Mumps
Parvovirus B19
Rubella

*Certain infections require more than one type of precaution From Centers for Disease Control and Prevention, Atlanta, GA.

---

of such diseases are indicated in Box 4-1. Droplet precautions include performing hand hygiene and wearing a mask when within 3 feet of a patient.

Contact Precautions

In addition to standard precautions, **contact precautions** are used for patients known or suspected to have diseases or conditions transmitted by direct patient contact or by contact with items in the patient's environment. Examples are listed in Box 4-2. Contact precautions include performing hand hygiene, donning gloves, and wearing a gown before entering the room if contact with patient or patient's environment or potentially contaminated equipment is anticipated.

In all cases, the phlebotomist should not take anything into the room except the specific equipment needed, including the phlebotomy tray. Only the specimen should come back out, and it should be placed in a biohazard labeled bag. Remove gloves and gown and perform hand hygiene before leaving the room. Contaminated items should be disposed of in the appropriate receptacle in the patient room. For used needles, the safety device should be activated, and it should be disposed of into the needle box in the room. There should be a dedicated tourniquet in the patient room, or the tourniquet should be discarded or disinfected after use.

BOX 4-2 Diseases for Which Contact Precautions
            Should Be Used

Gastrointestinal, respiratory, skin, or wound infections or
    colonization with multidrug-resistant bacteria judged by
    the infection control program, based on current state,
    regional, or national recommendations, to be of special
    clinical and epidemiologic significance
Enteric infections with a low infectious dose or prolonged
    environmental survival, including *Clostridium difficile*
In diapered or incontinent patients: enterohemorrhagic
    Escherichia coli O157:H7, *Shigella*, hepatitis A, or
    rotavirus
In infants and young children: respiratory syncytial virus,
    parainfluenza virus, or enteroviral infections
Skin infections that are highly contagious or that may
    occur on dry skin, including:
Diphtheria (cutaneous)
Herpes simplex virus (neonatal or mucocutaneous)
Impetigo
Major (noncontained) abscesses, cellulitis, or decubitus
Pediculosis
Scabies
Staphylococcal furunculosis in infants and young children
Zoster (disseminated or in an immunocompromised host)
    (also airborne)
Viral or hemorrhagic conjunctivitis
Viral hemorrhagic infections (Ebola, Lassa, or Marburg)

From Centers for Disease Control and Prevention, Atlanta, GA.

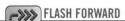 **FLASH FORWARD**

*You will learn about needle safety devices and procedures
in Chapter 8.*

BLOOD-BORNE PATHOGENS

Blood-borne pathogens (BBPs) are infectious agents
carried in the blood, certain body fluids, and unfixed
(unpreserved) tissues as defined in OSHA's Blood-
borne Pathogens Standard. Contracting a blood-borne
pathogen infection from an accidental needle stick is
the principal occupational risk for a phlebotomist.
The most common BBPs are listed in Box 4-3.

Contact with Blood-Borne Pathogens

The phlebotomist may be exposed to BBPs in a
number of ways. Exposures to blood or body fluids
can occur through:

• Percutaneous injury via needle-stick or puncture.
  Percutaneous contact occurs through the surface of

BOX 4-3 Blood-Borne Pathogens

Hepatitis B, C, and D
HIV
Human T-cell lymphotropic virus (HTLV) types I and II
Syphilis
Malaria
Babesiosis
Colorado tick fever

---

the skin, such as by scalpel cuts, transfusions,
sharps injuries, or other means that penetrate the
skin. Inoculation by accidental needlestick can
occur any time a needle is unsheathed. In Chapters
8 and 9, you will learn important safety techniques
to minimize the chances of a needle stick.
• Contact of mucous membranes (eyes, nose, mouth)
via splashes or touching eyes, nose, or mouth with
contaminated glove or hands.
• Contact of nonintact skin via splashes or contact
with contaminated gloves or hands. Nonintact
skin contact occurs through preexisting wounds,
scratches, abrasions, burns, or hangnails.
• Human bite.
• Contact with equipment or lab instruments contaminated with body fluid, as well as contact
through nail biting, smoking, eating, or contact
lens manipulation.
• Droplet transmission can occur by removal of
rubber stoppers; centrifuge accidents; splashing
or spattering, especially during transfer of blood
or other body fluids between containers; or failure
to wear a proper face shield.

Viral Survival

Blood-borne viruses have been shown to survive
outside the body for much longer than was once
believed possible. Viable HIV has been detected for
1 to 3 days after drying and can survive even longer
if it is frozen or lyophilized (freeze-dried). Hepatitis
B virus may be stable in dried blood and blood
products at 25°C for at least 7 days.

   This prolonged survival means that, as a phlebotomist, you must be even more aware of potential
sources of infection in your environment. Lab equipment such as centrifuges or quality-control products
that use human blood or body fluids should be handled with appropriate precautions. *Always* use PPE
when handling samples. Learn the procedures in
your lab for minimizing risk, including equipment-
related precautions, work practice controls, and spill

cleanup procedures. Disinfect your phlebotomy tray on a routine basis and whenever there is contamination with blood/body fluids. A 10% bleach solution, freshly made, can be used for this purpose.

CLEANING UP A SPILL

Despite careful techniques, spills do occur. Careful and thorough cleanup protects you and your coworkers from exposure to infectious agents and potential infection. Although each lab has its own detailed procedures, general guidelines include the following:

- Wear gloves.
- Use 10% bleach as a disinfectant. Bleach solutions must be made fresh every day.
- Clean up the visible blood first, and then disinfect the entire area of potential contamination.
- Allow the bleach to remain in contact with the contaminated area for 20 minutes to ensure complete disinfection.

Kits that contain powder or gels for absorption are available for large spills.

REVIEW FOR CERTIFICATION

Infection transmission can occur by contact (either direct or indirect), droplet, air, common vehicle, or vector. Hand hygiene is the single most important means of preventing spread of infection and should be done before and after patient contact; before donning gloves and after removing gloves, before performing procedures, after removing PPE, after touching potentially contaminated equipment, before eating, and whenever you enter or leave a patient's room, as well as at other times.

Breaking the chain of infection is accomplished through the use of standard and expanded precau-

tions and by following practices outlined in your facility's exposure control plan. The goal of standard precautions is to protect both the health care worker and patient from infectious agents through hand hygiene, use of PPE (gowns, gloves, face protection), engineering controls, and respiratory etiquette. Expanded precautions are used to guard against the transmission of specific organisms or types of diseases or conditions that require more than standard precautions.

Phlebotomists are particularly at risk for exposure to infection from blood-borne pathogens, which can occur by an accidental needle stick or other routes of exposure to blood. Use of appropriate PPE, engineering controls, and safe work practices can reduce your exposure to blood-borne pathogens and other infectious agents. Cleaning up spills properly and according to protocol reduces the risk of infection transmission should a spill occur.

BIBLIOGRAPHY

APIC Text of Infection Control & Epidemiology, ed 2. January 2005

Baron EJ, Finegold SM: Diagnostic Microbiology. St. Louis, Mosby, 1990.

Brzeicki LA: Safety First Staff Input Essential in Selection of PPE. Advance for Medical Laboratory Professionals. March 13, 2000.

CDC Guidelines for Isolation Precautions: Preventing Transmission of Infectious Agents in Healthcare Settings http://www.cdc.gov/ncidod/dhqp/gl_isolation.html

Clinical and Laboratory Standards Institute: M29-A3: Protection of Laboratory Workers from Occupationally Acquired Infections, ed 3. 2005.

Safe Needle Compliance Report. The POL Answer Book. Rockville, MD, 1999.

Weinstein S: Preventing blood-borne exposures in laboratory and phlebotomy staff. Advance for Medical Laboratory Professionals. September 6, 1999.

STUDY QUESTIONS

1. Define infection.
2. Name four classifications of pathogens.
3. List the infectious organisms that cause each of the following diseases:
   AIDS
   Hepatitis
   Tuberculosis
   Strep throat
   Syphilis
   Gonorrhea
   Malaria
   Trichomoniasis
   Oral and genital herpes
4. What are health care–associated infections, and how are they typically caused?
5. What three main elements make up the chain of infection?
6. List three ways in which one can break the chain of infection.
7. Explain the difference between direct and indirect contact transmission.
8. What is the difference between a vector and a fomite?
9. What is the most important and effective way of preventing the spread of infection?
10. Name four items included in PPE.
11. Explain what standard precautions are and why they are used.
12. Name three blood-borne pathogens.
13. Hepatitis B may be stable in dried blood for at least _____ days.
14. Bleach should be in contact with a contaminated area for _____ minutes for complete disinfection.
15. Explain the possible reasons behind the 1992 OSHA standards and give the policies set within this standard.

CERTIFICATION EXAM PREPARATION

1. Which of the following would not be considered a pathogen?
   a. bacteria
   b. viruses
   c. fungi
   d. vectors

2. Varicella-zoster is the cause of:
   a. syphilis
   b. chickenpox
   c. malaria
   d. hepatitis

3. HIV is the causative agent of:
   a. gonorrhea
   b. food poisoning
   c. AIDS
   d. hepatitis B

4. Vectors include:
   a. doorknobs
   b. medical instruments
   c. needles
   d. insects

5. Some types of *Escherichia coli* are normal flora of the:
   a. urinary tract
   b. respiratory tract
   c. colon
   d. circulatory system

6. The single most important way to stop the spread of infection is:
   a. isolation procedures
   b. standard precautions
   c. hand hygiene
   d. PPE

7. In putting on and removing PPE, the first article that is put on, and the last article that is taken off is/are the:
   a. mask
   b. shoe covers
   c. gown
   d. gloves

8. Which of the following is not an OSHA standard?
   a. All biohazard material must be labeled.
   b. Employees must practice standard precautions.
   c. Employers must have written airborne pathogen exposure control plans in the workplace.
   d. Employers must provide immunization against hepatitis B virus free of charge.

9. While standard precautions apply to all potentially infectious situations, expanded precautions are chosen based on:
   a. whether isolation is employed
   b. the potential means of transmission of the disease or condition
   c. airborne transmission
   d. the risk to the health care worker from accidental needle sticks

10. Ten percent bleach as a cleaning agent should be made fresh every:
    a. week
    b. 3 hours
    c. day
    d. 6 hours

11. The continuous links in the chain of infection are, in order:
    a. means of transmission, susceptible host, source
    b. source, means of transmission, susceptible host
    c. susceptible host, source, means of transmission
    d. none of the above

12. The purpose of a protective environment for highly immunosuppressed patients is to:
    a. prevent transmission of infection to the patient
    b. protect the general public from disease
    c. prevent transmission of infection from the patient
    d. protect the patient from spores in the environment

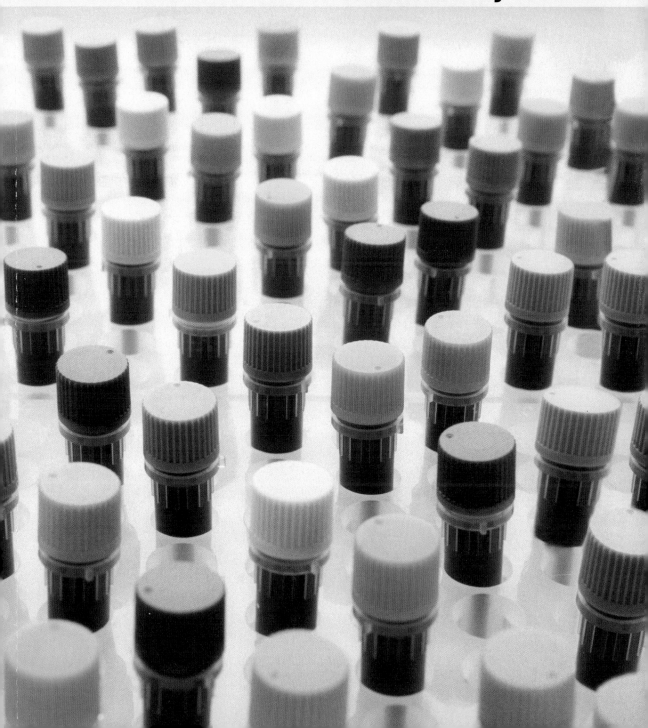

UNIT 2

Phlebotomy Basics

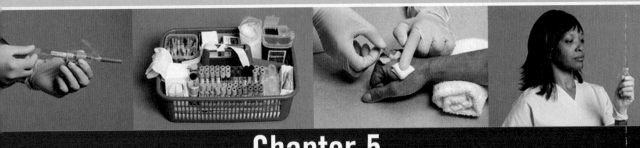

Chapter 5

Medical Terminology

OUTLINE

Parts of a Word

Abbreviations

Review for Certification

OBJECTIVES

After completing this chapter, you should be able to:

1. Define selected roots, suffixes, and prefixes.
2. Translate the English or common word for a condition or system into the appropriate medical form.
3. Use selected medical terms or expressions in their proper context.
4. Define and use correctly specific medical terms that apply to phlebotomy.
5. Define selected medical abbreviations and use them correctly.

KEY TERMS

combining form
combining vowel
prefix

root
suffix

The practice of medicine requires many specialized words whose meanings may at first seem impenetrably mysterious. In fact, however, most medical terms are formed from Latin or Greek and use prefixes, roots, combining vowels, and suffixes. Understanding the way in which words are constructed and memorizing the meanings of some of the most common word parts will allow you to decipher many terms encountered in the workplace. Abbreviations are also very common and should become familiar to you.

PARTS OF A WORD

Most medical terms have several parts. For instance, *phlebotomy* is a combination of two parts, *phlebo-* and *-tomy*. *Phlebo-* means "vein," and *-tomy* means "cutting into," so phlebotomy literally means "to cut into a vein." Similarly, *phlebitis* is a combination of two parts, *phlebo-* and *-itis*. Once you know that *-itis* means "inflammation," you can deduce that phlebitis is inflammation of a vein.

The parts of a word include the **root**, or main part; a **prefix**, or part at the beginning; and a **suffix**, or part at the end (Figure 5-1). For instance, *antecubital* includes the prefix *ante-*, meaning "forward of" or "before"; the root *cubit*, meaning "elbow"; and the suffix *-al*, meaning "pertaining to." Therefore, the word means "pertaining to the region forward of the elbow." Tables 5-1, 5-2, and 5-3 list commonly used prefixes, suffixes, and roots.

Words may also contain a combining vowel, added to make pronunciation easier. For instance, *leuk* is a root meaning "white," and *cyte* means "cell." An *o* is added to make *leukocyte*, a white blood cell. Similarly, *cyt* and *-logy*, meaning "study of," are joined with a combining vowel to form

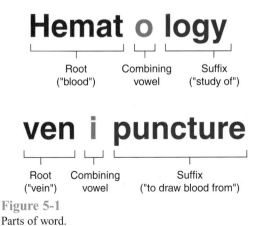

Figure 5-1
Parts of word.

TABLE 5-1 Prefixes

Prefix	Meaning	Examples
a-, an-	without	anemia (lack of blood)
ambi-, ampho-	both	ambidextrous (using both hands equally)
ante-	before, forward of	antecubital (forward of the elbow)
anti-	against	anticoagulant (coagulation preventer)
brady-	slow	bradycardia (slow heartbeat)
cryo-	cold	cryoagglutinins (proteins that clump in the cold)
dys-	bad, difficult	dyspnea (difficulty breathing)
ecto-, exo-	outside	exogenous (originating from outside)
endo-	inside	endoscope (apparatus for looking inside the body)
epi-	on, over	epicardium (the outermost layer of the heart)
hyper-	above, more, increased	hyperbilirubinemia (excess bilirubin in the blood)
hypo-	below, less, decreased	hypodermic needle
inter-	between	interstitial (relating to spaces between tissues)
intra-	within	intramuscular injection
iso-	same	isoagglutinin (a protein that causes clumping when it encounters other similar proteins)
macro-	large	macrophage
mega-	large	megakaryocyte
micro-	small	microcyte
neo-	new	neoplasm
para-	beside	parathyroid gland
per-	throughout, through	percutaneous (through the skin)
peri-	around	pericardium (the sac surrounding the heart)
poly-	many	polycythemia (elevated levels of blood cells)
post-	after	postprandial (after a meal)

Continued

TABLE 5-1 Prefixes—cont'd

Prefix	Meaning	Examples
pre-	before	preexisting
pro-	for, in front of	prothrombin
tachy-	fast	tachycardia (fast heartbeat)

Prefixes for Numbers

hemi-, semi-	half	hemiplegia (paralysis of half the body)
mono-, uni-	one	mononuclear (having a round [one-lobed] nucleus)
bi-, di-	two	bilaterally (on both sides)
tri-	three	tricuspid valve
tetra-, quad-	four	quadriceps (muscles of the anterior thigh)

Metric Prefixes

deca-	ten	decaliter (10 liters)
kilo-	thousand	kilogram (1000 grams)
deci-	tenth	deciliter (one tenth of a liter)
centi-	hundredth	centimeter (one hundredth of a meter)
milli-	thousandth	milliliter (one thousandth of a liter)
micro-	millionth	microgram (one millionth of a gram)
nano-	billionth	nanogram (one billionth of a gram)

Prefixes for Color

albi-	white	albino
cirrho-	tawny yellow	cirrhosis
cyan-	blue	cyanotic
erythro-	red	erythrocyte
leuko-	white	leukocyte
lute-	yellow	corpus luteum
melano-	black	melanoma
nigr-	black	substantia nigra
rube-	red	rubella

TABLE 5-2 Suffixes

Suffix	Meaning	Examples
-ectomy	surgical removal	appendectomy
-emia	blood condition	anemia, bacteremia
-gen, -genic, -genous	originating from	iatrogenic (caused by medical treatment)
-itis	inflammation	arthritis
-oma	tumor, growth	hematoma
-osis	condition	tuberculosis
-pathy	disease	cardiopathy
-penia	deficiency	thrombocytopenia
-plasty	shape or form	angioplasty (surgical repair or reshaping of a blood vessel)
-plegia	paralysis	tetraplegia (paralysis of all four limbs)
-stasis	stopping, control	hemostasis
-stomy	opening	colostomy
-tomy	cut	phlebotomy

TABLE 5-3 Word Roots

Root	Meaning	Examples
agglut-	clump together	agglutinin
angio-	vessel	angioplasty (reshaping a blood vessel)
arterio-	artery	arteriosclerosis
arthro-	joint	arthritis
bili-	bile	bilirubin
cardio-	heart	cardiologist (one who treats heart disease)
cephal-	head	encephalitis
colo-	colon	colostomy
cubit-	elbow	antecubital fossa
cyst-	bladder	cystitis, cystogram
derm-	skin	dermal puncture
gastr-	stomach	gastrostomy (opening into the stomach)
heme-	blood	hematology, hemagglutinins
hepato-	liver	hepatitis
necro-	death	necrosis (cell or tissue death)
nephr-	kidney	nephron
oste-	bone	osteoma
phago-, -phage	eat	phagocyte, macrophage
phlebo-	vein	phlebotomy
pneu-, -pnea	breath	pneumatic, apnea (lack of breathing)

TABLE 5-3 Word Roots—cont'd

Root	Meaning	Examples
pulmon-	lung	pulmonary insufficiency
ren-	kidney	renal artery
spleno-	spleen	splenomegaly (enlarged spleen)
thromb-	clot	thrombin, thrombosis
tox-, toxico-	poison	toxicology, detoxification
veno-	vein	venopressor

cytology, the study of cells. The combination of the word root and the combining vowel (usually an *o*) is called the combining form of the root. Combining vowels are not used when the suffix begins with a vowel. For instance, no combining vowel is used to form *leukemia*, which combines the root *leuk* and the suffix *-emia*, meaning "blood condition."

The spelling of roots can also change slightly when they are combined with different suffixes. For instance, *erythema*, meaning "redness of the skin," uses a slightly modified form of the root *erythro*.

The plurals of some medical terms are formed by changing the end of the word rather than adding an *s*. For instance, words ending in *-us* typically change to *-i* for the plural, as in *nucleus* and *nuclei*, or *thrombus* and *thrombi*. A list of such plurals is given in Table 5-4.

By memorizing some of the most common roots and remembering these simple guidelines, you should be able to deduce the meanings of many common medical terms. Keeping a medical dictionary handy allows you to learn terms you do not know. Medical dictionaries often have tables of word roots.

TABLE 5-4 Plurals

Singular Word Ending	Plural Form	Examples
-a	-ae	axilla, axillae fossa, fossae
-en	-ina	lumen, lumina
-is	-es	naris, nares
-ix	-ices	fornix, fornices cervix, cervices
-nx	-nges	pharynx, pharynges
-on	-oa	spermatozoon, spermatozoa
-um	-a	ovum, ova
-us	-i	articulus, articuli nucleus, nuclei
-ux	-uces	hallux, halluces

ABBREVIATIONS

Abbreviations are used widely in the health care field. In most cases, a particular abbreviation has only one widely used meaning within the medical field. For instance, MD, HIV, and Rx have unambiguous meanings in virtually any medical context (meaning "doctor of medicine," "human immunodeficiency virus," and "prescription," respectively). A few abbreviations are more context specific. For instance, AE may mean "above the elbow" to a phlebotomist reading a chart about a burn victim's scars, but it may mean "adverse effects" to a pharmacist comparing side effects of two drugs. Table 5-5 lists many of the abbreviations you will encounter. Abbreviations of medical tests are found in later chapters as they are covered.

TABLE 5-5 Commonly Encountered Abbreviations

Abbreviation	Definition
AC	accommodation
AC, ac	before meals
AD	right ear (auris dextra)
ad lib	as desired
adeno-CA	adenocarcinoma
AE	above the elbow; adverse effects
AGN	acute glomerulonephritis
AIDS	acquired immunodeficiency syndrome
AK	above the knee
ALL	acute lymphocytic leukemia
AMA	American Medical Association; against medical advice
AMI	acute myocardial infarction
AML	acute myelocytic leukemia
ARDS	adult respiratory distress syndrome
ASAP	as soon as possible
BID, bid	twice a day
BIN, bin	twice a night
BK	below the knee
BM	bowel movement
BP	blood pressure
Bx	biopsy
C	Celsius, centigrade
$\bar{c}$	with
CA, Ca	cancer
CAD	coronary artery disease
CAT	computerized axial tomography
CC	chief complaint
cc	cubic centimeter
CCU	coronary care unit
CDC	Centers for Disease Control and Prevention

Continued

TABLE 5-5 Commonly Encountered Abbreviations—cont'd

Abbreviation	Definition	Abbreviation	Definition
CGN	chronic glomerulonephritis	Gyn, gyn	gynecology
CHF	congestive heart failure	H	hypodermic
CLL	chronic lymphocytic leukemia	h	hour
cm	centimeter	HCl	hydrochloric acid
CML	chronic myelocytic leukemia	Hg	mercury
CNS	central nervous system	HIV	human immunodeficiency virus
CO_2	carbon dioxide	hs	at bedtime
COLD	chronic obstructive lung disease	hypo	hypodermically
contra	against	I&D	incision and drainage
COPD	chronic obstructive pulmonary disease	ICU	intensive care unit
		ID	intradermal
CPR	cardiopulmonary resuscitation	Ig	immunoglobulin
CS, C-section	cesarean section	IM	intramuscular
CT	computed tomography	IQ	intelligence quotient
CV	cardiovascular	IS	intercostal space
CVA	cerebrovascular accident	IU	international unit
CVD	cardiovascular disease	IUD	intrauterine device
CXR	chest x-ray; chest radiograph	IV	intravenous(ly)
d	day; 24 hours	IVC	intravenous cholangiography
/d	per day	IVP	intravenous pyelogram
D&C	dilation and curettage	KD	knee disarticulation
D&E	dilation and evacuation	kg	kilogram
db	decibel	KUB	kidney, ureter, bladder
DM	diabetes mellitus	L	liter
DNA	deoxyribonucleic acid	LAT, lat	lateral
DO	doctor of osteopathy	lb	pound
DOB	date of birth	LE	lupus erythematosus (also SLE, systemic lupus erythematosus)
DPT	diphtheria-pertussis-tetanus		
DVT	deep vein thrombosis	LMP	last menstrual period
Dx	diagnosis	LPN	licensed practical nurse
ECG, EKG	electrocardiogram	M, m	meter
EEG	electroencephalogram	mcg	microgram
EENT	eye, ear, nose, and throat	MD	doctor of medicine
ENT	ear, nose, and throat	mets	metastases
ER	emergency room	MH	marital history
et	and	MI	myocardial infarction
F	Fahrenheit	MICU	medical intensive care unit
FACP	Fellow of the American College of Physicians	mL	milliliter
		mm	millimeter
FACS	Fellow of the American College of Surgeons	MRI	magnetic resonance imaging
		MS	multiple sclerosis
FDA	Food and Drug Administration	MVP	mitral valve prolapse
FHR	fetal heart rate	NB	newborn
FHT	fetal heart tone	NICU	neonatal intensive care unit
FS	frozen section	NPO	nothing by mouth
FTND	full-term normal delivery	O_2	oxygen
FUO	fever of undetermined origin	OA	osteoarthritis
Fx	fracture	OB	obstetrics
g, gm	gram	OC	oral contraceptive
GC	gonorrhea	od	once a day
GI	gastrointestinal	OHS	open heart surgery
gr	grain	OR	operating room
gt, Gtt, gtt, gtts	drop, drops	Ortho, ORTH	orthopedics; orthopaedics

TABLE 5-5 Commonly Encountered Abbreviations—cont'd

Abbreviation	Definition	Abbreviation	Definition
OS	left eye (oculus sinister)	qn	every night
os	mouth	qns	quantity not sufficient
OT	occupational therapy (or therapist)	qs	quantity sufficient
Oto	otology	R	respiration
O2, OU	both eyes (oculi unitas)	RD	respiratory disease
OU	each eye (oculus uterque)	REM	rapid eye movement
oz	ounce	RN	registered nurse
P	pulse	RNA	ribonucleic acid
Pap	Papanicolaou (smear)	ROM	range of motion
paren	parenterally	Rx	prescription
Path	pathology	$\bar{s}$	without
PC, pc	after meals	SICU	surgical intensive care unit
PD	postprandial (after meals)	SOB	short(ness) of breath
PE	physical examination	SOS	if necessary
Peds	pediatrics	sp. gr.	specific gravity
pH	hydrogen ion concentration	Staph	*Staphylococcus*
PICU	pulmonary intensive care unit; pediatric intensive care unit	stat	immediately
		STD	sexually transmitted disease
PID	pelvic inflammatory disease	Strep	*Streptococcus*
PMP	previous menstrual period	subcu., SC	subcutaneous
PO	orally (per os)	T	temperature
post-op, p/o	after operation	T&A	tonsillectomy and adenoidectomy
pp	postprandial	TB	tuberculosis
pre-op	before operation	THR	total hip replacement
prep	prepare	TIA	transient ischemic attack
prn	as required	TID, tid	three times a day
PT	physical therapy (or therapist)	TPN	total parenteral nutrition
pt	patient	TPR	temperature, pulse, and respiration
PVC	premature ventricular contraction		
q	every	URI	upper respiratory infection
qd	every day	UTI	urinary tract infection
qh	every hour	VA	visual acuity
q2h	every two hours	VD	venereal disease
QID, qid	four times a day	wt	weight
qm, qam	every morning	x	multiplied by

REVIEW FOR CERTIFICATION

Medical terms are most commonly formed from Greek or Latin. Each term contains a root and may contain a prefix, suffix, combining vowel, or other root. A combining vowel, usually an *o*, is used with a root to create a combining form for ease of pronunciation. A large number of abbreviations are used in the health care environment. Most, but not all, abbreviations have unique meanings within a medical context.

BIBLIOGRAPHY

Davis NM: Medical Abbreviations: Conveniences at the Expense of Communication and Safety, ed 10. Neil M Davis Associates, 2001.

Dorland Illustrated Medical Dictionary, ed 29. Philadelphia, WB Saunders, 2000.

Smith GL, et al: Quick Medical Terminology. New York, Wiley, 1992.

STUDY QUESTIONS

1. The parts of a word always include a _____ and may include a _____ or _____.
2. Give the meaning of the following prefixes:
   ante-
   anti-
   brady-
   hyper-
   hypo-
   inter-
   intra-
   neo-
   micro-
   poly-
   post-
   tachy-
   cirrho-
   cyan-
   erythro-
   hemi-
   nano-
   epi-
   rube-
   peri-
   tetra-
   lute-
3. Give the meaning of the following roots:
   agglut-
   angio-
   bili-
   cardio-
   derm-
   heme-
   hepato-
   oste-
   phago-
   pnea-
   pulmon-
   ren-
   thromb-
   tox-
4. Give the meaning of the following suffixes:
   -emia
   -plasty
   -tomy
   -oma
   -penia
   -pathy
   -plegia
   -stasis
   -itis
   -genous

STUDY QUESTIONS—cont'd

5. List what each abbreviation stands for.
   SOB
   q
   DOB
   ASAP
   IV
   NPO
   OR
   UTI
   stat
   qns
   FUO
   CVA
   COLD
   hypo
   OB
   MI
   Rx
   STD
   O_2
   P
   NB
   TB
   AIDS
   prep

6. Write the plural form of each of the following words:
   papilla
   testis
   larynx
   scapula
   vertebra
   appendix

CERTIFICATION EXAM PREPARATION

1. *Hepato-* refers to:
   a. liver
   b. kidney
   c. heart
   d. blood

2. *Cyan-* refers to:
   a. red
   b. yellow
   c. black
   d. blue

3. *Hemi-* means:
   a. many
   b. half
   c. whole
   d. two

4. *-tomy* refers to:
   a. study of
   b. to cut
   c. shape or form
   d. opening

5. *Anti-* means:
   a. between
   b. among
   c. against
   d. for

6. *Leuko-* refers to:
   a. red
   b. yellow
   c. blue
   d. white

7. *-emia* refers to:
   a. blood condition
   b. tumor
   c. opening
   d. paralysis

8. *Pulmon-* refers to:
   a. liver
   b. lung
   c. colon
   d. heart

9. *Thromb-* refers to:
   a. hemolysis
   b. clotting
   c. lymphostasis
   d. tumor

10. *Derm-* refers to:
    a. death
    b. bone
    c. skin
    d. blood

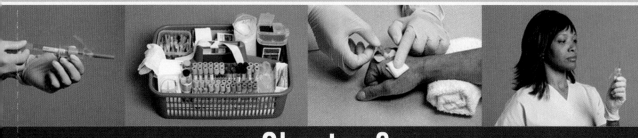

Chapter 6
Human Anatomy and Physiology

OUTLINE

OBJECTIVES

After completing this chapter, you should be able to:

1. Describe the three levels of organization of the human body.
2. Name four structures of the cell and describe the functions of each.
3. Name four kinds of tissue and explain the roles of each.
4. Define each anatomic term discussed and use it to locate various structures and position a patient.
5. Describe the eight major body cavities and list at least one organ contained in each.
6. For each of the following body systems, describe its major features, organs, and functions and list

diseases and common laboratory tests associated with each:
   a. skeletal
   b. muscular
   c. integumentary
   d. nervous
   e. digestive
   f. urinary
   g. respiratory
   h. endocrine
   i. reproductive

KEY TERMS

abdominal cavity
abduction
adduction
adrenal cortex
adrenal medulla
adrenocorticotropic
  hormone
afferents
agonist
aldosterone
alveoli
amino acid derivatives
amphiarthrosis
anatomic position
antagonist
anterior
anticitrullinated protein
antidiuretic hormone
arachnoid
articular cartilage
autonomic motor system
bile
Bowman's capsule
brain stem
bronchi
bronchioles
bulbourethral glands
calcitonin
carbohydrases
cardiac (striated
  involuntary) muscle
central nervous system
cerebellum
cerebral cortex
cerebrospinal fluid
cerebrum
cervix
chyme
cilia
collecting duct
connective tissue
corticosterone
cortisol

cortisone
cranial cavity
cytoplasm
dermis
diarthrosis
distal
distal convoluted tubule
dorsal
dura mater
efferents
epidermis
epididymis
epinephrine
epithelial tissue
esophagus
estrogens
extension
external respiration
fallopian tube
feedback loops
flexion
follicle-stimulating
  hormone
frontal plane
glomerulus
glucagons
glucocorticoids
gonads
ground substance
growth hormone
hematopoiesis
homeostasis
hormones
human chorionic
  gonadotropin
hypothalamus
inferior
insulin
internal respiration
interneuron
larynx
lateral
ligaments

lipases
loop of Henle
luteinizing hormone
medial
melanocyte-stimulating
  hormone
meninges
mineralocorticoids
mitochondria
motor neurons
myelin
nephron
nerves
neuromuscular junction
neurons
neurotransmitter
norepinephrine
nucleus
osteoblasts
osteoclasts
ovaries
ovulation
oxyhemoglobin
oxytocin
parathormone
pelvic cavity
penis
peptides
pericardial cavity
peripheral nervous
  system
peristalsis
peritoneal cavity
pharynx
pia mater
plasma membrane
pleural cavity
posterior
progesterone
prolactin
prone
prostate
proteases

proximal
proximal convoluted
  tubule
sagittal plane
scrotum
section
semen
seminal vesicles
skeletal (striated
  voluntary) muscle
smooth (nonstriated
  involuntary) muscle
somatic motor system
sphincter
spinal cavity
steroid hormones
superior
supine
synaptic cleft (synapse)
synarthrosis
synovial cavity
tendons
testosterone
thalamus
thermoregulation
thoracic cavity
thymosin
thyroid-stimulating
  hormone
thyroxine
tissues
trachea
tracts
transverse plane
triiodothyronine
ureter
urethra
uterus
vagina
vas deferens
ventral
ventricles
villi

ABBREVIATIONS

ABG: arterial blood gas
ACE: angiotensin converting enzyme
ACTH: adrenocorticotropic hormone
ADH: antidiuretic hormone
ALP: alkaline phosphatase

ALS: amyotrophic lateral sclerosis
ALT: alanine aminotransferase
ANA: antinuclear antibody
AST: aspartate aminotransferase
ATP: adenosine triphosphate

ABBREVIATIONS—cont'd

BUN: blood urea nitrogen
C&S: culture and sensitivity
CBC: complete blood count
CK: creatine kinase
CNS: central nervous system
COPD: chronic obstructive pulmonary disease
CSF: cerebrospinal fluid
CT: computed tomography
ENT: ear, nose, and throat
ESR: erythrocyte sedimentation rate
FBS: fasting blood sugar (glucose)
FSH: follicle-stimulating hormone
FTA-ABS: fluorescent treponemal antibody absorption test
GGT: γ-glutamyltransferase
GH: growth hormone
HBsAG: hepatitis B surface antigen
HCG: human chorionic gonadotropin
HCV: hepatitis C virus
HIV: human immunodeficiency virus
IRDS: infant respiratory distress syndrome

KOH: potassium hydroxide
LH: luteinizing hormone
MRI: magnetic resonance imaging
MSH: melanocyte-stimulating hormone
O&P: ova and parasites
PID: pelvic inflammatory disease
PMS: premenstrual syndrome
PSA: prostate-specific antigen
PTH: parathyroid hormone
RA: rheumatoid arthritis
RF: rheumatoid factor
RPR: rapid plasma reagin
SLE: systemic lupus erythematosus
STD: sexually transmitted disease
T$_3$: triiodothyronine
T$_4$: thyroxine
TSH: thyroid-stimulating hormone
TSS: toxic shock syndrome
URI: upper respiratory infection
UTI: urinary tract infection

An understanding of human anatomy and physiology allows the phlebotomist to interact more knowledgeably with both patients and other health care professionals. The tissues, organs, and body systems work together to create and maintain homeostasis, the integrated control of body function that is characteristic of health. Each body system is prone to particular types of diseases and is subject to particular tests that aid in diagnosing those diseases. As a phlebotomist, many of the patients you collect samples from will be undergoing diagnosis or treatment for diseases or other disorders. Others may require blood collection for reasons not related to illness, such as pregnancy or blood donation. In this chapter, we discuss all aspects of human anatomy and physiology except the circulatory system. Because of its special importance to phlebotomy, it is covered separately in the next chapter.

LEVELS OF ORGANIZATION

Just as a complex institution such as a hospital has different levels of organization, so does the human body. At the most basic level, the body is composed of cells. Cells of similar type join to form tissues, and tissues interact to form discrete units of function called organs. When different organs interact to carry out common tasks, they form an organ system. Organ systems themselves interact, making an integrated, functioning body.

At each level, the body acts to maintain **homeostasis**, or the dynamic steady state we think of when we refer to good health. Homeostasis requires many different functions: nutrition, materials processing, and waste elimination; repair of injury, defense against infection, and regulation of growth; and communication and coordination among the parts of the body.

Cells

Cells are the smallest living units in the body. Cells are much like small factories, using raw materials to produce products for internal use or export. For cells, the raw materials include oxygen from the air and food molecules such as sugars and amino acids; the products are often more complex molecules such as hormones or proteins. Muscle cells use up large amounts of sugar and oxygen to power their own movement, and neurons (nerve cells) use these same raw materials to create electrical and chemical signals.

The structures within cells that allow these functions to occur are complex (Figure 6-1). Among the most important are the following.

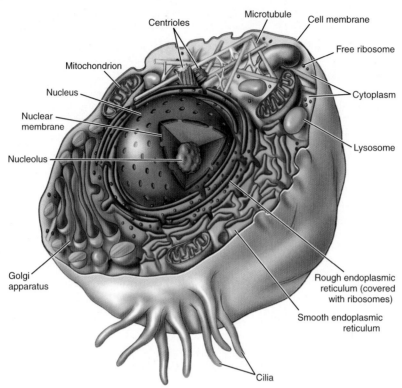

Figure 6-1
Cell structures include the plasma membrane, nucleus, mitochondria, and other organelles responsible for maintaining cellular homeostasis. (From Herlihy B, Maebius N: The Human Body in Health and Illness. Philadelphia, Saunders, 2000.)

Nucleus. The **nucleus** contains DNA. DNA is arranged in functional units called genes, and genes are linked together in long strings called chromosomes. Genes perform two functions. During the normal life of the cell, they act as blueprints for making proteins. During cell reproduction, they act as the material of heredity, forming copies of themselves so that each new cell formed has a complete and identical set of blueprints. Defects in genes are responsible for hereditary diseases such as hemophilia and sickle cell disease. All cells in the body begin with a nucleus, but red blood cells extrude theirs at maturity.

Mitochondria. **Mitochondria** are the cell's power plants, burning fuels such as sugar and fat with oxygen to supply energy for the cell in the form of adenosine triphosphate (ATP). Neurons and muscle cells contain very high numbers of mitochondria.

Cytoplasm. **Cytoplasm** refers to all the cellular material except the plasma membrane and the nucleus. Cytosol refers to the fluid portion of the cytoplasm.

Plasma Membrane. The **plasma membrane** encloses the cell and tightly regulates the flow of materials in and out of it. Membranes are flexible, allowing cells to change shape if necessary. For instance, the red blood cell must squeeze through tiny capillaries that are thinner than its normal diameter, a feat made possible by the flexibility of the membrane.

Tissues

Cells of similar structure and function combine to form **tissues**. The human body is composed of four basic types of tissues: epithelial, muscle, nerve, and connective.

Epithelial Tissue

Epithelial tissue forms flat sheets and is most often found on surfaces where exchange with the environment takes place, such as the lining of the gut (Figure 6-2), or where rapid regeneration must occur to protect internal structures, such as the skin or the surface of the eye. Epithelium may contain glands, which produce and secrete substances such as saliva, sweat, or insulin.

Stratified squamous

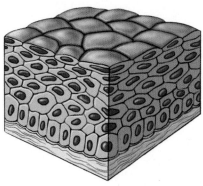

Figure 6-2 An example of epithelial tissue.
(From Herlihy B, Maebius N: The Human Body in Health and Illness. Philadelphia, Saunders, 2000.)

Muscle Tissue

Muscle tissue is contractile, meaning that it can shorten its length. Muscle cells contain long fibers of the proteins actin and myosin, whose movements produce muscle contraction. Muscles receive the stimulus to contract when the axon terminals of motor neurons (neurons that stimulate muscle) make contact with the muscle. The neuron releases a chemical (called a neurotransmitter) onto the muscle cell surface at the **neuromuscular junction**, causing the chemical changes within the muscle that lead to contraction.

Muscle tissue occurs in three forms, which differ in both structure and function (Figure 6-3):

1. **Skeletal, or striated voluntary, muscle** is the most widespread type, constituting all the muscles that move the skeleton. Under the microscope, striated muscle has a striped appearance.
2. **Cardiac,** or **striated involuntary, muscle** is found in the heart. It looks similar to skeletal muscle but has features that are unique to it. Cardiac muscle cells do not need stimulation by the nervous system to start a contraction. However, electrical stimulation is required to maintain the coordinated rhythm of the cells. This function is performed by the heart's physiologic pacemaker, found in the right atrium.
3. **Smooth,** or **nonstriated involuntary, muscle** lines blood and lymph vessels within the body just below the epithelial tissue, such as around the gut, the lungs, and the circulatory and reproductive systems. Constriction of smooth muscle regulates the passage of materials through the vessel. Smooth muscle also is found in the skin, where it is responsible for hair erection.

⇢>>> FLASH FORWARD

As you will learn in Chapter 7, primary hemostasis (bleeding control) involves smooth muscle constriction.

Nerve Tissue

Nerve tissue is specialized for intercellular communication by the conduction of electrical impulses and release of chemical messages. Nerve tissue is

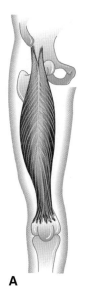

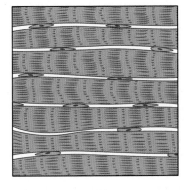

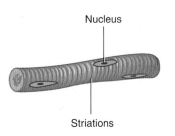

Nucleus

Striations

A

Figure 6-3
The three forms of muscle tissue. **A,** Skeletal.

Continued

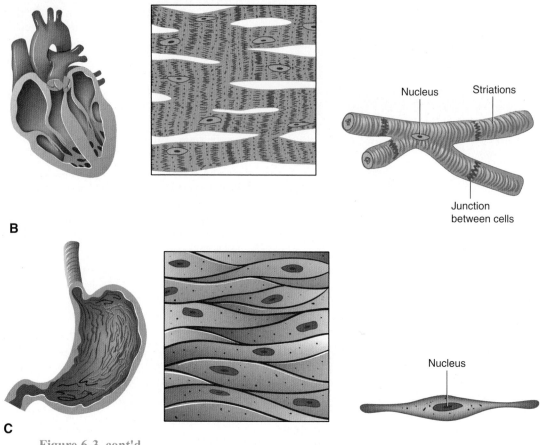

B

C

Figure 6-3, cont'd
The three forms of muscle tissue. **B**, Cardiac. **C**, Smooth.

composed of neurons and neuroglial cells. **Neurons** are excitable cells, meaning that they can be stimulated to undergo electrical and chemical changes. Neurons are found in the brain, the spinal cord, and throughout the body. Neuroglial cells nourish and support neurons in the brain and spinal cord.

The three major portions of the neuron are the dendrite, the cell body, and the axon (Figure 6-4). Axons can be extremely long—each of the motor neurons controlling the toes, for instance, has an axon that stretches from the spinal cord down the leg, through the ankle, to the muscles of the foot. Axons are insulated by a fatty sheath of **myelin**.

One neuron conveys information to another by releasing a chemical, called a **neurotransmitter**, at the small gap where they meet, called the **synaptic cleft**, or **synapse**. The neurotransmitter leaves the axon of the first neuron, crosses the synaptic cleft, and lands on a receptor on the dendrite of the second neuron, beginning a cascade of chemical changes down the length of the neuron. This may ultimately cause the second neuron to release its own neurotransmitter, thereby conveying information further along the neural chain.

Connective Tissue

The general function of **connective tissue** is to bind and support the other three types of tissue. Connective tissue is characterized by a relative scarcity of cells and a relative abundance of extracellular **ground substance** secreted by the cells. Bone is a connective tissue—its ground substance is collagen, impregnated with mineral crystals. Blood is also a connective tissue, with plasma as its ground substance.

Organs

An organ is a distinct structural unit in the body, specialized for some complex function. Organs such as the heart, lungs, and kidneys incorporate all four tissue types. In the lungs, for instance, epithelial tissue lines the airways, cleaning and moistening them and providing a barrier to infection. Smooth muscle constricts or relaxes to regulate the size of

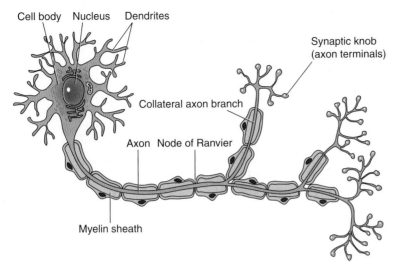

Cell body   Nucleus   Dendrites

Synaptic knob
(axon terminals)

Collateral axon branch

Axon   Node of Ranvier

Myelin sheath

Figure 6-4
Neurons are specialized for communication. Signals travel from dendrite to cell body to axon, causing the release of neurotransmitters into the synaptic cleft separating the two neurons.

the airway. Neurons in the bronchi detect the presence of excess mucus or other irritants and provoke a cough. Cartilage—a type of connective tissue—supports the larger airways to prevent collapse.

Body Systems

Body systems are groups of organs functioning together for a common purpose. The respiratory system, for instance, involves not only the lungs but also the upper airway, including the nasal passages and throat. It also includes the muscles that inflate the lungs, such as the diaphragm, the rib muscles, and the muscles of the neck.

After a brief discussion of anatomic terminology, we review the structure and function of the body systems, discuss how they may be involved in disease, and indicate what tests can be ordered to monitor their function.

ANATOMIC TERMINOLOGY

Medical anatomists describe the location and direction of body structures with reference to the **anatomic position** (Figure 6-5). In this position, the body is erect and facing forward, and the arms are at the side with palms facing forward. When referring to left and right, we use the person's, not the picture's, left and right. This is important, especially when discussing internal structures, such as the heart.

Directional Terms

Directional terms are used to describe the relation of one body part to another or to describe a motion in relation to some part of the body. These terms

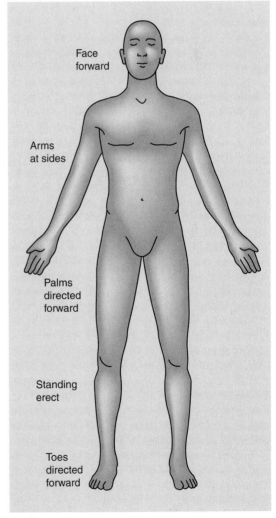

Face
forward

Arms
at sides

Palms
directed
forward

Standing
erect

Toes
directed
forward

Figure 6-5
The body in the anatomic position.

remove any ambiguity that might ensue from such phrases as "Insert the needle below the elbow," which could be interpreted to mean on the underside of the elbow rather than on the forearm. Understanding and careful use of these terms will allow you to perform procedures correctly and improve your ability to communicate with other health professionals. Refer to Figure 6-6 as you learn the following pairs of terms.

Ventral and **anterior** refer to the front surface of the body. Routine venipuncture is performed on the ventral surface of the forearm. **Dorsal** and **posterior** refer to the back surface of the body. Hand venipuncture is usually performed on the dorsal surface of the hand.

Lateral means more toward the side, away from the body's central axis. In the anatomic position, the thumb is lateral to the other fingers. **Medial** means more toward the middle.

Distal means further away from the point of attachment of the structure in question. The elbow is distal to the shoulder, and the hand is distal to the wrist. **Proximal** means closer to the point of attachment.

Inferior means below. The mouth is inferior to the nose. **Superior** means above. The eyebrows are superior to the eyes.

Prone means lying on the abdomen with the face down. **Supine** means lying on the back. Patients may be placed in this position during venipuncture if they are likely to faint.

Flexion refers to a movement that bends a joint. **Extension** straightens the joint.

Abduction is a movement that takes a body part further away from the central axis, and **adduction** brings it closer.

Body Planes

Depicting internal organs is often best done by slicing through them to make a **section,** or an imaginary flat surface. There are three sectional planes, two vertical and one horizontal (Figure 6-7):

Frontal plane—a vertical plane dividing the body into front and back.
Sagittal plane—a vertical plane dividing the body into left and right.
Transverse plane—a horizontal plane dividing the body into top and bottom.

Body Cavities

Body cavities are spaces within the body that contain major organ systems. There are two large body cavities, the ventral cavity and the dorsal cavity. These are subdivided to form the eight major body cavities (Figure 6-8).

Ventral Cavities

Thoracic cavity—contains the heart (within the **pericardial cavity**) and lungs (within the **pleural cavity**).
Abdominal cavity—contains the stomach, small and large intestines, spleen, liver, gallbladder, pancreas, and kidneys (all but the kidneys are within the **peritoneal cavity**).

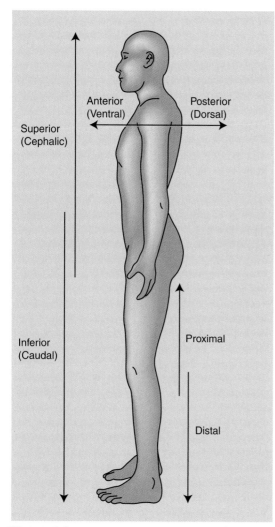

Figure 6-6
Directional terms are used to indicate relative positions and direction on the body.

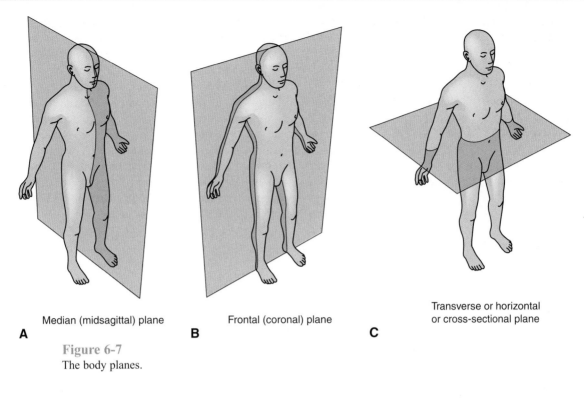

Median (midsagittal) plane

A

Frontal (coronal) plane

B

Transverse or horizontal or cross-sectional plane

C

Figure 6-7
The body planes.

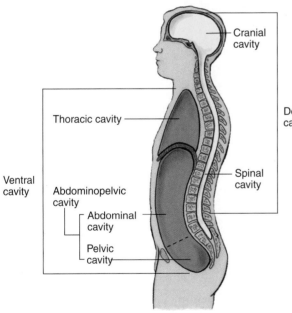

Figure 6-8
The body cavities. Note that some smaller cavities are within others. (From Applegate E: The Anatomy and Physiology Learning System, ed 3. Philadelphia, Saunders, 2006.)

Pelvic cavity—contains the bladder, rectum, ovaries, and testes.

Dorsal Cavities

Cranial cavity—contains the brain.
Spinal cavity—contains the spinal cord.

SKELETAL SYSTEM

The skeletal system includes all the bones, plus the connective tissue at the joints. It functions to support the body, provide movement, and protect the internal organs. Bones also store the minerals phosphorus and calcium, and the marrow of certain bones is the site of **hematopoiesis**, formation of blood cells.

Features of Bone

Bone is formed by **osteoblasts**. These cells produce collagen fibers and deposit calcium salts (principally calcium phosphate). This mixture of protein and mineral gives bone its unique combination of hardness and resiliency. Bone growth and development involve a complex balance between the action of osteoblasts and that of other cells, called **osteoclasts**, whose job is to break down bone and release

stored minerals. This dynamic balance allows the growth of bone despite its rigidity and allows it to be remodeled to accommodate changing stresses.

Bones are classified by their shapes as long, short, flat, sesamoid, or irregular. Long bones include those in the arms and legs. Short bones are found in the wrists and ankles. Flat bones protect inner organs such as the heart and brain. *Sesamoid* means "shaped like a sesame seed"; the patella (kneecap) is an example. Irregular bones are those that are not classified as one of the other types, for example, the vertebrae. The principal bones of the skeleton are illustrated in Figure 6-9.

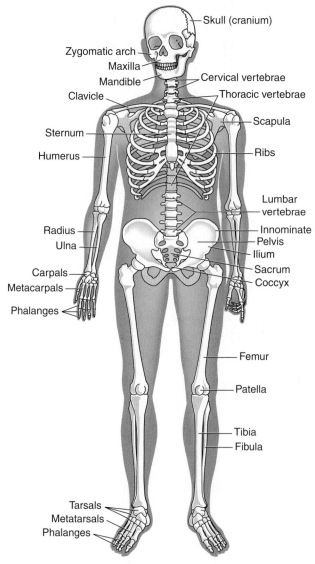

Figure 6-9
The major bones of the human skeleton.

Features of Joints

Joints connect one bone to another. There are three types of joints: immovable (**synarthrosis**), partially movable (**amphiarthrosis**), and free moving (**diarthrosis**). Fixed, or immovable, joints include the sutures of the cranium and facial bones. The vertebral joints are partially movable, restrained to protect the spinal cord from trauma. The appendicular joints, such as the shoulder, elbow, and knee, are free moving.

The structure of a typical free-moving joint is shown in Figure 6-10. The two bones are held together with **ligaments**, a type of tough, fibrous connective tissue. The fluid-filled **synovial cavity** is enclosed within the synovial membrane. The bearing surfaces of the bones are lined with smooth **articular cartilage**. The combination of synovial fluid and articular cartilage allows the two bone surfaces to slide against each other without becoming damaged or irritated.

Bone and Joint Disorders

Bone disorders include fractures, metabolic diseases, infections, neoplastic diseases, and developmental abnormalities (Box 6-1). Joint disorders include trauma, inflammation, degenerative changes, and metabolic diseases. An orthopedist is a specialist who treats bone disorders. Joint disorders are treated by a rheumatologist. Common lab tests ordered for these disorders are listed in Table 6-1.

MUSCULAR SYSTEM

Skeletal muscles move the skeleton, allowing the vast range of activities that make up daily life. Cardiac muscle pumps the blood for the circulatory system. The primary function of smooth muscle is to regulate the passage of materials through vessels.

Features of Skeletal Muscle

Skeletal muscles are those attached to the skeleton. Skeletal muscles account for 45% of the weight of the body. Muscles attach to the skeleton by means of **tendons**, a type of fibrous connective tissue. A muscle's two points of attachment are on opposite sides of a joint, so that contraction of the muscle bends the joint. In general, the bone on one side of a joint remains stationary while the other moves. Skeletal muscles often occur in pairs, called antagonistic pairs, whose actions are opposed. The biceps, for example, flexes the elbow, and the triceps extends it (Figure 6-11). During flexion, the biceps is called the **agonist**, and the triceps the **antagonist**. During extension, the triceps is the agonist, and the biceps is the antagonist.

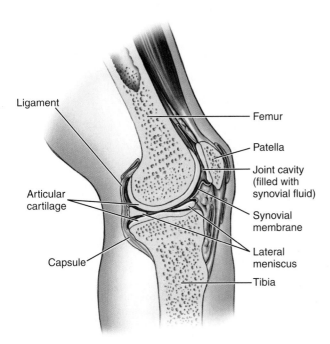

Ligament

Femur

Patella

Joint cavity (filled with synovial fluid)

Articular cartilage

Synovial membrane

Capsule

Lateral meniscus

Tibia

Figure 6-10

A typical joint in cross section. (Modified from Herlihy B, Maebius N: The Human Body in Health and Illness. Philadelphia, Saunders, 2000.)

BOX 6-1   Disorders of Bones and Joints

Bones
Fractures
Simple—no puncture through the skin
Compound—bone protrudes though the skin
Complicated—broken bone plus injured soft tissue
Comminuted—break that has splintered into many pieces
Impacted—broken bone is driven into another bone
Greenstick—bone is bent or partially broken
Pathologic—fracture due to disease, not stress

Metabolic Disease
Osteomalacia—softening of the bone from lack of calcium;
    can be due to vitamin D deficiency, calcium deficiency, or
    parathormone hypersecretion; childhood rickets is one
    form; can cause bowlegs
Osteoporosis—loss of bone mass and decrease in bone
    density; can be due to deficiency of estrogen, protein,
    calcium, or vitamin D; common in postmenopausal
    women; can lead to brittle and broken bones

Neoplastic Disease
Osteoma—usually benign
Sarcoma—malignant

Infectious Disease
Osteomyelitis—bone inflammation caused by a bacterial
    infection; can be caused by improper phlebotomy tech-
    nique; very difficult to treat

Developmental Disease
Scoliosis—spine is curved side to side; can be congenital or
    develop in teens

Spina bifida—congenital disease; abnormal closing of the
    vertebrae, causing malformation of the spine
Acromegaly—excess growth of extremities, caused by over-
    production of growth hormone

Joints
Trauma
Overextension, compression, or shear of ligaments—common
    sports injury; slow to heal

Infectious Disease
Lyme disease—inflammation of the synovial membrane,
    caused by a bacterial infection; transmitted through tick
    bites

Autoimmune Disease
Rheumatoid arthritis—swelling and irritation of the synovial
    membrane
Systemic lupus erythematosus (SLE)—affects cartilage, bones,
    ligaments, and tendons; more common in females

Degenerative Disease
Osteoarthritis (also called degenerative joint disease)—results
    from cumulative wear and tear on joint surfaces; affects
    ~20% of the population older than 60 years

Metabolic Disease
Gout—uric acid crystals form in the joints, causing pain and
    inflammation

TABLE 6-1   Common Lab Tests for Bone and Joint Disorders

Test	Disorder or Purpose
Alkaline phosphatase (ALP)	Bone metabolism marker
Calcium	Mineral calcium imbalance
Magnesium	Mineral magnesium imbalance
Fluorescent antinuclear antibody (ANA)	Systemic lupus erythematosus (SLE)
Rheumatoid factor (RF)	Rheumatoid arthritis (RA)
Synovial fluid analysis	Arthritis
Uric acid	Gout
Erythrocyte sedimentation rate (ESR)	General inflammation test

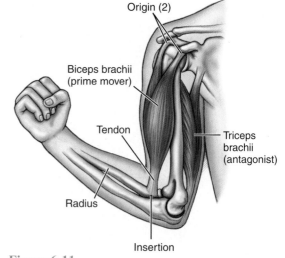

Figure 6-11
Muscles usually occur in antagonistic pairs, such as the triceps and biceps of the upper arm. (From Herlihy B, Maebius N: The Human Body in Health and Illness. Philadelphia, Saunders, 2000.)

Disorders of Skeletal Muscle

Disorders affecting skeletal muscle include trauma, genetic diseases of muscle proteins, metabolic diseases, autoimmune disorders, and motor neuron infection or degeneration (Box 6-2). Muscle disorders may be treated by an orthopedist, a rheumatologist, or a neurologist. Common lab tests ordered for these disorders are listed in Table 6-2.

BOX 6-2 Disorders of the Muscular System

Trauma
Contusions
Tendon injuries
Tendonitis—from overuse or overexertion; repetitive strain injuries

Genetic Disease
Muscular dystrophies—inherited defects in the proteins of the muscle cell; Duchenne's muscular dystrophy is the most common type

Metabolic Disease
Inherited defects in metabolic function, especially of the mitochondria; most are rare

Autoimmune Disease
Myasthenia gravis—antibodies form against the receptor for acetylcholine, preventing nerve-muscle communication
Polymyositis and dermatomyositis

Motor Neuron Disease
Poliomyelitis—viral infection that has been virtually eradicated; new cases caused by vaccine virus; can cause paralysis
Amyotrophic lateral sclerosis (ALS; also called Lou Gehrig's disease)—degeneration of motor neurons; cause unknown

---

TABLE 6-2 Common Lab Tests for Muscle Disorders

Test	Disorder or Purpose
Aldolase	Muscle disease
Aspartate aminotransferase (AST)	Muscle disease
Creatine kinase (CK-MM)	Muscle damage
CK isoenzymes (CK-MM, CK-MB)	Cardiac muscle damage
Lactate dehydrogenase	Cardiac muscle damage
Troponin	Cardiac muscle damage
Myoglobin	Muscle damage

INTEGUMENTARY SYSTEM

The integumentary system forms the outer covering of the body and includes the skin, hair, nails, and sweat glands. The principal functions of the integumentary system are protection, **thermoregulation** (control of body temperature), and sensation. The skin forms an effective barrier against invasion by microbes and chemicals. Evaporation of sweat from the surface of the skin is the major means by which humans cool themselves. Sensory cells embedded in the skin allow the brain to receive information about the environment.

Features of the Integumentary System

Skin is a layered structure that forms by continual division of its innermost layer, the **dermis** (Figure 6-12). Cells of the **epidermis** gradually die and slough off as they move toward the outermost layers. Callus is epidermis that has extra amounts of the structural protein keratin, which provides a tough protective layer in regions subject to frequent abrasion or impact. Keratin is also the principal component of hair and nails, which are dead tissues formed from living follicles within the skin. Below the dermis is a subcutaneous layer of connective tissue, including the fat layer that provides padding and insulation. Capillary beds that lie within the dermis supply the blood for a dermal puncture.

Two main types of glands are found in the skin. Sweat glands are located in the dermis, with ducts reaching up through the epidermis to form pores on the surface of the skin. Sweat cools the body by evaporation. Salt is excreted at the same time. Sebaceous glands produce an oily substance called sebum that lubricates the skin and hair.

Disorders of the Integumentary System

Disorders affecting the integumentary system include trauma, infection, neoplastic disease, and inflammation (Box 6-3). Integumentary disorders are treated by a dermatologist. Common lab tests ordered for these disorders are listed in Table 6-3.

NERVOUS SYSTEM

The nervous system includes the **central nervous system** (the brain and spinal cord) and the **peripheral nervous system** (all the neurons outside the central nervous system) (Figure 6-13). Sensory information from the periphery is received by the

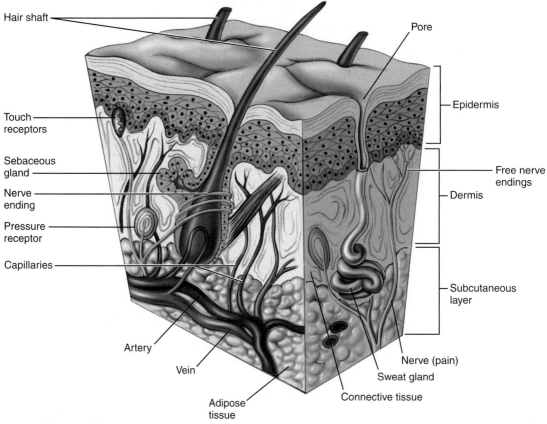

Figure 6-12
The integumentary system covers and protects the body. It permits sensation of the environment, and regulates the internal temperature. (Modified from Herlihy B, Maebius N: The Human Body in Health and Illness. Philadelphia, Saunders, 2000.)

BOX 6-3 Disorders of the Integumentary System

Infection
Fungal Infection
Ringworm
Athlete's foot

Bacterial Infection
Staphylococcus infection—impetigo
Streptococcus infection—necrotizing fasciitis ("flesh-eating" bacteria)

Neoplastic Disease
Carcinoma
Melanoma

Inflammation
Psoriasis
Acne

TABLE 6-3 Common Lab Tests for Integumentary Disorders

Test	Disorder or Purpose
Culture and sensitivity (C&S)	Bacterial or fungal infection
Potassium hydroxide (KOH) prep	Fungal infection
Skin biopsy	Malignancy

central nervous system (CNS), where it is integrated and processed to form an understanding of experience. The CNS directs movement by sending commands to the muscles through the motor portion of the peripheral nervous system. The CNS also directs some actions of other organs, including secretion by some glands.

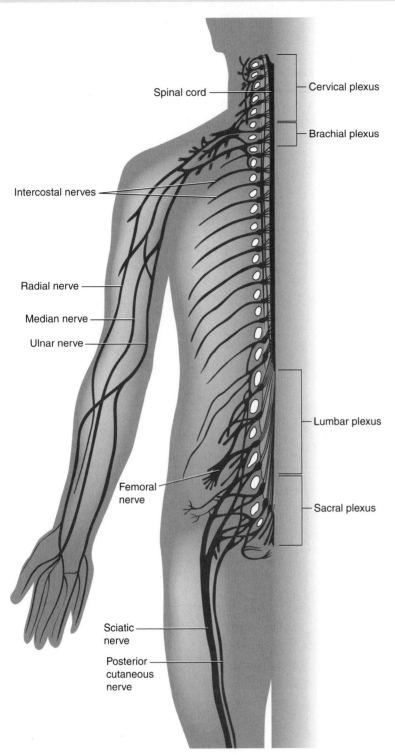

Spinal cord

Cervical plexus

Brachial plexus

Intercostal nerves

Radial nerve

Median nerve

Ulnar nerve

Lumbar plexus

Femoral nerve

Sacral plexus

Sciatic nerve

Posterior cutaneous nerve

Figure 6-13
The nervous system receives sensations and controls motor responses, as well as helping to maintain homeostasis.

Peripheral Nervous System

The peripheral nervous system is composed of two major divisions, the sensory and somatic systems. Sensory neurons, called **afferents**, receive stimulation from specialized cells within their sensory organ—the eyes, nose, mouth, ears, skin, and subcutaneous tissue such as joints, muscle, and internal organs. Afferents transmit information to spinal cord neurons, allowing sensory information to ascend to the brain. Motor neurons, called **efferents**, receive information from spinal cord neurons and carry it to the target organ, either a muscle or a gland. (A third type of neuron, the **interneuron**, conveys information between afferents and efferents and is located in the CNS.)

Neurons are bundled together in the periphery for protection. These bundles are called **nerves**. A nerve may contain only motor or only sensory neurons, or it may be a mixed nerve, containing both. Nerves also contain blood vessels, which nourish the neurons within.

Motor System

The motor system is divided into two branches, the **somatic** and the **autonomic**. Somatic **motor neurons** innervate skeletal muscles and can be consciously controlled. Autonomic motor neurons innervate cardiac and smooth muscle and normally cannot be consciously controlled (although indirect control is possible through focused relaxation techniques

such as meditation and biofeedback). Digestive secretions are also partly controlled by the autonomic system, as are secretions from the adrenal medulla.

Motor commands of both types originate in the brain and descend through the spinal column. Spinal neurons make synapses with lower motor neurons, which branch out through the gaps between vertebrae to reach their target.

Central Nervous System

Within the CNS, bundles of neurons are called **tracts**. The spinal cord has both ascending and descending tracts. The top of the spinal cord merges into the **brain stem**, a region at the base of the skull that is vital for basic life processes, including respiration (Figure 6-14). The brain stem also connects with the **thalamus**, a major relay station for incoming sensory information. Posterior to the brain stem

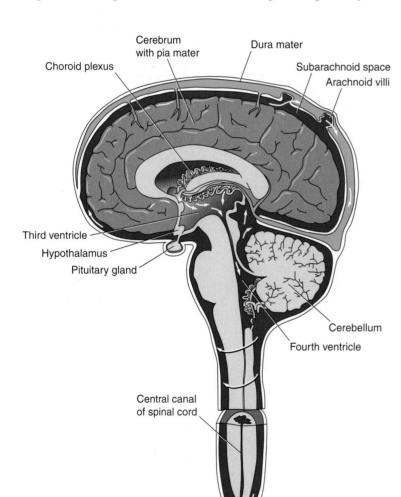

Cerebrum
with pia mater

Choroid plexus

Dura mater

Subarachnoid space
Arachnoid villi

Third ventricle
Hypothalamus
Pituitary gland

Central canal
of spinal cord

Cerebellum

Fourth ventricle

Figure 6-14
This sagittal section of the brain and cranium shows the brain's internal organization, plus the ventricles and three protective membranes.

is the **cerebellum**, a principal site for fine-tuning of motor commands. Superior to the brain stem and partially covering the cerebellum is the **cerebrum**, which contains the **cerebral cortex**, divided into left and right hemispheres. The cerebral cortex is the site of thought, emotion, and memory. Motor control of the left side of the body begins in the right cerebral

---

TABLE 6-4 Common Lab Tests for Neurologic Disorders

Test	Disorder or Purpose
Cerebrospinal fluid (CSF) analysis Cell count and differential Culture and Gram's stain Protein and glucose	Meningitis, other neurologic disorders
Creatine kinase isoenzymes (CK-BB)	Brain damage (causes elevations)

---

hemisphere, and the right side of the body is controlled by the left cerebral hemisphere.

In addition to the nutrients received from blood, the brain is nourished and cushioned by **cerebrospinal fluid** (CSF), which is secreted by the brain and circulates within the **ventricles** (see Fig. 6-14). The brain is surrounded by three membranes—the **pia mater**, the **arachnoid**, and the **dura mater**—that lubricate and protect the brain. Together, these constitute the **meninges**. The spinal cord is also surrounded by meninges.

Disorders of the Nervous System

Disorders affecting the nervous system include trauma, stroke, infection, neoplastic diseases, degeneration, autoimmune diseases, developmental disorders, and psychiatric illnesses (Box 6-4). Neurologic disorders are treated by a neurologist, and psychiatric disorders are treated by a psychiatrist or other mental health professional. Common lab tests ordered for these disorders are listed in Table 6-4. Disorders of the CNS are most often diagnosed using imaging techniques such as magnetic resonance imaging (MRI) and computed tomography (CT) scanning.

DIGESTIVE SYSTEM

The digestive system is responsible for the absorption of nutrients and elimination of waste from the digestive tract. The digestive system includes the mouth, esophagus, stomach, small and large intestines, rectum, and anus, plus the accessory digestive organs, including the liver, gallbladder, and pancreas (Figure 6-15). The purpose of digestion is to break down food into molecules small enough to be absorbed by the intestines. This process includes both mechanical and chemical digestion.

BOX 6-4 Disorders of the Central Nervous System

Trauma
Concussion
Subdural hemorrhage
Subarachnoid hemorrhage
Penetrating wound

Stroke
Embolic stroke—blood clot lodges within a cerebral vessel
Hemorrhagic stroke—blood vessel bursts; usually preceded by aneurysm

Infection
Meningitis
Shingles—peripheral infection, caused by varicella-zoster
Herpes—peripheral infection, caused by varicella-zoster
Polio

Neoplastic Disease
Neuroma—benign tumor of neural tissue
Neurosarcoma—malignant tumor of neural tissue

Degenerative Disease
Alzheimer's disease—most common neurodegenerative disease, causing widespread degeneration of cortex
Amyotrophic lateral sclerosis (ALS; also called Lou Gehrig's disease)
Parkinson's disease—degeneration of the basal ganglia, important for movement control

Autoimmune Disease
Multiple sclerosis—progressive attack on myelin sheath surrounding CNS neurons
Guillain-Barré syndrome—short-term but life-threatening postinfectious attack on motor neurons
Myasthenia gravis

Developmental Disorders
Cerebral palsy—perinatal damage to motor centers of the brain, often accompanied by other impairments
Epilepsy

Psychiatric Illness
Schizophrenia
Depression
Bipolar disorder

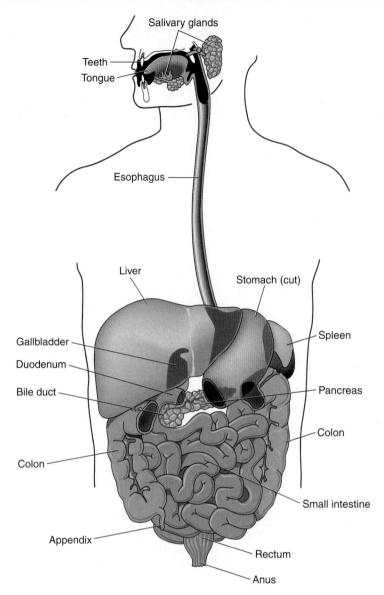

Salivary glands

Teeth

Tongue

Esophagus

Liver

Stomach (cut)

Gallbladder

Duodenum

Bile duct

Spleen

Pancreas

Colon

Colon

Small intestine

Appendix

Rectum

Anus

Figure 6-15
The digestive system extends from the mouth to the anus and includes the accessory organs of digestion.

The Digestion Process

Mouth to Stomach

Mechanical digestion begins in the mouth. Chewing increases the surface area of food, allowing faster chemical attack by the enzymes of the stomach and intestines. Saliva lubricates the food, allowing it to pass smoothly down the **esophagus**. Smooth muscles of the esophagus constrict in a wavelike motion called **peristalsis**, forcing the bolus of food down into the stomach. A ring of smooth muscle at the stomach's opening, called a **sphincter**, relaxes to admit the bolus of food, and then contracts to prevent reflux of the stomach's contents.

The strong muscular walls of the stomach churn the food, and glands within the walls secrete hydrochloric acid and the enzyme pepsin, beginning the process of chemical digestion. This thick, soupy mixture is called **chyme**. Secretion is controlled hormonally, to prevent the release of enzymes when food is not available. The stomach itself is protected from digestion by a layer of mucus.

Small Intestine

The partially digested chyme is passed by peristalsis through another sphincter into the small intestine, where further chemical digestion occurs. The pancreas secretes a large array of digestive enzymes into the small intestine, including **proteases** for breaking proteins into amino acids, **lipases** for breaking fats into fatty acids, and **carbohydrases** for breaking complex carbohydrates into simple sugars. The gallbladder releases **bile**, which also aids in the breakdown of fat. Glands in the intestinal wall release enzymes as well. The high internal surface area of the small intestine is made up of numerous finger-like projections called **villi**. These allow for rapid and efficient absorption of the digested molecules, and the rich blood supply allows nutrients to be carried away quickly to the liver for further processing and storage. Fat is absorbed by the lymphatic system instead of the blood system. You will learn about the lymphatic system in Chapter 7.

Large Intestine and Elimination

The remaining material is passed through another sphincter past the appendix into the large intestine, or colon. Here, much of the water is reabsorbed, and the indigestible solid material is compacted to form feces. Feces are eliminated through the anus, by strong peristaltic contraction of the smooth muscle of the rectum.

Liver

The liver is a central organ in both digestion and, more importantly, nutrient processing and storage. The liver produces the bile that is stored in the gallbladder. After nutrients are absorbed by the small intestine, they pass in the bloodstream directly to the liver for further chemical action and storage. Carbohydrates are stored in the liver for immediate use, and numerous harmful substances are detoxified there as well. The liver has a central role in the elimination of bilirubin, a hemoglobin breakdown product. A damaged liver leads to jaundice, a condition in which unprocessed bilirubin gives a yellowish color to the skin.

Disorders of the Digestive System

Disorders affecting the digestive system include infection, inflammation, chemical damage, and autoimmune disease (Box 6-5). Digestive disorders are treated by an internal medicine specialist or gastroenterologist. Common lab tests ordered for these disorders are listed in Table 6-5.

BOX 6-5 Disorders of the Digestive System

Infection

Ulcer—infection by *Helicobacter pylori*, treated with antibiotics; relation to stress largely discredited

Gastroenteritis—can be viral or bacterial

Hepatitis—inflamed liver due to infection or injury; commonly viral (A, B, or C)

Appendicitis—infection and inflammation by resident bacteria; can be life-threatening if appendix bursts

Giardiasis

Tapeworm

Inflammation

Cholecystitis—inflamed gallbladder

Colitis—inflamed colon; causes diarrhea

Pancreatitis—inflamed pancreas due to injury, alcohol, drugs, or gallstones

Peritonitis—inflamed abdominal cavity caused by a ruptured appendix, perforated ulcer, or other infectious process

Chemical Damage

Cirrhosis of the liver—often due to prolonged alcohol consumption

Gallstones

Autoimmune Disease

Crohn's disease—causes intestinal cramping

TABLE 6-5 Common Lab Tests for Digestive Disorders

Test	Disorder or Purpose
Complete blood count (CBC)	Appendicitis
Amylase, lipase	Pancreatitis
Liver tests	Liver disease
Alkaline phosphatase (ALP)	
Alanine aminotransferase (ALT)	
Aspartate aminotransferase (AST)	
γ-Glutamyltransferase (GGT)	
Bilirubin	
Hepatitis B surface antigen (HBsAG)	
Hepatitis C antibody	
HCV by PCR	
Ammonia	
Gastrin	Gastric malignancy
Carotene	Steatorrhea (malabsorption syndrome causing fatty stools)
Occult blood	Gastrointestinal bleeding
Ova and parasites (O&P)	Parasitic infection
Stool culture	Stool pathogens

URINARY SYSTEM

The urinary system includes the kidneys, the bladder, and the urethra (Figure 6-16). Through the production of urine, it functions to remove metabolic wastes from the circulation, maintain acid-base balance, and regulate body hydration. The kidneys also produce hormones that control blood pressure (renin) and regulate the production of red blood cells (erythropoietin).

The Kidney

Blood flows into the kidney through the renal artery. Within the kidney, capillaries form into tight balls, called glomeruli (Figure 6-17). Each **glomerulus** is enclosed within a glove-like structure known as **Bowman's capsule**. Blood pressure forces fluid out of the glomerulus into Bowman's capsule, and then into the renal tubule. This fluid is similar in composition to the plasma it is derived from, but without most of the proteins. As it flows—first through the **proximal convoluted tubule**, around the **loop of Henle**, and through the **distal convoluted tubule**—its composition changes according to the needs of the body at the time. Salts, sugar, and other small molecules are reclaimed, along with water, and returned to the capillary bed surrounding the tubule.

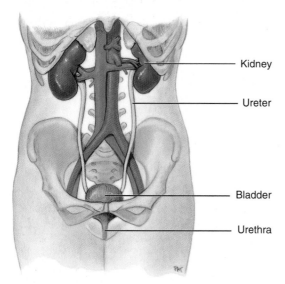

— Kidney

— Ureter

— Bladder

— Urethra

Figure 6-16
The urinary system collects urine from the kidneys for storage and elimination. (From Applegate E: The Anatomy and Physiology Learning System, ed 3. Philadelphia, Saunders, 2006.)

Transport of these substances is accomplished by a combination of active transport, osmosis, and diffusion. Other substances are actively secreted back into the tubule from the capillaries. The fluid remaining in the tubule at the far end—urine—enters the **collecting duct** and drains into the bladder through the **ureter**. The entire structure, from glomerulus to collecting duct, is known as a **nephron**.

Disorders of the Urinary System

Disorders affecting the urinary system include infection, inflammation, and chemical disorders (Box 6-6). Renal failure—the inability of the kidneys to maintain blood homeostasis—is life-threatening and must be treated with dialysis or transplantation. Urinary disorders are treated by a urologist. Common lab tests ordered for these disorders are listed in Table 6-6.

RESPIRATORY SYSTEM

The respiratory system includes the upper airways (nasal passages and throat) and the lower airways (trachea, larynx, bronchi, and lungs). It also involves the muscles of respiration in the abdomen, chest, and neck. The function of the respiratory system is to obtain oxygen for use by the body's cells and to expel the carbon dioxide waste from metabolic processes. The respiratory system relies on the circulatory system to transport gases to and from the lungs. **External respiration** refers to the exchange of gases in the lungs, and **internal respiration** refers to the exchange of oxygen and carbon dioxide at the cellular level.

Features of the Respiratory System

External Respiration
External respiration begins with the expansion of the chest cavity through the combined actions of the diaphragm, intercostal muscles, and accessory muscles of respiration (Figure 6-18). This expansion lowers the internal air pressure, so that the higher external pressure forces air into the airways. Air entering the nostrils is warmed, moistened, and filtered by passing over mucus-covered ciliated membranes. It then passes through the throat, or **pharynx**, and enters the **trachea**, passing through the **larynx** and past the vocal cords. The trachea branches into left and right **bronchi**, which branch further as they enter the lungs (see Fig. 6-18). These smaller branches, called **bronchioles**, continue to

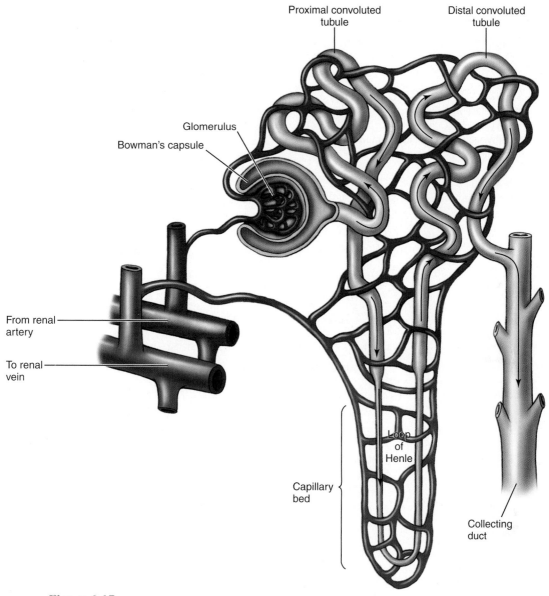

Figure 6-17
The nephron is the functional unit of the kidney. (Modified from Herlihy B, Maebius N: The Human Body in Health and Illness. Philadelphia, Saunders, 2000.)

branch until they form blind sacs called **alveoli**. Oxygen from the air passes by diffusion through the thin walls of each alveolus into the capillaries that surround it. Carbon dioxide from the blood passes out by diffusion at the same time. Exhalation is accomplished principally by relaxation of the respiratory muscles, with some additional force supplied by contraction of the abdominal muscles.

The trachea contains C-shaped rings of cartilage to prevent collapse of the airway during inspiration. Trachea, bronchi, and bronchioles are lined with epithelial tissue, which secretes thin mucus for moistening

and cleaning the air. This mucus traps dust, bacteria, and other particles entering the airways. Tiny hair filaments on the cell surfaces, called **cilia**, continually sweep this mucus up the airway to the throat, where it is swallowed. During infection, mucus production increases, and the mucus becomes thicker as well. A cough is then required to clear it.

Internal Respiration

Oxygen binds to hemoglobin in the red blood cells, forming **oxyhemoglobin**. In this form, it is carried through the circulatory system to all the body's

BOX 6-6 Disorders of the Urinary System

Infection or Inflammation

Urinary tract infection (UTI)—bacterial infection of the urinary tract

Cystitis—inflammation of the bladder

Glomerulonephritis—inflammation of the glomerulus due to infection or immune disorder

Pyelonephritis—inflammation of kidney tissue due to a bacterial infection

Chemical Disorders

Renal calculi (kidney stones)—crystals of calcium oxalate, uric acid, or other chemicals form within the tubules

TABLE 6-6 Common Lab Tests for Urologic Disorders

Test	Disorder or Purpose
Blood urea nitrogen (BUN)	Kidney disease
Creatinine	Kidney disease
Creatinine clearance	Glomerular filtration
Culture and sensitivity (C&S)	Urinary tract infection
Electrolytes	Fluid balance
Osmolality	Fluid balance
Protein/microalbumin	Kidney disorders
Renin/ACE	Hypertension
Routine urinalysis	Screening tests for renal or metabolic disorders

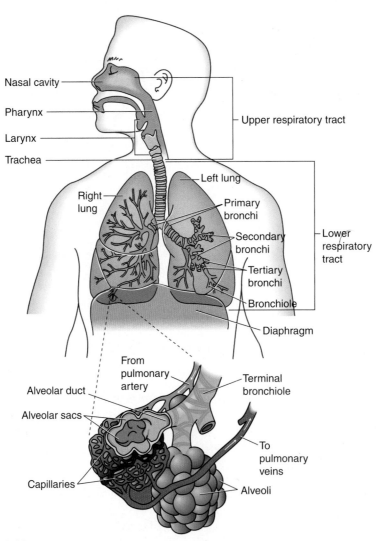

Figure 6-18

Structure of the lungs. The bronchial tree branches until it terminates in alveoli, where gas exchange occurs.

tissues. Because oxygen is being used in the tissues, its concentration there is decreased in relation to its concentration in the blood, and oxygen flows by diffusion out of the blood into the tissues. It passes into cells and finally to the mitochondria, which use it to react with carbon and hydrogen from food molecules, supplying energy to the cell. The waste products—carbon dioxide and water—then diffuse out of the cell. Carbon dioxide dissolves in the blood and is carried back to the lungs.

Disorders of the Respiratory System

Disorders affecting the respiratory system include infection, inflammation, obstruction, insufficient ventilation, developmental disorders, and neoplastic diseases (Box 6-7). Respiratory failure occurs when

TABLE 6-7 Common Lab Tests for Respiratory Disorders

Test	Disorder or Purpose
Arterial blood gases (ABGs): pH (acidity), P_{O_2} (oxygen), P_{CO_2} (carbon dioxide)	Most respiratory disorders; assess lung function
Cold agglutinins (test for antibodies that react with red blood cells at cold temperatures)	Atypical pneumonia
Electrolytes	Impaired gas exchange
RSV	Viral pneumonia
Microbiologic tests	Microbial infection—
Cultures	pneumonia or pharyngitis
Throat swabs	
Bronchial washings	

the respiratory system cannot supply adequate gas exchange to maintain body function. It is a life-threatening condition and is treated by temporary or permanent mechanical devices to aid ventilation. Diseases of the upper respiratory tract are commonly treated by a primary care physician or an ear, nose, and throat (ENT) specialist. Disorders of the lower respiratory tract are most often treated by a pulmonologist. Common lab tests ordered for these disorders are listed in Table 6-7.

ENDOCRINE SYSTEM

The endocrine system comprises the glands and other tissues that produce hormones, which are released from glandular tissue directly into the circulatory system (Figure 6-19). The endocrine system functions with the nervous system to tightly regulate body function, maintaining homeostasis. Because of the fine degree of control required, endocrine glands are themselves regulated by other endocrine glands, in multiple control systems known as **feedback loops**. Many of these feedback loops involve the brain as well, especially the small portion of the brain known as the **hypothalamus**.

Hormones

Hormones are chemical substances released into the circulation by one group of cells that affect the function of other cells. Hormones exert their effects by binding to receptors at the target cell. Receptors may be on the surface of the target cell, in its cytoplasm,

---

BOX 6-7 Disorders of the Respiratory System

Infection
Upper respiratory infection (URI)—infection of the nose, throat, or larynx; can be viral, fungal, or bacterial
Pneumonia—infection of the lower airway; can be viral, fungal, bacterial, or mycobacterial
Strep throat—infection of the throat by *Streptococcus* bacteria
Tuberculosis—infection by *Mycobacterium tuberculosis*

Inflammation
Bronchitis—inflammation of the bronchi, due to irritation or infection
Emphysema—chronic inflammation of alveoli and bronchioles; can be caused by smoking
Pleurisy—inflammation of the pleural membrane

Obstruction
Asthma—obstructed bronchi due to airway constriction
Chronic obstructive pulmonary disease (COPD)—due to emphysema
Pulmonary edema—fluid in the lungs

Insufficient Ventilation
Spinal cord injury
Muscular dystrophy
Polio
ALS

Developmental Disorder
Infant respiratory distress syndrome (IRDS)—collapsed alveoli; common in premature infants

Neoplastic Disease
Lung cancer

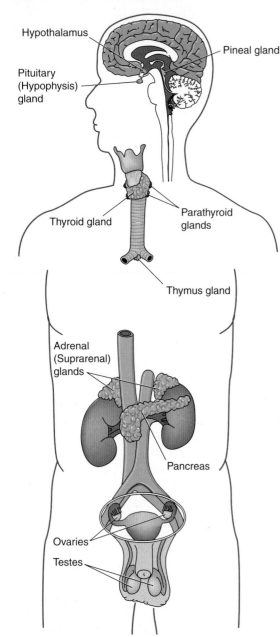

Figure 6-19
The glands of the endocrine system.

or in its nucleus. There are three principal types of hormones: **steroid hormones** (including testosterone and progesterone), **amino acid derivatives** (including thyroxine and epinephrine, which is also called adrenaline), and **peptides** (including insulin). Each type has its own mechanisms of action and duration of response. For instance, epinephrine works quickly to produce a short-lived response, whereas steroid hormones such as testosterone work slowly to produce long-lasting effects.

Endocrine Glands

Pituitary Gland

The pituitary gland is located at the base of the brain, just outside the cranium. It is involved in virtually every feedback loop in the endocrine system, sending hormones out and receiving hormonal messages from every other endocrine gland, including the thyroid, the adrenals, and the ovaries. For this reason, it is often called the master gland of the endocrine system. The hypothalamus secretes a variety of hormones that directly influence pituitary function.

The pituitary has two lobes, the anterior and the posterior. The anterior pituitary secretes **thyroid-stimulating hormone** (TSH); **adrenocorticotropic hormone** (ACTH); and **follicle-stimulating hormone** (FSH) and **luteinizing hormone** (LH), which act on the ovaries and testes. In addition, the anterior pituitary secretes **growth hormone** (GH), which regulates the rate of growth throughout the body; **melanocyte-stimulating hormone** (MSH), which increases melanin pigment production in skin cells; and **prolactin**, which increases milk production in the mammary glands.

The posterior pituitary produces **antidiuretic hormone** (ADH), which regulates water reabsorption by the kidney, and **oxytocin**, which stimulates smooth muscle contraction in the uterus during labor and in the mammary glands during nursing.

Thyroid Gland

The thyroid gland wraps around the trachea, just below the larynx. The thyroid secretes **thyroxine**—also called T_4, because it contains four atoms of iodine—and small amounts of **triiodothyronine**, or T_3. These two hormones regulate the basal metabolic rate, or energy consumption rate, of virtually every cell in the body. The thyroid also secretes **calcitonin**, which lowers calcium levels in body fluids.

Parathyroid Gland

The parathyroid gland is located behind the thyroid. It secretes **parathormone**, which regulates the amount of calcium and phosphorus in the circulation.

Thymus Gland

The thymus sits behind the sternum and plays a key role in the early development of the immune system. Among other functions, it secretes **thymosin**, which develops and maintains immunity. The thymus shrinks throughout life, and its function in adults, if any, is not clear.

Pancreas

The pancreas is located behind the stomach. It has two distinct functions. As discussed earlier, it produces digestive enzymes that are secreted into the small intestine. As an endocrine gland, it produces two hormones that regulate the level of the sugar glucose in the blood: insulin and glucagon.

Insulin promotes the uptake of glucose by the body's cells, thereby lowering blood sugar levels. It also promotes the conversion of glucose into glycogen, a storage carbohydrate, in the liver and skeletal muscles. **Glucagon** promotes the breakdown of glycogen back into glucose and increases its release into the blood, thereby elevating blood sugar levels. The antagonistic effects of these two hormones allow tight regulation of blood glucose levels.

Adrenal Glands

There are two adrenal glands, one located above each kidney (the word *adrenal* means "*above the kidney*"). Each adrenal gland is composed of two parts.

The inner **adrenal medulla** secretes the catecholamines **epinephrine** and **norepinephrine** under the direct control of the autonomic nervous system. These hormones have the familiar effects of increasing the heart rate, increasing blood flow to the skeletal muscles, and producing a subjective feeling of heightened awareness and anticipation. They are a crucial part of the "fight or flight" response.

The outer **adrenal cortex** secretes steroid hormones. These include the **glucocorticoids**, which influence glucose metabolism; the **mineralocorticoids**, which control electrolyte balance; and androgens, or male sex hormones.

The principal glucocorticoids are cortisol, cortisone, and **corticosterone**, which decrease glucose consumption and promote fat usage. They also reduce inflammation, accounting for their use on skin rashes and other irritations. **Aldosterone** is the principal mineralocorticoid, helping to regulate sodium and water balance in the kidneys.

Gonads

The gonads are the ovaries and testes. The testes produce **testosterone**, the principal male sex hormone. Testosterone promotes sperm maturation, increases protein synthesis in skeletal muscle, and causes the development of male secondary sex characteristics, including facial hair and a deep voice. The ovaries produce **estrogens** and **progesterone**, whose functions include regulation of the menstrual cycle, development of the uterus, and development

---

BOX 6-8 Disorders of the Endocrine System

Hyposecretion
Addison's disease—loss of adrenal cortex function
Diabetes insipidus—lack of ADH
Diabetes mellitus—lack of insulin production; autoimmune destruction of pancreatic islet cells
Pituitary dwarfism—lack of GH
Hypothyroidism—lack of thyroxine; can be caused by iodine deficiency (goiter); can lead to myxedema, death

Hypersecretion
Acromegaly or gigantism—excess GH, commonly due to pituitary tumor
Cushing's disease—excess cortisol and ACTH
Graves' disease—excess thyroid hormone
Hyperinsulinism—most often due to insulin overdose or tumor

---

of the mammary glands and other female secondary sex characteristics.

Disorders of the Endocrine System

Disorders affecting the endocrine system most often involve either hypersecretion or hyposecretion (Box 6-8). Hypersecretion is most often caused by a tumor of the glandular tissue or excess administration (as with insulin); hyposecretion may be due to genetic disease, autoimmunity, or nutritional deficiency. Diseases of the endocrine system are treated by an endocrinologist. Common lab tests ordered for these disorders are listed in Table 6-8.

REPRODUCTIVE SYSTEMS

The reproductive systems include the **gonads**—ovaries or testes—plus the accessory structures required for successful reproduction. The reproductive system in men serves the function of producing and ejaculating sperm. In women, the reproductive system produces mature eggs, allows for their fertilization, and hosts and nourishes the embryo as it develops.

Male Reproductive System

The testes are the site of sperm production as well as testosterone production (Figure 6-20). The testes are enclosed by the **scrotum**. Sperm pass from the testis into the **epididymis**, a coiled tube atop the testis, where they mature. Mature sperm pass into the **vas deferens**, where they are stored before ejaculation. Sexual arousal causes contraction of the smooth

TABLE 6-8 Common Lab Tests for Endocrine Disorders

Test	Disorder or Purpose
Parathyroid hormone (PTH)	Parathyroid function
Vitamin D	Parathyroid function
Calcium	Parathyroid function
Phosphorus	Parathyroid function
Catecholamines (epinephrine, norepinephrine)	Adrenal function
Cortisol	Adrenal cortex function; Addison's disease
Fasting glucose, fasting blood sugar (FBS)	Diabetes mellitus
Growth hormone (GH)	Pituitary function
Thyroid function studies	Thyroid disorder
T_3, T_4, and thyroid-stimulating hormone (TSH)	Graves' disease, Hashimoto's thyroiditis
Luteinizing hormone (LH)	Infertility
Follicle-stimulating hormone (FSH)	Infertility
Testosterone	Infertility

muscle lining, the vas deferens, propelling sperm into the **urethra**. Fluid from several glands is secreted into the urethra as well, to nourish and protect the sperm and provide a fluid medium for them to swim in. Glands supplying fluid are the **prostate**, the **seminal vesicles**, and the **bulbourethral glands**. The sperm and fluid together constitute **semen**. The urethra passes through the **penis**, whose spongy muscular tissue swells with blood during erection. Ejaculation occurs when strong peristaltic contractions of urethral smooth muscle propel the semen out of the urethra.

Female Reproductive System

The **ovaries** produce eggs during early development. Beginning at puberty, one or more eggs mature each month, under the influence of the pituitary hormones FSH and LH. At the same time, estrogens and progesterone produced by the ovaries induce changes in the uterine lining in preparation for implantation of a fertilized egg, including tissue buildup and increased blood flow. **Ovulation**, or release of the egg, is triggered by a sharp spike in LH levels. The egg enters the **fallopian tube** (Figure 6-21), where it is conveyed toward the **uterus** by cilia on the surface of the cells lining the tube. Fertilization occurs within the fallopian tube. Fertilization can occur only when a sperm swims up the **vagina**, through the **cervix**, through the uterus, and into the fallopian tube containing the egg and unites with the egg, all within the 2 to 4 days after ovulation in which the egg remains viable.

Implantation of the fertilized egg in the wall of the uterus induces changes that lead to the development of the placenta. Among other hormones, the placenta releases **human chorionic gonadotropin** (HCG), which can be detected by early pregnancy tests. Without HCG, the uterine lining begins to deteriorate shortly after ovulation, culminating in menstruation. An unfertilized egg passes out of the uterus at that time.

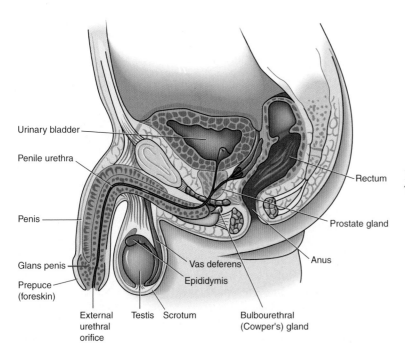

Urinary bladder

Penile urethra

Penis

Glans penis

Prepuce (foreskin)

External urethral orifice

Testis

Scrotum

Vas deferens

Epididymis

Bulbourethral (Cowper's) gland

Anus

Prostate gland

Rectum

Figure 6-20
The male reproductive system.

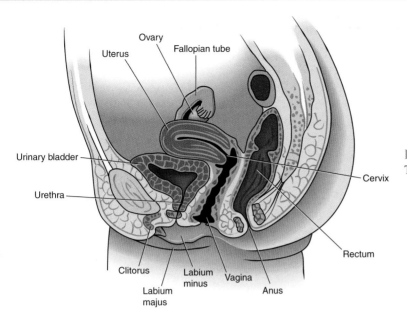

Figure 6-21
The female reproductive system.

Disorders of the Reproductive Systems

Disorders of the male reproductive system are treated by a urologist or an endocrinologist. Disorders of the female reproductive system are treated by an obstetrician-gynecologist or an endocrinologist (Box 6-9). Infertility may be treated by a specialist. Common lab tests ordered for these disorders are listed in Table 6-9.

TABLE 6-9 Common Lab Tests for Reproductive Disorders

Test	Disorder or Purpose
Semen analysis	Infertility; assess effectiveness of vasectomy
Testosterone	Evaluation of testicular function
Prostate-specific antigen (PSA)	Prostate cancer
Rapid plasma reagin (RPR)	Syphilis
Fluorescent treponemal antibody absorption test (FTA-ABS)	Syphilis
Culture and sensitivity (C&S)	Microbial infection
Pap smear	Cervical or vaginal carcinoma
Estradiol	Assess ovarian or placental function
Estrogen	Assess ovarian function
Human chorionic gonadotropin (HCG)	Assess for pregnancy or ectopic pregnancy

BOX 6-9 Disorders of the Reproductive Systems

Male Reproductive System
Sperm malformation
Sexually transmitted disease (STD):
    Gonorrhea
    Genital herpes
    Syphilis
    HIV
Benign prostatic hyperplasia
Prostate cancer

Female Reproductive System
Sexually transmitted disease (STD):
    Gonorrhea
    Genital herpes
    Syphilis
    HIV
    Chlamydia infection
    Trichomoniasis
Endometriosis—endometrial tissue migrates to areas outside the uterus
Fibroids—benign uterine tumors
Pelvic inflammatory disease (PID)—infections in the pelvic region that cause infertility; can be due to *Chlamydia or* other microorganisms
Toxic shock syndrome (TSS)—*Staphylococcus* infection associated with use of super-absorbent tampons
Premenstrual syndrome (PMS)
Cancer:
    Vaginal
    Cervical
    Uterine
    Ovarian

REVIEW FOR CERTIFICATION

Cells are the smallest unit of structure and function in the body and are made up of numerous subcellular structures, including the nucleus, the mitochondria, and the plasma membrane. Cells of similar function combine to make tissue. The four tissue types—epithelial, connective, muscle, and nerve—combine to create organs, which in turn combine to create organ systems and, ultimately, the functioning body. Anatomic terminology is used to describe the relationships of body parts. Each of the body systems—skeletal, muscular, integumentary, nervous, digestive, urinary, respiratory, endocrine, and reproductive—has its own set of organs and interactions that contribute to its function, as well as its own set of disorders. A summary table of common lab tests arranged by body system is presented in Table 6-10.

BIBLIOGRAPHY

Guyton AC: Textbook of Medical Physiology, ed 10. Philadelphia, WB Saunders, 2000.

Martini F: Fundamentals of Anatomy and Physiology, ed 4. Upper Saddle River, NJ, Prentice-Hall, 2001.

TABLE 6-10 Summary of Common Lab Tests by Body System

Test	Disorder or Purpose	Test	Disorder or Purpose
Bone and Joints		Culture and Gram's stain	
Alkaline phosphatase (ALP)	Bone metabolism marker	Protein and glucose	
Anti-citrullinated protein	Rheumatoid factor (rheumatoid arthritis)	Creatine kinase isoenzymes (CK-BB)	Brain damage (causes elevations)
Calcium	Mineral calcium imbalance	**Digestive System**	
Magnesium	Mineral magnesium imbalance	Complete blood count (CBC)	Appendicitis
		Amylase, lipase	Pancreatitis
Fluorescent antinuclear antibody (ANA)	Systemic lupus erythematosus (SLE)	Liver tests	Liver disease
Rheumatoid factor (RF)	Rheumatoid arthritis (RA)	Alkaline phosphatase (ALP)	
Synovial fluid analysis	Arthritis	Alanine aminotransferase (ALT)	
Uric acid	Gout	Aspartate aminotransferase (AST)	
Erythrocyte sedimentation rate (ESR)	General inflammation test	γ-glutamyltransferase	
		Bilirubin	
Muscle		Hepatitis B surface antigen (HBsAG)	
Aldolase	Muscle disease	Hepatitis C antibody	
Aspartate aminotransferase (AST)	Muscle disease	Ammonia	
		Gastrin	Gastric malignancy
Creatine kinase (CK-MM)	Muscle damage	Carotene	Steatorrhea (malabsorption syndrome causing fatty stools)
CK isoenzymes (CK-MM, CK-MB)	Cardiac muscle damage		
Lactate dehydrogenase	Cardiac muscle damage	Occult blood	Gastrointestinal bleeding
Troponin	Cardiac muscle damage	Ova and parasites (O&P)	Parasitic infection
Myoglobin	Muscle damage	Stool culture	Stool pathogens
Integument		**Urologic System**	
Culture and sensitivity (C&S)	Bacterial or fungal infection	Blood urea nitrogen (BUN)	Kidney disease
Potassium hydroxide (KOH) prep	Fungal infection	Creatinine	Kidney disease
		Creatinine clearance	Glomerular filtration
Skin biopsy	Malignancy	Culture and sensitivity (C&S)	Urinary tract infection
Nervous System		Electrolytes	Fluid balance
Cerebrospinal fluid (CSF) analysis	Meningitis, other neurologic disorders	Osmolality	Fluid balance
Cell count and differential		Protein	Kidney disorders

TABLE 6-10 Summary of Common Lab Tests by Body System—cont'd

Test	Disorder or Purpose	Test	Disorder or Purpose
Renin/ACE	Hypertension	Growth hormone (GH)	Pituitary function
Routine urinalysis	Screening tests for renal or metabolic disorders	Thyroid function studies	Thyroid disorder
		T_3, T_4, and thyroid-stimulating hormone (TSH)	Graves' disease
Respiratory System		Luteinizing hormone (LH)	Infertility
Arterial blood gases (ABGs):pH (acidity), Po_2 (oxygen),Pco_2 (carbon dioxide)	Most respiratory disorders; assess lung function	Follicle-stimulating hormone (FSH)	Infertility
		Testosterone	Infertility
Cold agglutinins (test for antibodies that react with red blood cells at cold temperatures)	Atypical pneumonia	**Reproductive System**	
		Semen analysis	Infertility; assess effectiveness of vasectomy
Electrolytes	Impaired gas exchange		
Microbiologic tests	Microbial infection—pneumonia or pharyngitis	Testosterone	Evaluation of testicular function
Cultures		Prostate-specific antigen (PSA)	Prostate cancer
Throat swabs		Rapid plasma reagin (RPR)	Syphilis
Bronchial washings		Fluorescent treponemal antibody absorption test (FTA-ABS)	Syphilis
Purified protein derivative (PPD)	Skin test for tuberculosis		
Endocrine System		Culture and sensitivity (C&S)	Microbial infection
Parathyroid hormone (PTH)	Parathyroid function	Pap smear	Cervical or vaginal carcinoma
Vitamin D	Parathyroid function		
Calcium	Parathyroid function	Estradiol	Assess ovarian or placental function
Phosphorus	Parathyroid function		
Catecholamines (epinephrine, norepinephrine)	Adrenal function	Estrogen	Assess ovarian function
		Human chorionic gonadotropin (HCG)	Assess for pregnancy or ectopic pregnancy
Cortisol	Adrenal cortex function; Addison's disease		
Fasting glucose, fasting blood sugar (FBS)	Diabetes mellitus		

STUDY QUESTIONS

1. What is homeostasis?
2. Name the four basic types of tissues that compose the human body, and give an example of each.

Matching:

3. nucleus
4. plasma membrane
5. mitochondria
6. cytoplasm

a. regulates the flow of materials in and out of the cell
b. "power plants" of the cell
c. contains DNA
d. cellular material

7. Describe the "anatomic position."
8. What are body cavities?

Matching:

9. ventral
10. posterior
11. lateral
12. medial
13. prone
14. supine
15. extension
16. inferior

a. lying on the abdomen facing down
b. toward the side
c. toward the middle
d. straightening the joint
e. front surface of the body
f. below
g. back surface of the body
h. lying on the back

17. Name and describe the three body planes.
18. What is hematopoiesis?
19. Name three lab tests, and the disorders they test for, that are used to assess for bone and joint disorders.
20. _____ is a bone infection that can be caused by improper phlebotomy technique.
21. Name four lab tests that are used to assess for muscle disorders.
22. What are the divisions of the central nervous system?
23. Name five lab tests that are used to assess for digestive disorders.
24. Describe the difference between external and internal respiration.
25. What does the endocrine system do?
26. Name the three types of joints, and give an example of each.

CERTIFICATION EXAM PREPARATION

1. The term to define the overall well-being of the body is:
   a. hemolysis
   b. hemostasis
   c. homeostasis
   d. hematopoiesis

2. The functional unit of the nervous system is:
   a. nephron
   b. neuron
   c. neoplasm
   d. nucleus

3. ATP is found in which part of the cell?
   a. mitochondria
   b. cytoplasm
   c. nucleus
   d. plasma membrane

4. Which type of muscle tissue is involved in hemostasis?
   a. skeletal
   b. smooth
   c. epithelial
   d. striated

5. Blood is considered to be which type of tissue?
   a. nerve
   b. connective
   c. muscle
   d. epithelial

6. In which system does hematopoiesis occur?
   a. skeletal
   b. nervous
   c. muscular
   d. digestive

7. Which is not a lab test that assesses for muscle disorders?
   a. AST
   b. troponin
   c. C&S
   d. aldolase

8. Which is not a lab test that assesses for disorders of the integumentary system?
   a. C&S
   b. KOH prep
   c. BUN
   d. skin biopsy

9. Hepatitis involves the:
   a. heart
   b. liver
   c. brain
   d. ovaries

10. Which is not a lab test to assess for liver problems?
    a. AST
    b. GGT
    c. ALP
    d. ESR

11. _____ promotes the breakdown of glycogen back to glucose.
    a. insulin
    b. glucagon
    c. thymosin
    d. calcitonin

12. Pancreatitis can be screened for by performing which lab test?
    a. amylase
    b. CSF
    c. myoglobin
    d. occult blood

13. The functional unit of the kidney is known as the:
    a. neuron
    b. medulla
    c. thalamus
    d. nephron

14. Microbiology may perform the following lab test for urologic disorders:
    a. BUN
    b. PPD
    c. C&S
    d. FBS

CERTIFICATION EXAM PREPARATION—cont'd

15. ABGs typically test for:
    a. digestive disorder
    b. urinary disorders
    c. respiratory disorders
    d. muscular disorders

16. The hormone that regulates the amount of calcium and phosphorus in the circulation is:
    a. insulin
    b. thymosin
    c. oxytocin
    d. parathormone

17. Which hormone regulates water reabsorption by the kidney?
    a. ACTH
    b. TSH
    c. ADH
    d. MSH

18. The hormone that can be detected by early pregnancy tests is:
    a. HCG
    b. ADH
    c. GH
    d. MSH

19. Thyroxine is otherwise known as:
    a. T_3
    b. T_4
    c. TSH
    d. T_1

20. Hormones are produced by which body system?
    a. integumentary
    b. endocrine
    c. digestive
    d. respiratory

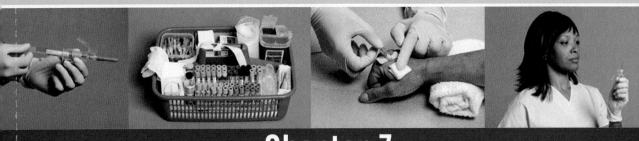

Chapter 7

Circulatory, Lymphatic, and Immune Systems

OUTLINE

Circulatory System
  The Heart
  Circulation through the Heart
  Contraction of the Heart
   and Blood Pressure
  Blood Vessels
  Blood

Hemostasis
Blood Disorders
Lymphatic System
  Lymphatic Vessels
  Lymph Organs
  Lymphatic System Disorders

Immune System
  Nonspecific Immunity
  Specific Immunity
  Immune System Disorders
Review for Certification

OBJECTIVES

After completing this chapter, you should be able to:

1. Describe the circulation of blood from the heart to the lungs and other body tissues.
2. Differentiate arteries, veins, and capillaries.
3. Locate the major arteries and veins of the human body.
4. Define systole, diastole, and sphygmomanometer.
5. List and define at least 10 diseases of the heart and blood vessels.
6. Describe the components of whole blood.
7. Describe the three cellular elements of the blood, including their major functions.
8. Explain the process of hemostasis.
9. For red blood cells, white blood cells, and hemostasis, list at least three diseases that affect each.
10. Describe laboratory tests that may be used to detect diseases of red and white blood cells and hemostasis.
11. Differentiate lymphatic circulation from that of blood.
12. Explain the functions of the lymphatic system.
13. Differentiate among nonspecific, humoral, and cellular immunity.
14. Describe the functions of T and B cells.

KEY TERMS

adhesion	aortic semilunar valve	bicuspid valve	cytokines
aggregation	arteries	CD4+ cells	cytotoxic T cells
AIDS	arterioles	cellular immunity	diastole
albumin	atria	cephalic vein	electrolytes
allergy	autoimmunity	coagulation	endocardium
antibodies	B cells	common pathway	eosinophils
antigens	basilic vein	complement	epicardium
aorta	basophils	coronary arteries	erythrocyte

Continued

KEY TERMS—cont'd

extrinsic pathway	leukocytes	plasmin	stroke
fibrin	lymphedema	plasminogen	systemic circulation
fibrin degradation	lymph nodes	platelets	systole
products	lymphocytes	polymorphonuclear	T cells
fibrinogen	lymphoma	leukocytes	terminal lymphatics
fibrin split products	major histocompatibility	primary hemostasis	thoracic duct
formed elements	complex	prothrombin	thrombin
granulocytes	median cubital vein	pulmonary arteries	thrombocytes
helper T cells	megakaryocytes	pulmonary circulation	tissue plasminogen
hemostasis	memory cells	pulmonary semilunar	activator
human leukocyte antigen	memory T cells	valve	tricuspid valve
humoral immunity	mitral valve	pulmonary trunk	tunica adventitia
immunization	monocytes	pulmonary veins	tunica intima
immunoglobulins	mononuclear leukocytes	reticulocyte	tunica media
inflammation	myocardial infarction	right atrioventricular valve	vascular spasm
interferons	myocardium	right lymphatic duct	veins
interleukins	natural killer cells	secondary hemostasis	venae cavae
interstitial fluid	neutrophils	segmented neutrophils	ventricles
intrinsic pathway	pericardium	serum	venules
ischemia	phagocytes	severe combined	
left atrioventricular valve	plasma	immune deficiency	
leukemia	plasma cells	sphygmomanometer	

ABBREVIATIONS

AIDS: acquired immunodeficiency syndrome
APTT: activated partial thromboplastin time
AST: aminotransferase
AV: atrioventricular
CBC: complete blood count
CK: creatine kinase
DIC: disseminated intravascular coagulation
FDP: fibrin degradation product
FSP: fibrin split product
HIV: human immunodeficiency virus
HLA: human leukocyte antigen

LD: lactate dehydrogenase
MHC: major histocompatibility complex
MI: myocardial infarction
NK: natural killer
PMN: polymorphonuclear leukocyte
RBC: red blood cell
SCID: severe combined immune deficiency
SEG: segmented neutrophil
TIBC: total iron-binding capacity
t-PA: tissue plasminogen activator
WBC: white blood cell

The circulatory system transports blood containing oxygen and nutrients throughout the body and picks up metabolic waste products for disposal. Beginning at the heart, blood passes from arteries to capillaries to veins, and then back to the heart. The structure of each type of blood vessel is adapted to its function within the system. In addition to its role in nutrient and waste transport, blood transports hormones and enzymes, as well as clotting factors that minimize blood leakage in the event of injury. Hemostasis ensures that a rupture in a blood vessel is repaired quickly. A separate but linked circulatory system, the lymphatic system, redistributes intercellular fluid and provides an important route of transport for cells of the immune system. The immune system fights foreign invaders through a combination of cellular and chemical defenses.

CIRCULATORY SYSTEM

The circulatory system is a system of closed tubes. Circulation occurs in two large loops—the pulmonary circulation and the systemic circulation. The **pulmonary circulation** carries blood between the heart and lungs for gas exchange, and the **systemic circulation** carries blood between the heart and the rest of the body's tissues. In both cases, **arteries** carry blood away from the heart to capillary beds, where exchange occurs. **Veins** return blood to the heart.

The Heart

The heart is a muscular double pump whose contractions push blood through the circulatory system. It is located in the thoracic cavity behind and slightly to the left of the sternum, between the lungs. The heart is surrounded by a thin membranous sac, the **pericardium**, which supports and lubricates the heart during contraction. The outer layer of the heart, the **epicardium**, consists of epithelial cells and underlying fibrous connective tissue. The **coronary arteries** that nourish the heart are embedded in this layer. The middle layer, the **myocardium**, is composed of cardiac muscle, whose cells make extensive contacts with adjacent cells to allow electrical activity to spread easily from one cell to the next. The innermost layer, the **endocardium**, is made up of endothelial cells, modified epithelium that is continuous with the endothelium lining the blood vessels that enter and exit the heart's chambers.

The four chambers of the heart are the left and right **atria** (singular: atrium) and the left and right **ventricles** (Figure 7-1). The atrial septum divides the two atria, and the interventricular septum divides the two ventricles.

The heart has four valves that prevent the backflow of blood. The **right atrioventricular** (AV) **valve**, also called the **tricuspid valve**, separates the right atrium and the right ventricle, and the **pulmonary semilunar** (pulmonic) **valve** separates the right ventricle from the **pulmonary arteries**. The **left atrioventricular valve**, also called the **bicuspid** or **mitral valve**, separates the left atrium from the left ventricle, and the **aortic semilunar valve** separates the left ventricle from the **aorta**.

Circulation through the Heart

Deoxygenated blood from the systemic circulation collects in the superior and inferior **venae cavae** (singular: vena cava), which empty into the right atrium (Figure 7-2). Contraction of the right atrium forces blood through the tricuspid valve into the right ventricle. Contraction of the right ventricle forces blood out through the pulmonary semilunar valve, through the **pulmonary trunk** and into the left and right pulmonary arteries. Blood then travels to the lungs, picking up oxygen and releasing carbon dioxide in the capillaries surrounding the alveoli. Returning to the heart via the left and right **pulmonary veins**,

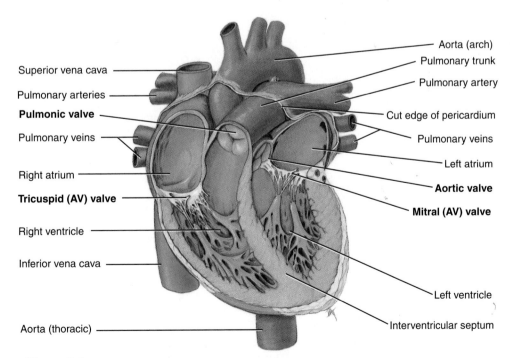

Figure 7-1
The heart is a muscle composed of four chambers, separated by valves. (From Applegate E: The Anatomy and Physiology Learning System, ed 3. Philadelphia, Saunders, 2006.)

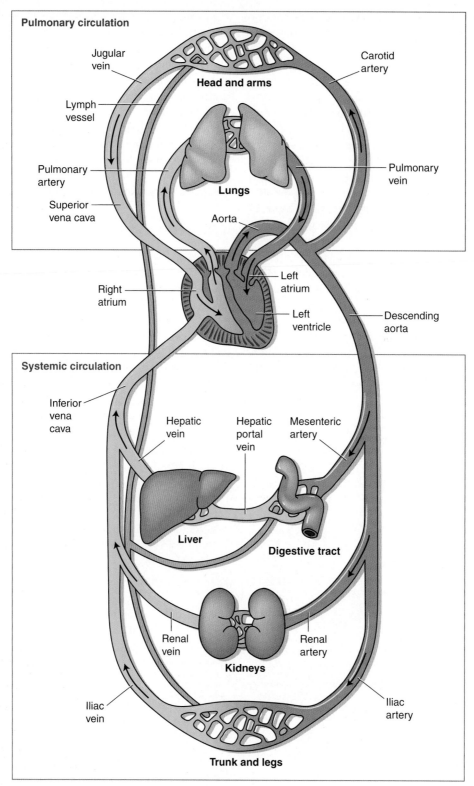

Figure 7-2
Blood flow through the heart. Blood from the body enters the right atrium and passes into the right ventricle, where it is pumped to the lungs. It reenters the left atrium and passes into the left ventricle, where it is pumped to the rest of the body.

oxygenated blood enters the left atrium. Contraction of the left atrium forces blood through the mitral valve into the left ventricle. Contraction of the left ventricle forces blood through the aortic semilunar valve into the aorta. The aorta rises up from the top of the heart before turning and descending through the thoracic and abdominal cavities. Many of the major arteries in the body branch directly from the aorta. Arteries branch further into arterioles, which lead to capillary beds within the tissues. Blood becomes deoxygenated as it passes through the capillaries and then enters venules, which link to form veins. Major veins empty into the venae cavae, which return blood to the right atrium, completing the cycle.

Contraction of the Heart and Blood Pressure

Each heartbeat cycle includes a contraction and a relaxation of each chamber. The contraction, called **systole**, develops pressure and forces blood through the system. The relaxation, called **diastole**, allows the chamber to fill again. The two atria contract together, as do the two ventricles. Atrial systole occurs slightly before ventricular systole and is not as forceful. The familiar "lubb-dupp" sound of the heartbeat is actually the sound of the valves closing—the "lubb" is the closing of the two AV valves at the start of ventricular systole, and the "dupp" is the closing of the two semilunar valves as arterial backpressure forces them shut at the start of ventricular diastole.

Blood in the circulatory system is under pressure, even during ventricular diastole. Blood pressure, measured by a **sphygmomanometer**, is the measure of the force of blood on the arterial walls. Blood pressure is given as the ratio of ventricular systole to diastole. Blood pressure differs markedly at different points in the circulatory system, and for this reason, it is always measured from the brachial artery at the upper arm.

Blood Vessels

In general, blood vessels (except for capillaries) have three discrete layers surrounding the lumen, or the space in which blood flows (Figure 7-3). The **tunica adventitia**, or outer layer, is composed of connective tissue; the **tunica media**, or middle layer, is made of smooth muscle; and the **tunica intima**, or inner layer, is composed of a single layer of endothelial cells.

Arteries

Arteries are built to withstand the high blood pressure generated by ventricular contraction. They have a thick muscular wall, which can expand when blood is pumped into them and then contract to maintain flow and pressure during diastole. Arteries are located deeper than veins are, but they can be found by feeling for the pulse. Arteries branch into smaller vessels called **arterioles**, which ultimately branch to form capillaries. Figure 7-4 indicates the names and locations of the major arteries.

A **myocardial infarction** (MI, or heart attack) occurs when the heart receives inadequate blood supply through the coronary arteries. This often occurs when the arteries become clogged with built-up atherosclerotic plaques. The resulting lack of oxygen, termed **ischemia**, causes damage to the muscle. The damaged cardiac muscle releases a number of proteins into the circulation, which can be used for diagnosis

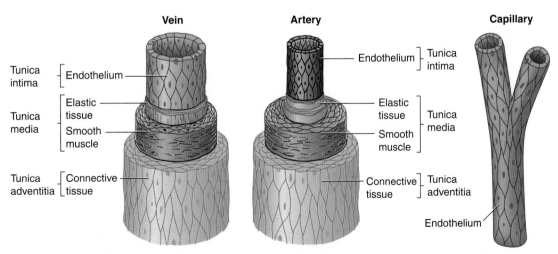

Figure 7-3
Arteries, veins, and capillaries have structures that correlate with their functions.

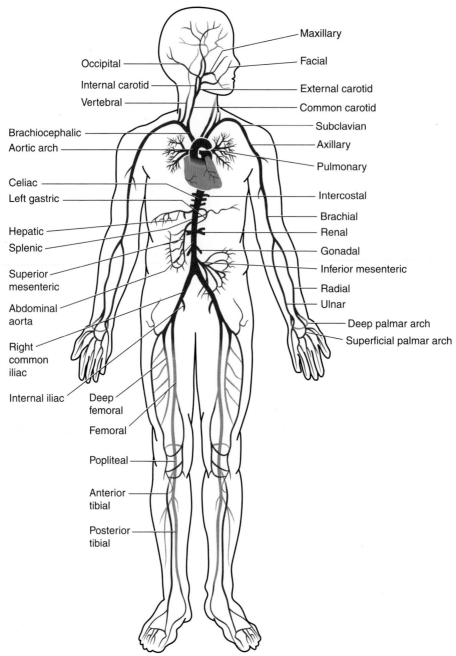

Figure 7-4
The major arteries of the body.

Capillaries

Capillaries are composed only of the tunica intima, a single layer of endothelial cells. This allows rapid diffusion of gases and nutrients between

and to determine the timing of the MI. Tests used are indicated in Box 7-1. Other disorders of the heart and blood vessels are listed in Table 7-1.

tissues and blood across the capillary membrane. Capillaries form meshworks, called *capillary beds,* which permeate the tissues. On average, no cell is farther than a few cells away from a capillary. In its chemical composition, capillary blood is more similar to arterial blood than to venous blood, especially in warmed tissue, where blood flow is rapid.

BOX 7-1   Tests Used to Diagnose a Myocardial
           Infarction

Aspartate aminotransferase (AST)
Creatine kinase total (CK total)
Creatine kinase MB fraction (CK-MB)
Lactate dehydrogenase total (LD total)
Isoenzyme LD_1
Isoenzyme LD_2
Myoglobin
Troponin T
Troponin 1

Veins

Capillary blood enters **venules**, the smallest veins. Venules join to form larger veins. Veins have thinner walls and less muscle than arteries do, because they do not experience large fluctuations in blood pressure. To help prevent backflow of blood, veins have valves within them at various points along their length that are pushed closed when blood flows back against them (Figure 7-5). Veins are closer to the surface than arteries are. Most blood tests are performed on venous blood because of the easier access and because venipuncture is safer than arterial puncture. The major veins are illustrated in Figure 7-6.

Circulatory Anatomy of the Antecubital Fossa

The antecubital fossa is the area just below the elbow joint where blood is usually drawn. This area is easily accessible and contains several prominent veins that are usually located a safe distance from nerves and arteries, making it an ideal location for venipuncture. Becoming familiar with the anatomy of this area will help you draw blood safely and confidently.

The capillary beds of the hand drain into a network of veins that pass into the forearm. These collect to form several major veins (Figure 7-7). On the anterior surface (where blood is drawn), the

---

TABLE 7-1   Disorders of the Heart and Blood Vessels

Arteries		Heart	
Aneurysm	A bulge in a vessel, usually an artery, caused by weakening of the wall or hypertension. Without surgical correction, aneurysms may burst.	Coronary artery disease	Any type of degenerative change in the coronary arteries, including coronary atherosclerosis.
Arteriosclerosis	Accumulation of fatty deposits on the tunica intima of arteries causing thickening and toughening of the arterial wall. Loss of elasticity increases strain on the artery and may lead to myocardial infarction or stroke.	Congestive heart failure	Inadequate heart output, leading to edema of the peripheral tissues.
		Myocardial infarction	Death of heart muscle cells due to an interruption in blood supply. Also known as a *heart attack*.
Stroke	A loss of blood to the brain, due to either hemorrhage or, more commonly, blocked circulation.	Bacterial infection	Pericarditis—infection of the pericardium; endocarditis—infection of the endocardium.
		Rheumatic heart disease	Autoimmune disease affecting cardiac tissue, caused by a previous streptococcal infection elsewhere in the body.
Veins			
Varicose veins	Veins that are tortuous and dilated because of swelling and loss of function of valves. Often due to prolonged sitting or standing.	Valvular heart disease	Thickening and calcification of a valve causes stenosis, or narrowing of the passage through the valve, and incomplete closure. Causes heart murmur and may lead to congestive heart failure.
Hemorrhoids	Swollen veins in the walls of the anus, often due to prolonged exertion or pressure during defecation.		

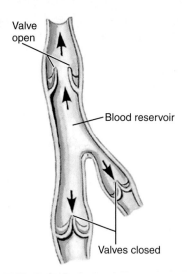

Valve open

Blood reservoir

Valves closed

Figure 7-5
Valves in veins prevent backflow of blood. (From Thibodeau GA, Patton KT: Anatomy and Physiology, ed 5. St. Louis, Mosby, 2003.)

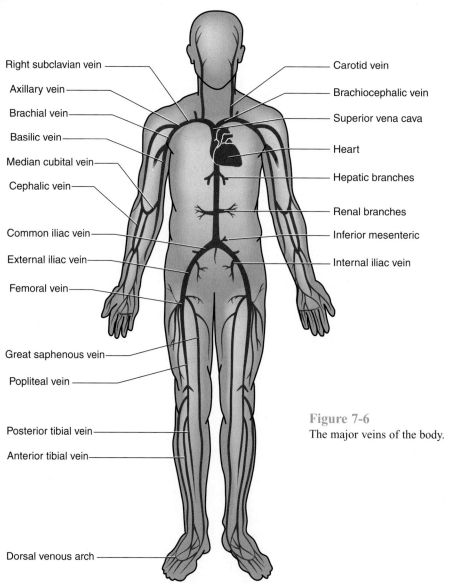

Right subclavian vein

Axillary vein

Brachial vein

Basilic vein

Median cubital vein

Cephalic vein

Common iliac vein

External iliac vein

Femoral vein

Great saphenous vein

Popliteal vein

Posterior tibial vein

Anterior tibial vein

Dorsal venous arch

Carotid vein

Brachiocephalic vein

Superior vena cava

Heart

Hepatic branches

Renal branches

Inferior mesenteric

Internal iliac vein

Figure 7-6
The major veins of the body.

most prominent of these are the **cephalic vein**, the **median cubital vein**, and the **basilic vein**. The median cubital vein splits just below the elbow, sending one branch to the basilic vein and one branch to the cephalic vein. Thus, these veins form a rough letter "M" in this region. Blood is typically drawn from one of the veins forming part of this M. In other patients, the veins will resemble the letter "H."

It is important to note that the exact anatomy of this region may vary considerably from person to person. Veins may branch multiple times, some smaller veins may be absent, or they may be located in unusual places. For the phlebotomist, this rarely causes problems, however, as long as a prominent vein can be found for drawing blood.

Problems can arise, however, from the location of other structures in the antecubital fossa. The brachial artery passes through the elbow, splitting into the radial and ulnar arteries. These are located deeper than the veins, though, and the skilled phlebotomist rarely has any trouble avoiding them. A more common (though still rare) complication arises from the position of two nerves that also

pass through this busy intersection. The external cutaneous nerve passes very close to the cephalic vein, and the internal cutaneous nerve passes very close to the basilic vein. In many patients, the nerves are no deeper than the veins, and in some patients the nerves may pass over, rather than under, the veins. Contacting the nerve with the needle causes an intense, sharp pain, and may lead to long-term nerve damage.

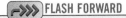 **FLASH FORWARD**

You will learn more about nerve and artery complications in Chapter 11.

Blood

Blood is composed of **plasma**—the fluid portion—and cellular components, called the **formed elements** (Figure 7-8). An average adult has 5 to 6 liters of blood.

 Clinical Tip: If 3 mL of plasma is needed for a test, 6 mL of whole blood should be drawn.

Plasma

Plasma constitutes 55% of the volume of blood. It is 90% water, with the rest made up of dissolved proteins, amino acids, gases, electrolytes, sugars,

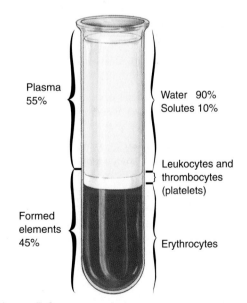

Figure 7-7

Veins of antecubital fossa. (From Bonewit-West K: Clinical Procedures for Medical Assistants, ed 6. Philadelphia, Saunders, 2004.)

Cephalic vein
Basilic vein
Median cubital vein

Plasma 55%
Water 90%
Solutes 10%
Leukocytes and thrombocytes (platelets)
Formed elements 45%
Erythrocytes

Figure 7-8

Composition of blood. (From Applegate E: The Anatomy and Physiology Learning System, ed 3. Philadelphia, Saunders, 2006.)

hormones, lipids, and vitamins, plus waste products such as urea, destined for excretion.

The most significant elements of plasma are **albumin**, a plasma protein responsible for osmotic pressure and transport of many types of molecules; the **immunoglobulins**, or **antibodies**, which are important parts of the immune system; and **fibrinogen**, responsible for blood clotting. Other proteins include hormones, such as insulin, and transport proteins, such as transferrin, which carries iron. Plasma also contains **complement**, a group of immune system proteins that, when activated, destroy target cells by puncturing their membranes. **Electrolytes** include the major ions of plasma— sodium (Na^+) and chloride (Cl^-), plus potassium (K^+), calcium (Ca^{2+}), magnesium (Mg^{2+}), bicarbonate (HCO_3^-), phosphate (PO_4^{3-}), and sulfate (SO_4^{2-}) ions.

Serum

Plasma without its clotting factors is called **serum**. Serum is formed when a blood sample is collected in a glass or plastic container and is induced to clot (a "serum separator tube" is used for this purpose). The conversion of fibrinogen to fibrin forms strands that trap all of the cellular elements. After clotting, the serum is separated from the clotted material by centrifugation. A serum sample is used for many types of tests, since clotting would interfere with the results. Serum is the most commonly analyzed sample in clinical pathology. Plasma samples are used for stat tests (because results are needed immediately) and for coagulation tests.

Formed Elements

The formed elements constitute 45% of blood volume. Ninety-nine percent of these are red blood cells (RBCs), with white blood cells (WBCs) and platelets making up the rest. All blood cells are formed in the bone marrow from the division of long-lived progenitors called *stem cells.*

Red Blood Cells

RBCs carry hemoglobin, the iron-containing oxygen transport protein that gives blood its red color (Figure 7-9). There are 5 million RBCs in a microliter (μL) of whole blood (1 microliter = 10^{-6} liter). An RBC initially contains a cell nucleus, but this is expelled shortly after formation, at which stage the RBC is known as a **reticulocyte**. (The reticulocyte count, a common laboratory test, provides the physician with an indirect measure of how well the bone marrow is producing RBCs.) Once released

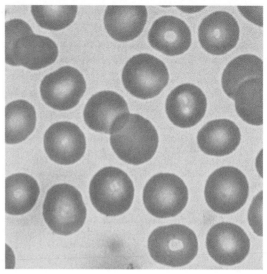

Figure 7-9
Wright-stained red blood cells as seen through a light microscope. (From Carr JH, Rodak BF: Clinical Hematology Atlas, ed 2. Philadelphia, Saunders, 2004.)

into the peripheral circulation, it matures in a day or two into an **erythrocyte**.

A single RBC remains in the peripheral circulation about 120 days before being removed by the liver, bone marrow, or spleen. RBC destruction results in three major breakdown products: iron, amino acids, and bilirubin. The iron and amino acids are recycled. The only waste product, bilirubin, is transported to the liver for elimination from the body. The iron-containing heme groups are recycled to make new hemoglobin for packing into new RBCs.

White Blood Cells

WBCs, or **leukocytes**, protect the body against infection. WBCs are produced in the bone marrow and lymph nodes and undergo a complex maturation process, which may involve the thymus and other organs. There are 5000 to 10,000 WBCs in a microliter of whole blood. At any one time, most WBCs are not in the blood but in the peripheral tissues and lymphatic system.

An important feature of all WBCs is their ability to recognize specific molecules on the surface of infectious agents and to distinguish them from markers on the body's own cells. This molecular recognition is responsible for the extraordinary ability of the immune system to protect the body against the daily threat of attack from bacteria, viruses, and other infectious organisms.

There are five types of leukocytes. Three (neutrophils, eosinophils, and basophils) are very similar and are often called the **granulocytes**, owing to the presence of visible granules in their cytoplasm. Lymphocytes and monocytes (which together are referred to as **mononuclear leukocytes**) contain different kinds of granules. Although the contents of the granules differ among the different cell types, they all contain powerful chemicals that destroy foreign cells and signal other parts of the immune system.

Neutrophils, so-called because their granules do not take up either acidic or basic dyes, make up 40% to 60% of all leukocytes in the blood (Figure 7-10, *A*). They are **phagocytes**, whose role is to attack and digest bacteria, and their numbers increase during a bacterial infection. They are often the first WBCs on the scene of an infection, and their rather short life span (approximately 3 to 4 days) is further shortened when they engulf and digest bacterial and cellular debris. Neutrophils are also called **polymorphonuclear leukocytes** (PMNs), or **segmented neutrophils** (segs), because of their highly divided and irregularly shaped nuclei.

Eosinophils take up the dye eosin, which stains their granules an orange-red (see Figure 7-10, *B*). They represent 1% to 3% of all circulating leukocytes. Eosinophils are also phagocytic, and their principal targets are parasites and antibody-labeled foreign molecules rather than cells. Their numbers increase in the presence of allergies, skin infections, and parasitic infections.

Basophils stain darkly with basic dyes and are deep purple in a standard blood smear (see Figure 7-10, *C*). They account for less than 1% of leukocytes in the blood. Increased numbers of basophils are usually associated with some kind of leukemia.

Lymphocytes make up 20% to 40% of all circulating leukocytes, but this is a small fraction of their total number, most of which reside in lymph nodes (see Figure 7-10, *D*). Lymphocytes circulate between the lymphatic system and the circulatory system, and their numbers may increase during viral infection. Lymphocytes include B cells, which produce antibodies; natural killer (NK) cells, which destroy both foreign cells and infected cells; and T cells, which control cellular immunity.

Monocytes are large phagocytic cells that make up 3% to 8% of all circulating leukocytes (see Figure 7-10, *E*). Monocytes pass from the circulatory system into the peripheral tissues, where they transform into macrophages and act as roving sentries. Their signals help activate B cells to make antibodies.

Platelets

Platelets are created in the bone marrow from **megakaryocytes**, which package and release them into the circulation. Although they are also called

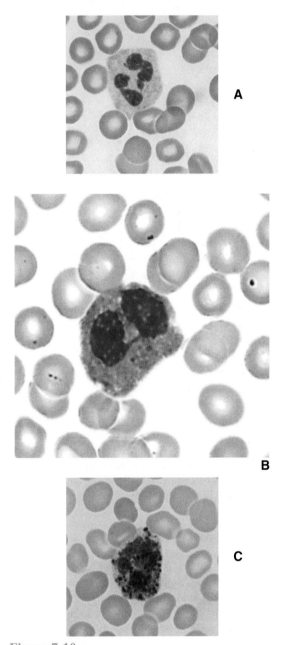

Figure 7-10
Wright-stained smears. **A,** Neutrophil. **B,** Eosinophil. **C,** Basophil. (From Carr JH, Rodak BF: Clinical Hematology Atlas, ed 2. Philadelphia, Saunders, 2004.)

Continued

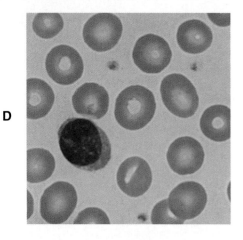

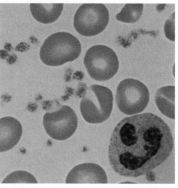

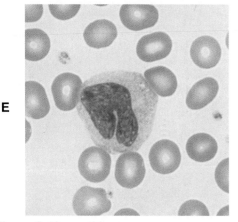

Figure 7-10, cont'd
Wright-stained smears. **D,** Lymphocyte. **E,** Monocyte. (From Carr JH, Rodak BF: Clinical Hematology Atlas, ed 2. Philadelphia, Saunders, 2004.)

thrombocytes, platelets are not actually cells; they are simply membrane-bound packets of cytoplasm (Figure 7-11). Platelets play a critical role in blood coagulation, as discussed later. There are approximately 200,000 in a microliter of blood, each of which remains in circulation for 9 to 12 days.

Hemostasis

Hemostasis refers to the processes by which blood vessels are repaired after injury. It occurs in a series of steps, from muscular contraction of the vessel walls, through clot formation, to removal of the clot when the vessel repairs itself.

Vascular Phase

Rupture of a vein or artery causes an immediate **vascular spasm,** or contraction of the smooth muscle lining the vessel. This reduces the vessel diame-

ter, substantially reducing the blood loss that would otherwise occur. This contraction lasts about 30 minutes. For capillaries, this may be enough to allow the wound to seal.

Platelet Phase

Exposure of materials beneath the endothelial lining causes platelets to stick to the endothelial cells almost immediately, a process known as **adhesion.** Additional platelets then stick to these, a process known as **aggregation.** Aggregating platelets become activated, releasing factors that promote fibrin accumulation in the next phase. The combination of the vascular phase and the platelet phase is called **primary hemostasis.** The next phase, coagulation, is known as **secondary hemostasis.**

Coagulation Phase

Coagulation involves a complex and highly regulated cascade of enzymes and other factors whose activation ultimately results in formation of a blood clot—a meshwork of fibrin, platelets, and other blood cells that closes off the wound. The coagulation cascade begins from 30 seconds to several minutes after the injury.

Coagulation is initiated through two different pathways that feed into a single common pathway (Figure 7-12). The **extrinsic pathway** begins with the release of tissue factor by endothelial cells, which combines with calcium ions and coagulation factor VII from the plasma to form an active enzyme. The **intrinsic pathway** is initiated when other plasma coagulation factors contact the materials exposed when the blood vessel is damaged

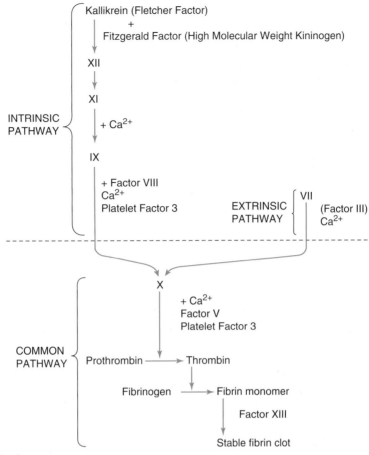

Figure 7-12
The two coagulation pathways.

(similar to platelet adhesion). A series of reactions takes place to form an enzyme that can initiate the **common pathway**.

Enzymes from both pathways then enter the common pathway, reacting with factors X and V to convert circulating inactive **prothrombin** (also called *factor II*) to active **thrombin**. Once activated, thrombin converts circulating fibrinogen to fibrin. **Fibrin** is a fibrous protein whose strands adhere to the platelets and endothelial cells at the wound, forming a dense fibrous network that, in turn, traps other cells. Platelets then contract and pull the edges of the wound closer together, allowing endothelial cells to grow across the wound and repairing the damaged lining.

Fibrinolysis

As the wound is closed and tissue repair commences, fibrin itself is broken down slowly by **plasmin**, an enzyme made from **plasminogen** by **tissue plasminogen activator** (t-PA). Synthetic t-PA is used to dissolve blood clots in **stroke**, MI, pulmonary embolism, and other conditions. Urokinase and streptokinase are also used to activate plasminogen in these conditions. The production of **fibrin degradation products** (FDPs) can be monitored to determine the rate of fibrinolysis. **Fibrin split products** (FSPs) are also used for this purpose.

Blood Disorders

Blood disorders and the tests for them are outlined in Table 7-2. Knowing these will improve your ability to interact with your professional colleagues. However, it is very important to remember that the phlebotomist may not know the actual reason any particular test is ordered for any particular patient. You should not discuss the purpose of a test with a patient—that is the role of the doctor.

TABLE 7-2 Blood Disorders

Disorder	Description	Tests
Red Blood Cells and Hemoglobin		
Anemia	Decrease in number of RBCs or amount of hemoglobin in the blood	Reticulocyte count Iron studies—ferritin and TIBC Vitamin B_{12} and folate levels CBC
Sickle-cell disease	Inherited hemoglobin disorder resulting in sickle-shaped RBCs; requires inheritance from both parents (autosomal recessive inheritance)	Sickle-cell solubility Hemoglobin electrophoresis CBC
Thalassemia	A group of inherited hemoglobin disorders resulting in decreased production of hemoglobin and anemia	Hemoglobin electrophoresis CBC
Polycythemia	Increase in total number of blood cells, especially RBCs; treated with therapeutic phlebotomy	CBC
White Blood Cells		
Bacterial infection	WBCs respond to many kinds of infection and inflammations	CBC with differential Bacterial cultures
HIV infection	Infection of helper T cells by HIV; can lead to AIDS	Anti-HIV antibody Western blot T-cell count—CD 3, 4,& 8
Leukemia	Malignant neoplasm in the bone marrow, causing increased production of WBCs	CBC with differential Cell marker studies
Mononucleosis	Increased numbers of reactive lymphocytes in response to infection with the Epstein-Barr virus	CBC Monospot or heterophile antibody
Hemostasis, Platelets, and Clotting		
Thrombocytopenia	Decreased number of platelets	CBC
Hemophilias	A group of inherited disorders marked by deficient clotting factor production and increased bleeding; the most common is hemophilia A, a deficiency in clotting factor VIII	APTT/PT and clotting factor activity (Factor VIII activity)
Disseminated intravascular coagulation (DIC)	Activation of the clotting system throughout the circulatory system in response to bacterial toxins, trauma, or other stimuli; fibrin is eventually degraded, but small clots may form, damaging tissue; fibrinogen deficiency may follow	FDP D-dimer Fibrinogen
Thrombosis	Localized activation of the clotting system; called thrombophlebitis in veins; an embolus is a piece of clot that has broken off and entered the circulation	Protein C Protein S

Clinical Tip: Don't discuss the purpose of tests with your patient—leave that to the doctor.

returns tissue fluid to the circulatory system—in the process, screening it for signs of infection—and provides a passageway for lymphocytes patrolling the tissues.

LYMPHATIC SYSTEM

The lymphatic system includes the lymphatic vessels, the lymph nodes, and several associated organs, plus the lymph fluid flowing in the lymphatic vessels and the leukocytes that reside in the lymph nodes and elsewhere (Figure 7-13). The lymphatic system

Lymphatic Vessels

In contrast to arteries and veins, which form a complete circulatory loop, lymphatic vessels are closed at their distal ends. These closed-end tubes, called **terminal lymphatics**, are slightly larger than capillaries and permeate the tissues (except for the central

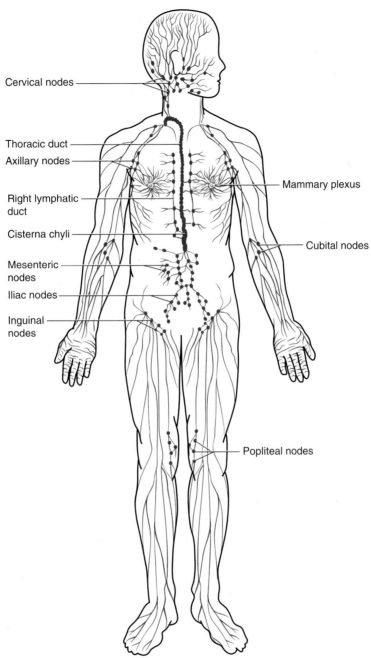

Cervical nodes

Thoracic duct
Axillary nodes

Right lymphatic
duct

Cisterna chyli

Mesenteric
nodes

Iliac nodes

Inguinal
nodes

Mammary plexus

Cubital nodes

Popliteal nodes

Figure 7-13
The lymphatic system permeates the body, collecting interstitial fluid and returning it to the circulation.
Lymph nodes are important components of the immune system.

nervous system), although not as extensively as capillaries do. The wall of a terminal lymphatic vessel is an endothelial layer, one cell thick. Small lymphatic vessels feed into larger ones, and finally into the **thoracic duct** and **right lymphatic duct**. These empty into the venous system just distal to the superior vena cava. Along the way, valves within the lymphatic vessels keep fluid moving in one direction.

Lymphatic fluid is derived from the fluid between cells, called **interstitial fluid**. Interstitial fluid is a combination of plasma that has been forced out of capillaries by blood pressure and cellular fluid exiting the cells through osmosis. Lymphatic fluid thus carries the chemical signature of the peripheral fluid as a whole. Most importantly, it contains proteins or other molecules released by infectious agents, which are carried to the lymph nodes for examination by WBCs. Lymphatic fluid is also important for the transport of fat—terminal lymphatics in the intestine absorb dietary fat, keeping it out of the capillary circulation.

Lymph Organs

Lymph nodes are chambers located along the lymphatic vessels and are populated by lymphocytes. Lymph nodes are especially common in the digestive, respiratory, and urinary tracts. The tonsils are particularly large lymph nodes. Lymphocytes in the nodes screen the lymph fluid for signs of infection. In addition, macrophages journey to the lymph nodes from infection sites, carrying molecular samples for examination by B and T cells.

The other organs of the lymphatic system include the spleen and the thymus. In the spleen, worn-out RBCs are recycled by macrophages, and blood is examined by resident B and T cells. The thymus is principally involved in maturation of the immune system during development and early life.

Lymphatic System Disorders

Lymphedema is an accumulation of interstitial fluid in tissues due to a blocked lymphatic vessel. Elephantiasis is a severe form of lymphedema, caused by a mosquito-borne parasite that colonizes the lymphatic vessels. **Lymphoma** is a tumor of a lymph gland. Hodgkin's disease is a type of lymphoma.

Because they provide passageways for mobile cells, lymphatic vessels provide a route for the spread of metastatic cancer cells, which may either take up residence in a lymph node or pass out of the lymphatic system to invade surrounding tissue. For this reason, biopsy of nearby lymph nodes is often performed to determine whether a cancer has metastasized.

IMMUNE SYSTEM

The immune system involves the coordinated action of many different cell types, along with the circulating proteins of antibodies and complement. In addition, it includes the physical barriers to the entry of infection, such as the skin and the epithelial lining of the lungs, gut, and urinary tract.

Nonspecific Immunity

Nonspecific immunity refers to defense against infectious agents independent of the specific chemical markers on their surfaces. This includes physical barriers, the complement system, and phagocytes (monocytes and neutrophils), which engulf and destroy foreign cells without regard to their exact identity.

Inflammation is a coordinated nonspecific defense against infection or irritation. It combines increased blood flow and capillary permeability, activation of macrophages, temperature increase, and the clotting reaction to wall off the infected area. These actions also activate the mechanism of specific immunity.

Specific Immunity

Specific immunity involves the molecular recognition of particular markers, called **antigens**, on the surface of a foreign agent. Recognition of these antigens in the appropriate context triggers activation of T cells and B cells, as well as increasing the activity and accuracy of nonspecific defenses such as complement and macrophages.

In one form of antigen recognition, antigens are taken up by a macrophage, which displays them on its surface in a receptor complex controlled by genes in the **major histocompatibility complex** (MHC). The proteins in these complexes are also known as **human leukocyte antigens** (HLAs). The antigen complex is presented to T cells, which are activated when they recognize the HLA-antigen combination. Activated T cells influence the production of **cytotoxic T cells**, which recognize antigens and destroy both foreign cells and infected host cells, and **memory T cells**, which are primed to respond more rapidly if the antigen is encountered again later in life. Other T cells, called **helper T cells**, are important regulators of the entire immune response. They are needed to make both antibodies and cytotoxic T cells. Helper T cells are also known as T4 or **CD4+ cells**, after one of their surface receptors; these are the cells infected by human immunodeficiency virus (HIV). T cell–based immunity is also called **cellular immunity**.

Antigens can also be recognized in another way. An antigen can bind to an antibody, a product of a B cell. Each B cell makes a slightly differently shaped antibody, allowing recognition of an enormous variety of antigens. If the antibody shape is complementary to the antigen shape, it will activate the B cell under the influence of helper T cells and macrophages to undergo rapid cell division. Most of the offspring are **plasma cells**, which produce and release large numbers of antibodies into the lymphatic system and, ultimately, into the circulation.

These antibodies bind to antigens at the site of infection and elsewhere, directly inactivating them; they also act as flags for targeting by macrophages. The remainder of the B-cell offspring become **memory cells**, which serve a similar function to memory T cells. This is the basis of **immunization**. Antibody-based immunity is also called **humoral immunity**, after *humor*, the antiquated term for a body fluid.

In addition to the direct contact between cells, immune cells communicate through **cytokines**, chemical messengers that include **interferons**, **interleukins**, and others. Functionally, these molecules are hormones, released by one cell to influence the behavior of another.

Immune System Disorders

Autoimmunity is an attack by the immune system on the body's own tissues. Autoimmune disorders include rheumatoid arthritis, systemic lupus erythematosus, myasthenia gravis, and multiple sclerosis. **Allergy** is an inappropriately severe immune reaction to an otherwise harmless substance. **Severe combined immune deficiency** (SCID) is an inherited disorder marked by an almost total lack of B and T cells. Acquired immunodeficiency syndrome **(AIDS)** is due to HIV infection.

REVIEW FOR CERTIFICATION

The pulmonary circulation carries blood between the heart and lungs for gas exchange, and the systemic circulation carries blood between the heart and the rest of the body's tissues.

The heart is a muscular double pump located in the thoracic cavity. It is surrounded by the pericardium. The epicardium, myocardium, and endocardium are the three layers of the heart. Blood from the systemic circulation passes from the venae cavae into the right atrium, and through the tricuspid valve into the right ventricle. From there, blood passes out through the pulmonary semilunar valve, through the pulmonary trunk, into the left and right pulmonary arteries, and on to the lungs. It returns via the pulmonary veins to the left atrium, and then through the mitral valve into the left ventricle. It passes out through the aortic semilunar valve into the aorta, which branches to form the major arteries. Arteries branch further into arterioles, which lead to capillary beds within the tissues, where oxygen exchange occurs. Blood then enters venules and veins, which empty into the venae cavae. Blood pressure is higher in the arteries than in the veins. Arteries are thick and muscular; veins are thinner and contain valves to prevent backflow. Capillaries are composed of a single layer of endothelial cells.

Blood is composed of plasma and cellular components. RBCs carry hemoglobin. WBCs protect the body against infection. There are five types of WBCs: neutrophils, eosinophils, basophils, lymphocytes, and monocytes. Platelets play a critical role in blood coagulation. Serum is plasma minus its clotting factors. Hemostasis occurs in four phases: the vascular phase (muscular contraction of the vessel walls), the platelet phase, the coagulation phase (clot formation), and fibrinolysis (removal of the clot). The coagulation phase includes the intrinsic and extrinsic pathways, which unite to enter the common pathway.

The lymphatic system returns interstitial fluid to the circulatory system through lymphatic ducts, screening it for signs of infection at lymph nodes. Lymph organs include the tonsils, the spleen, and the thymus.

Nonspecific immunity includes physical barriers, the complement system, inflammation, and phagocytes. Specific immunity involves recognition of antigens, which triggers activation of T cells (cellular immunity) and B cells (humoral immunity).

BIBLIOGRAPHY

Guyton AC: Textbook of Medical Physiology, ed 10. Philadelphia, WB Saunders, 2000.

Horowitz SH: Venipuncture-induced Causalgia: Anatomic Relations of Upper Extremity Superficial Veins and Nerves, and Clinical Considerations. Transfusion. September 2000.

Stiene-Martin AE, Lotspeich-Steininger CA, Koepke JA: Clinical Hematology: Principles, Procedures, Correlations, ed 2. Philadelphia, Lippincott Williams & Wilkins, 1998.

STUDY QUESTIONS

1. Describe the different functions of the circulatory system.
2. Discuss the difference between pulmonary and systemic circulation.
3. Explain the functional difference between veins and arteries.
4. Name the four valves of the heart.
5. Contraction of the heart is known as _____, and relaxation is known as _____.
6. Name the three layers surrounding the lumen of veins and arteries.
7. The yellow liquid portion of whole blood, containing fibrinogen, is known as _____.
8. The formed elements constitute _____% of blood volume.
9. What is the role of a phagocyte?
10. Which type of lymphocyte produces antibodies?
11. Describe the two pathways in the coagulation cascade.
12. Define and give an example of autoimmunity.
13. Describe the lymph organs and their functions. Give one lymphatic system disorder and explain its due process.
14. Name the types of immunity, how they differ, and how they are similar.
15. Explain the function of enzymes in the coagulation process.

CERTIFICATION EXAM PREPARATION

1. In the circulatory system, gas exchange occurs in the:
   a. capillaries
   b. veins
   c. arteries
   d. venules

2. Which blood vessels are a single cell in thickness?
   a. capillaries
   b. veins
   c. arteries
   d. arterioles

3. Veins and arteries are composed of how many layers?
   a. 1
   b. 2
   c. 3
   d. 4

4. A characteristic of arteries is:
   a. They are composed of a single layer of endothelial cells.
   b. They have a thick muscle layer lining the lumen.
   c. They have valves along the lumen.
   d. They carry blood toward the heart.

5. An average adult has:
   a. 1 to 2 liters of blood
   b. 7 to 8 liters of blood
   c. 3 to 4 liters of blood
   d. 5 to 6 liters of blood

6. Plasma constitutes ____% of total blood volume.
   a. 80
   b. 92
   c. 55
   d. 45

7. Another name for a WBC is:
   a. leukocyte
   b. reticulocyte
   c. erythrocyte
   d. electrolyte

8. The main function of leukocytes is to:
   a. transport hemoglobin
   b. transport lipids

c. protect the body against infection
d. recycle RBCs

9. Which leukocyte is known as a phagocyte?
   a. lymphocyte
   b. neutrophil
   c. eosinophil
   d. basophil

10. Platelets remain in the circulation for:
    a. 2 to 5 days
    b. 9 to 12 days
    c. 10 to 20 days
    d. 1 month

11. Which cellular component is responsible for the transport of hemoglobin?
    a. WBCs
    b. RBCs
    c. electrolytes
    d. plasma

12. Which lab test does not assist in diagnosing HIV infection?
    a. Western blot
    b. T-cell count
    c. APTT
    d. anti-HIV antibody

13. A group of inherited disorders marked by increased bleeding times is known as:
    a. anemias
    b. leukemias
    c. polycythemias
    d. hemophilias

14. Which organ is not included in the lymphatic system?
    a. liver
    b. spleen
    c. thymus
    d. tonsils

15. Helper T cells are needed to make:
    a. antigens
    b. antibodies
    c. cytokines
    d. interleukins

UNIT 3

Specimen Collection

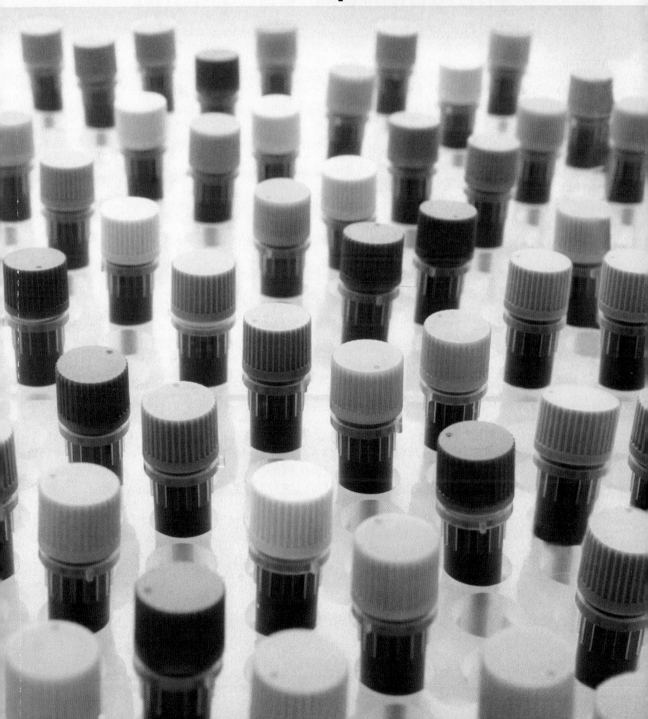

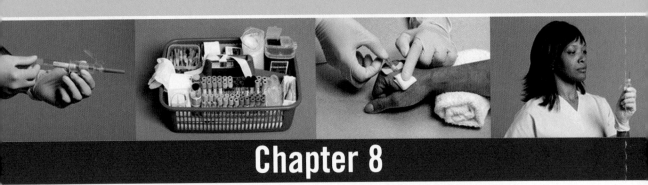

Chapter 8

Venipuncture Equipment

OUTLINE

Phlebotomy Equipment
Organizing and Transporting
  Equipment
Locating Veins
Cleaning the Puncture Site
Protecting the Puncture Site
Needles
  Features of Needles
  Multisample Needles

Safety Syringes and Safety
  Syringe Needles
Winged Infusion Sets
  or Butterflies
Needle Safety
Needle Adapters
Evacuated Collection Tubes
Types of Blood Specimens

Tube Additives
  Anticoagulants
  Clot Activators
  Thixotropic Gel
Color-Coded Tops
Order of Draw
Needle Disposal Containers
Review for Certification

OBJECTIVES

After completing this chapter, you should be able to:

1. List the equipment that should be available for venipuncture.
2. Describe the purpose of a tourniquet; list types that may be used to locate a vein.
3. Differentiate between an antiseptic and a disinfectant. List those that may be used for blood collection.
4. Locate the bevel, shaft, hub, and point of a needle. Describe safety features that may be included.
5. Define gauge.
6. Name the parts of a syringe, and describe how the syringe system differs from the evacuated tube system.

7. Explain when a syringe system or winged infusion set (butterfly) is used in blood collection.
8. Describe the proper use of the tube holder (needle adapter).
9. Differentiate whole blood, serum, and plasma. List at least one use for each.
10. Describe at least nine additives, including their mode of action and uses.
11. List at least ten different colors for tube stoppers. Identify the additive(s) in each, and state one use for each.
12. State the correct order in which various types of tubes should be collected.
13. Describe the proper disposal of a used needle.

KEY TERMS

additives
anticoagulants
antiseptic
bacteriostatic
butterfly
clot activators
disinfectant

gauge
glycolysis
inpatients
Luer adapter
lumen
multisample needle
needle adapter

order of draw
outpatients
plasma
sepsis
serum
thixotropic gel
tourniquet

tube advancement mark
tube holder
whole blood
winged infusion set

ABBREVIATIONS

APTT: activated partial thromboplastin time
CBC: complete blood count
CLSI: Clinical and Laboratory Standards Institute
EDTA: ethylenediaminetetraacetic acid
FBS: fasting blood sugar (glucose)
HLA: human leukocyte antigen

OSHA: Occupational Safety and Health
  Administration
PST: plasma separator tube
SPS: sodium polyanetholesulfonate
SST: serum separator tube

Equipment for routine venipuncture includes material needed for the safe and efficient location of a vein and collection of a blood sample, plus equipment to ensure the safety and comfort of both the patient and the user. Most venipuncture procedures are performed with a double-ended multisample needle that delivers blood into an evacuated tube with a color-coded stopper. The stopper indicates the additives used in the tube. Learning what each color signifies, and in what order different-colored tubes should be drawn, is essential for a phlebotomist.

PHLEBOTOMY EQUIPMENT

As a phlebotomist, your primary duty is to collect blood and prepare it for delivery to the lab. Your collection equipment includes the needles and tubes that allow you to collect a patient's blood, plus materials to ensure that a vein can be located, the puncture site is sterile, and the sample is labeled and transported correctly. In addition, your equipment includes materials that protect you from potential blood hazards and that allow you to dress the puncture site after collection. A list of commonly stocked equipment is provided in Box 8-1.

ORGANIZING AND TRANSPORTING EQUIPMENT

Phlebotomists use a portable tray to carry all necessary equipment. Like a carpenter's toolbox, the tray is a compact, efficient way to store and transport the tools of your trade to your work site (Figure 8-1).

You are responsible for making sure that your tray is well stocked, clean, and organized at all times. You should empty the tray and disinfect it with a bleach solution once a week. A mixture of one part bleach to nine parts water works well as a disinfectant.

You will encounter patients in two primary settings: inpatient and outpatient. **Inpatients** have been admitted to a hospital, and you usually draw their blood at the bedside. A cart is sometimes used to transport large quantities of supplies when you are scheduled to collect samples from many patients, but the cart should remain in the hospital corridor, to reduce the risk of spreading infection from one patient to another. Bring only the tray into the room. Once in the patient's room, do not place your tray on the patient's bed, where it could easily be overturned. Instead, *place the tray on a flat, solid surface such as a night stand*. Always keep extra supplies within reach, however. You may need them during a draw; for instance, you may need to replace a tube while the needle is still

---

BOX 8-1 Equipment Used in Routine Venipuncture

Needles
Needle disposal containers
Needle holders
Collection tubes
Syringes
Winged infusion sets (butterflies)
Marking pens
Tourniquets
Antiseptic cleaning solution
Gauze pads
Bandages
Gloves

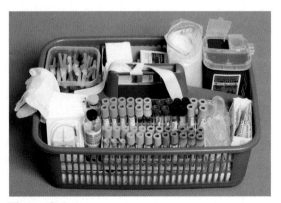

Figure 8-1
Phlebotomy tray.

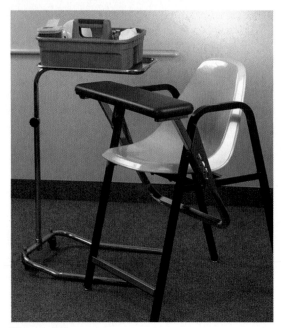

Figure 8-2
Phlebotomy drawing station.

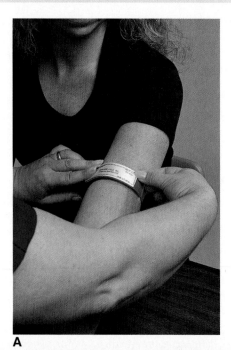

A

in the patient's arm (which can happen if you get a defective tube).

 Clinical Tip: Never place your tray on the patient's bed.

Outpatients usually come to you at a phlebotomy drawing station in a clinic or hospital. The drawing station includes a special phlebotomy chair with an adjustable armrest (Figure 8-2). The armrest locks to prevent the patient from falling out in the event of fainting. A bed may also be available for patients with a history of fainting. Supplies may be available at the drawing station, or you may need to bring your tray to it.

LOCATING VEINS

To draw blood, you first need to locate a vein. Applying a **tourniquet** is the most common way to do this. A tourniquet prevents venous blood flow out of the arm, causing the veins to bulge. Various types of tourniquets are shown in Figure 8-3.

The most common type of tourniquet is a simple strip of latex tied around the upper arm. Both flat and round latex strips are available, in adult and pediatric sizes. Latex has the advantage of being inexpensive and therefore disposable. Once used, a tourniquet should be disposed of to reduce the risk

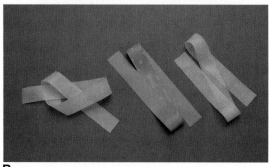

B

Figure 8-3
Various types of tourniquets. (*A* from Bonewit-West K: Clinical Procedures for Medical Assistants, ed 6. Philadelphia, Saunders, 2004.)

of pathogen transmission between patients. In the rare cases in which the tourniquet is not disposed of after a single use, latex is still a good choice, since it is easy to clean and does not support bacterial growth well. Disposable nonlatex tourniquets are also available and may be a good option to reduce the risk of latex sensitivity reactions. Tourniquets with Velcro® closures are easy to apply and are often more comfortable for the patient, although they are more expensive and more difficult to disinfect than latex. The Seraket (Propper Manufacturing Co., Long Island City, NY) has a Velcro® closure and allows pressure to be partially relieved, and then reapplied, during a prolonged draw. This can reduce some lab test errors that occur with long tourniquet use.

A blood pressure cuff may also be used as a tourniquet. It too allows you to temporarily relieve pressure and then reapply it. The cuff is inflated to a pressure above the diastolic but below the systolic reading. Using the cuff requires special training beyond your normal phlebotomy training, and should only be done with approval of your supervisor.

A Venoscope Transilluminator (Applied Biotech, Lafayette, LA) shines a bright light through the patient's skin. When it is positioned properly, veins are visible as dark lines within the tissue. This works especially well for finding veins in the hand and foot.

CLEANING THE PUNCTURE SITE

Antiseptics and disinfectants are used to reduce the risk of infection. By convention, **antiseptic** refers to an agent used to clean living tissue. **Disinfectant** refers to an agent used to clean a surface other than living tissue. However, these definitions are not clear-cut and the terms are often used interchangeably.

An antiseptic prevents **sepsis**, or infection. Antiseptics are used to clean the patient's skin before routine venipuncture collection to prevent contamination by normal skin bacteria. The most commonly used antiseptic is 70% isopropyl alcohol (rubbing alcohol). Isopropyl alcohol is **bacteriostatic**, meaning that it inhibits the growth or reproduction of bacteria but does not kill them. For maximal effectiveness, the antiseptic should be left in contact with the skin for 30 to 60 seconds. Prepackaged alcohol "prep pads" are the most commonly used product.

Other antiseptics are often used for blood cultures or arterial punctures, although recent research indicates isopropyl alcohol may be equally effective for blood cultures. Povidone-iodine solution (Betadine) is commonly used. However, iodine interferes with some chemistry test results and cannot be used routinely. For patients who are allergic to iodine, chlorhexidine gluconate or benzalkonium chloride (Zephiran Chloride) is available. Because these are harsher chemicals, they should be washed off the skin with alcohol after collection. Chlorhexidine gluconate should not be used on infants less than two months of age.

PROTECTING THE PUNCTURE SITE

After drawing blood, you need to stop the bleeding by applying pressure to the puncture site. This is done with a 2- by 2-inch gauze pad, folded into quarters. When the bleeding stops, usually within several minutes, the gauze can be replaced with an adhesive bandage. Alternatively, you can tape the gauze in place using surgical tape or an adhesive bandage.

NEEDLES

In routine venipuncture, a needle inserted into a vein allows blood to flow out into an evacuated collection tube or syringe. A critical part of your job as a phlebotomist is knowing which needle and which tube to use in each situation.

All needles used for phlebotomy are sterile, disposable, and used only once. Inspect each needle package before opening it to be sure that the seal has not been broken. If it has, discard it. Next inspect the needle itself, to be sure that it has no manufacturing defects. The needle should be straight, sharp, beveled, and free of nicks or burrs. Discard any defective needle.

Features of Needles

All needles have several features you should be familiar with (Figure 8-4).

Point
A sharp needle provides smooth entry into the skin with a minimum of pain.

Bevel
The bevel, or angle, eases the shaft into the skin and prevents the needle from coring out a plug of tissue.

Shaft
Shafts differ in both length and gauge. The needles used for routine venipuncture range from ¾ to 1½ inches long. The choice is mainly one of personal preference. Some phlebotomists prefer a longer needle because it is easier to manipulate; others prefer a shorter needle because it makes patients less uneasy.

The **gauge** describes the diameter of the needle's **lumen**, the hollow tube within the shaft. The

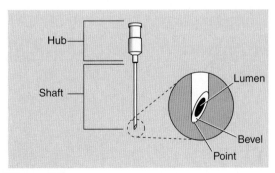

Figure 8-4
Parts of a needle.

smaller the gauge number, the larger the lumen diameter; the larger the number, the smaller the lumen. Needle packs are color-coded by gauge for easy identification. The choice of gauges is not a matter of personal preference; it depends on the type of collection and the condition of the patient. The largest-diameter needles routinely used in phlebotomy are 16 gauge. The blood bank uses 16-gauge needles to collect blood from donors for transfusions. The smallest are 23 gauge, for collection from small, fragile veins. A typical gauge for routine adult collection is 20 to 21 gauge. Large needles deliver blood more quickly but are more damaging to the tissue and may collapse the vein. Small needles are less damaging to tissue, but collection is slower, and the blood cells may be hemolyzed as they pass through the narrower opening. Learning the most appropriate gauge for each clinical situation is part of your training as a phlebotomist.

Hub

The needle attaches to the collecting tube or syringe at its hub.

Multisample Needles

For most collections, you use a double-ended needle. While one tip of the needle penetrates the patient's skin, the second tip pierces the rubber cap of an evacuated collection tube. The most common double-ended needle is the **multisample needle** (Figure 8-5), which has a retractable rubber sleeve that covers the second tip when it is not inserted into a tube. A multisample needle remains in place in the patient's vein while one tube is replaced with another. The sleeve keeps blood from leaking onto or into the adapter or tube holder while changing tubes.

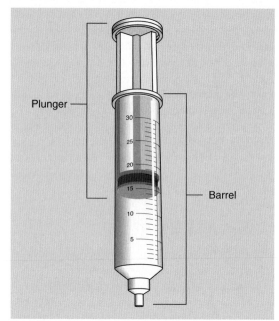

Figure 8-6
A syringe.

Safety Syringes and Safety Syringe Needles

A syringe (Figure 8-6) is useful for patients with fragile or small veins, when the vacuum of the collection tube is likely to collapse the vein. Because suction can be applied gradually, by slowly drawing back the plunger, a syringe provides a controlled, gentle vacuum for fragile veins. A syringe needle (also called a hypodermic needle; see Figure 8-4) fits onto the syringe barrel. The needles come in a wide range of sizes. The most common size is 22 gauge, 1 inch long. Syringe needles have an advantage over multisample needles, in that blood appears in the hub when the vein has been entered. A safety device for syringe needle must be used whenever drawing with a syringe.

> **⏩ FLASH FORWARD**
>
> *The use of syringes for venous collection is discussed in Chapter 9.*

Winged Infusion Sets or Butterflies

The **winged infusion set** (Figure 8-7), or **butterfly**, is widely used for the delivery of intravenous medications. In phlebotomy, it is used for venipuncture on small veins, such as those in the hand, and in elderly or pediatric patients. Without the bulk of a syringe or collection tube in the way, the butterfly

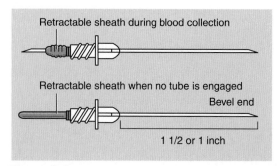

Figure 8-5
Multisample needle. The cap has been removed for clarity.

Hub adapter

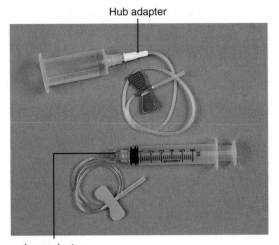

Luer adapter

Figure 8-7

Winged infusion set attached to an evacuated tube holder with a Luer adapter. (From Bonewit-West K: Clinical Procedures for Medical Assistants, ed 6. Philadelphia, Saunders, 2004.)

needle allows you great flexibility in placing and manipulating the needle.

The most common needle size is 23 gauge, ½ to ¾ inch long. The needle is held by a plastic butterfly-shaped grip and is connected to flexible latex tubing. By using an appropriate adapter, when necessary, the tubing can be connected to either an evacuated collection tube or a syringe. Many styles of safety needle are available that cover the needle tip when it is not in use.

Most, but not all, butterflies are now designed to be used with an evacuated tube system. Those that are not can be fitted using a Luer adapter.

NEEDLE SAFETY

Accidental needle sticks are a major concern in health care. A recent study by the Centers for Disease Control and Prevention estimated that approximately 1000 accidental needle sticks a day occur nationwide. Although most of these injuries are to nurses, phlebotomists are at risk too. To respond to this problem, the Occupational Safety and Health Administration (OSHA) issued a directive in November 1999, stressing the use of safety devices to help reduce the number of sharps injuries. The Needle Safety and Prevention Act specified types of "engineering controls" mentioned in the Bloodborne Pathogens Standard to increase needle safety. Federal legislation enforces the use of safety devices, and many states have also passed legislation related to safety devices.

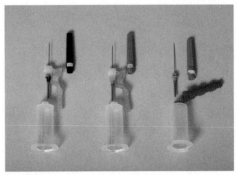

Figure 8-8

Recapping safety devices. (Courtesy of Zack Bent. From Garrels M, Oatis CS: Laboratory Testing for Ambulatory Settings: A Guide for Health Care Professionals. Philadelphia, Saunders, 2006.)

Several standard strategies are used to increase needle safety. Internally self-blunting needles are rendered safe before they are removed from the patient's vein. Retractable needles have a blunt cannula inside the needle tip, which is advanced beyond the tip before the needle is removed from the patient's arm. Retractable technologies cause the needle to retract into the syringe, tube holder, or other device (Figure 8-8).

NEEDLE ADAPTERS

For most collections, you will use a multisample needle and an evacuated collection tube. To ensure a firm, stable connection between these two essential parts, a **needle adapter** (also called a **tube holder**) is used (Figure 8-9). A needle adapter is a translucent plastic cylinder. One end has a small opening that accepts the multisample needle. The other end has a wide opening that accepts the collection tube. Adapters come in different sizes to fit tubes of different diameters, and it is important to choose an adapter that fits the tube you are using. Some manufacturers have standardized their tubes so that they all fit one adapter; others provide inserts that allow one adapter to fit a variety of tube sizes.

To ensure the proper connection between the needle and the tube, adapters have a **tube advancement mark** indicating how far the tube can be pushed in without losing the vacuum.

 Clinical Tip: Be careful not to push the tube past the tube advancement mark.

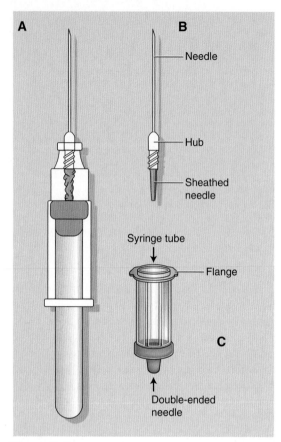

Figure 8-9

The evacuated tube system **(A)**, consisting of a multi-sample needle **(B)** attached to a needle adapter **(C)**.

Like a needle, an adapter is used only once, and it is discarded while still attached to the needle. By disposing of the needle and adapter together, you reduce the risk of accidental needle stick while trying to separate them. Also, once it is used, the adapter may be contaminated with blood that was aerosolized while switching tubes.

EVACUATED COLLECTION TUBES

Color-coded, evacuated collection tubes are at the center of modern phlebotomy. Tubes hold blood for later testing in the lab, and each type of tube may contain different sets of **additives**, which are chemicals designed to promote or prevent certain changes in the blood sample. Which tube to use depends on what tests have been ordered. A critical part of your training is learning and memorizing which tube to use for each test.

As shown in Figure 8-10, tube tops are either thick rubber stoppers or rubber stoppers with plastic tops (such as in the BD Vacutainer® Hemogard

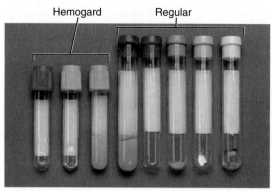

Figure 8-10
Types of tube tops.

system). The plastic top minimizes the chance of an aerosol spray forming when the stopper is removed. The tubes themselves are made either of glass or shatter-resistant plastic. Most tubes are plastic, which is not only safer for transportation, but can also withstand the extremely high forces inside a centrifuge. Unlike glass, plastic does not strongly activate platelets. Serum samples, which require platelet activation, are collected in plain glass tubes, or plastic tubes that contain a platelet activator.

Tubes are evacuated so that a measured amount of blood will flow in easily. They are available in a variety of sizes, from 2 to 15 mL. Be sure to match the needle gauge to the tube: A 23-gauge needle on a 15-mL tube will likely cause hemolysis, for instance. If you need a small needle, use two small tubes instead. "Partial-draw" tubes are also available. These have a smaller vacuum, and will pull a smaller volume of blood into the tube than a fully evacuated tube.

The best tube size to use depends on several factors. Each test requires a particular minimum sample volume, which may range from less than 1 mL to 10 mL or more. Your lab has a manual that states the volume required for each test. You may choose to draw a greater volume, however, perhaps because smaller tubes are more expensive, or because testing equipment works better with a certain size tube.

For example, for an activated partial thromboplastin time (APTT), a type of coagulation test, the minimum sample size is 0.5 mL plasma. As you learned in Chapter 7, whole blood is slightly more than half plasma. Routinely, you might use a 5-mL tube for convenience and cost. However, you could choose a 2.7-mL tube for a pediatric patient or for someone with small veins, knowing that the minimum test requirements would be met because this would give you about 1.5 mL of plasma.

Each tube carries an expiration date, and unused tubes must be discarded when they expire. Out-of-date tubes may have decreased vacuum, preventing a proper fill, or they may have additives that degrade with time. Use of an expired tube can lead to the need to redraw blood or to improper test results. A computerized stock monitoring system may be available where you work, making the task easy. Even with such a system, however, it is ultimately the phlebotomist's duty to use only tubes with a valid date.

TYPES OF BLOOD SPECIMENS

Three types of blood specimens are used for analysis:

1. **Whole blood** is blood collected and mixed with an anticoagulant, so that it will not clot. Whole blood is used for most hematology tests, including blood type and cell counts, and to determine the level of certain hormones and metals.
2. **Serum** is the fluid portion of blood that remains after clotting. No anticoagulant is used when collecting a serum sample. Complete clotting takes 30 to 60 minutes, after which the sample can be centrifuged to separate the serum. Serum is used for many lab tests, including most chemistry and immunology tests. Unlike plasma, serum does not contain fibrinogen or some other clotting factors (which are left behind or used up in forming the clot) and thus cannot be used for coagulation studies.
3. **Plasma** is the fluid portion of blood, including fibrinogen and other clotting factors. Plasma is obtained from whole blood by first adding an anticoagulant and then centrifuging. It is used for coagulation studies. It is also used for stat chemistry tests, when there is no time to wait for clotting to occur before centrifuging.

TUBE ADDITIVES

Except for the glass red-topped tube, which has no additives, all tubes contain one or more additives. Additives include anticoagulants to prevent clotting, clot activators to promote it, thixotropic gel to separate components, and preservatives and inhibitors of various cellular reactions to maintain the integrity of the specimen.

Any tube containing an additive must be inverted and mixed well immediately after removal from the adapter. Turning the tube over, and then back upright again, equals one inversion. The exact number of inversions needed varies with tube type; most need five to eight inversions. Many tubes are coated inside with silicone, in order to prevent blood from adhering to the wall of the tube and to slow down the clotting process.

Anticoagulants

Anticoagulants prevent blood from clotting. Sodium or potassium ethylenediaminetetraacetic acid (EDTA) binds calcium, thereby inhibiting the coagulation cascade. Other additives that bind calcium include sodium citrate, potassium oxalate, and sodium polyanetholesulfonate (SPS). Another anticoagulant, heparin (linked with sodium, lithium, or ammonium), inhibits clotting by preventing the conversion of prothrombin to thrombin. Having the correct ratio of blood to anticoagulant is important, so you must take care to fill the tube completely. Anticoagulants must be mixed well by gently and repeatedly inverting the tube.

The choice of anticoagulant is determined by the tests to be done. EDTA preserves blood cell integrity well, prevents platelet clumping, and is compatible with blood staining, but it interferes with coagulation studies. Citrate is used for coagulation studies. SPS is used for blood cultures because it inhibits certain immune system components that could otherwise destroy blood-borne bacteria and neutralizes antibiotics that the patient may be taking. Heparin is preferred for plasma chemistry determinations and for blood gas determinations. Potassium oxalate, combined with sodium fluoride or iodoacetate, is used for glucose determination.

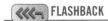 **FLASHBACK**

You learned about the coagulation cascade in Chapter 7.

Sodium fluoride inhibits **glycolysis** and is used for glucose determination. Glycolysis is a cellular reaction used to harvest energy from glucose. Lithium iodoacetate is an alternative antiglycolytic agent.

Clot Activators

Clot activators promote coagulation. Thrombin directly increases clotting and is used for stat serum chemistry determinations or if the patient is on anticoagulants (often prescribed to prevent a recurrence of stroke, for example). Inert substances such as glass or silica promote clotting by providing more surface area for platelet activation. Other inert substances are siliceous earth, clay, and celite. Clot activators may be adhered to the side of the tube, and therefore the sample must be inverted five times to allow the blood to come in contact with the activator. Some inert substances may interfere with certain tests (e.g., blood bank procedures) and therefore cannot be used.

Thixotropic Gel

Thixotropic gel is an inert, synthetic substance whose density is in between that of cells and that of blood serum or plasma. When the specimen is centrifuged, the gel becomes a liquid and moves between the lower cell layer and the upper serum or plasma layer. It hardens again after standing and forms a barrier between the two layers, thus preventing contamination and allowing easy separation. For instance, in the light green-topped tube used for determining potassium, the gel prevents the plasma from being contaminated by potassium released by red blood cells. (*Thixo-* means "related to touch" and refers to the gel's ability to liquefy when shaken.)

COLOR-CODED TOPS

Each combination of additives is distinguished by a different colored top. However, different manufacturers may use slightly different color-coding schemes. In some situations, the requisition indicates the color tube to use; in other cases, the name of the test is specified, and you need to determine the correct tube. This information is found in the lab's directory of services.

> **Clinical Tip:** Any tube with an additive should be inverted gently and repeatedly to mix the contents immediately after collection. Do not shake tubes, as this can cause cells to become damaged, resulting in hemolysis.

Red (Glass Tube)

Tests: Chemistry, serology, blood bank
Additives: None
Specimen: Serum
Notes: Blood collected in a red-topped glass tube takes 30 minutes to clot. Serum is separated by centrifugation after clotting.

Red (Plastic Tube)

Tests: Chemistry and serology
Additives: Clot activators
Specimen: Serum

Light Blue

Tests: Coagulation tests
Additives: Sodium citrate
Specimen: Plasma
Notes: Fill the tube completely to maintain the ratio of nine parts blood to one part sodium citrate (4.5 mL of blood to 0.5 mL of citrate).

Lavender

Tests: Complete blood count (CBC)
Additives: EDTA. Dipotassium EDTA (K_2 EDTA) is spray-dried onto the sides of the tube. This is the form preferred by CLSI (see below). Tripotassium EDTA (K_3 EDTA) is in liquid form, and disodium EDTA (Na_2 EDTA) is in powdered form.
Specimen: Whole blood

Pearl
Tests: Viral loads
Additives: Gel with EDTA
Specimen: Plasma

Gold BD Hemogard™ Closure; Red/Gray Stopper

Tests: Most chemistry tests
Additives: Clot activators, thixotropic gel
Specimen: Serum
Notes: Also called serum separator tubes (SSTs), "stat" tubes, and tiger-top or jungle-top tubes. Invert gently five times.

Gray

Tests: Lactic acid measurement, glucose tolerance test, fasting blood sugar (FBS), blood alcohol levels

Additives: Antiglycolytic agent that preserves glucose, either iodoacetate (preserves glucose 24 hours) or sodium fluoride (preserves glucose 3 days); may also have the anticoagulant potassium oxalate or heparin.

Specimen: Plasma

Black

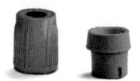

Tests: Sedimentation rate
Additives: Sodium citrate
Specimen: Whole blood
Notes: Fill the tube completely to maintain the ratio of four parts blood to one part citrate.

Green

Tests: Stat chemistry tests, ammonia, electrolytes, arterial blood gases
Additives: Heparin
Specimen: Plasma

Light Green; Green/Gray Stopper

Tests: Stat potassium
Additives: Heparin; thixotropic gel
Specimen: Plasma
Notes: Also called plasma separator tubes (PSTs)

Orange BD Hemogard™ Closure; Yellow/Gray Stopper

Tests: Stat chemistry
Additives: Thrombin
Specimen: Serum
Notes: Allows for 5-minute clotting time. Used for patients on anticoagulant therapy.

Royal Blue

Tests: Toxicology, trace metals, nutritional analysis
Additives: Heparin or EDTA, or none
Specimen: Plasma or serum
Notes: These tubes are chemically clean, and the stoppers are specially formulated to prevent the release of small amounts of materials that could contaminate the sample and give erroneous test results.

Tan

Tests: Lead analysis
Additives: Heparin
Specimen: Plasma
Notes: The tube is formulated to contain less than 0.1μg/mL of lead.

Yellow, Sterile

Tests: Blood culture
Additives: SPS (sodium polyethanol sulfonate) to inhibit complement and phagocytosis
Specimen: Whole blood
Notes: Used to recover microorganisms that are causing blood infection

Yellow, Nonsterile

Tests: Human leukocyte antigen (HLA) studies (paternity testing and tissue typing)
Additives: Acid citrate dextrose
Specimen: Whole blood
Notes: The dextrose nourishes and preserves red blood cells, and the citrate is an anticoagulant.

Pink

Tests: Antibody screen, compatibility test. This tube is similar to the standard lavender top tube, but its closure and label meet the standards set by the American Association of Blood Banks.

Additives: K_2 EDTA
Specimen: Plasma, whole blood

ORDER OF DRAW

Patients often need to have more than one test performed and therefore more than one tube filled. Because the same multisample needle is used to fill all the tubes, material from an earlier tube could be transferred into a later tube if it contacts the needle. Good technique can reduce this risk somewhat (discussed in more detail in the next chapter); however, it cannot eliminate it entirely. For this reason, the Clinical and Laboratory Standards Institute (CLSI) has developed a set of standards dictating the proper **order of draw** for a multitube draw. The order is the same for syringe samples as for direct filling from a multisample needle. The order-of-draw standards have undergone several revisions within the past decade, and not all institutions have adopted the most recent set of standards (termed H3-A5). It is important for you to follow the order of draw used at your institution, even if it differs from the order below.

1. Blood culture tubes (which are sterile) are drawn first. This prevents the transfer of unsterilized material from other tubes into the sterile tube.
2. Light blue-topped tubes (for coagulation tests) are next. These tubes are always drawn before tubes containing other kinds of anticoagulants, because other additives could contaminate this tube and interfere with coagulation testing.
3. Red/gray (gold BD Hemogard™) tubes and plastic red-top tubes are next. These contain clot activators, which would interfere with many other samples if passed into other tubes. Glass red-top tubes, which do not contain additives, may also be drawn now.
4. Green tubes are drawn next. The heparin from the green tube is less likely to interfere with EDTA-containing tubes than vice versa.
5. Lavender tubes are next. EDTA binds many metals in addition to calcium, so it can cause problems with many test results, including giving falsely low calcium and falsely high potassium readings. For this reason, lavender tubes are drawn near the end.
6. The gray-topped tube is last. This tube contains potassium oxalate. The potassium would elevate the potassium levels measured in electrolyte analysis, and oxalate can damage cell membranes. Also, another additive, sodium

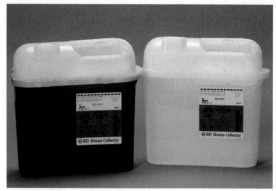

Figure 8-11
Needle disposal systems reduce the risk of accidental injury while removing the needle. (From Bonewit-West K: Clinical Procedures for Medical Assistants, ed 6. Philadelphia, Saunders, 2004.)

fluoride, elevates sodium levels and inhibits many enzymes.

Other color tubes are typically drawn after these six, but you should check the instructions on the manufacturer's package insert, and your lab procedures manual, for specific information. The glass red-top tube (but not the plastic red-top tube) may be drawn after the sterile tube, if your institution allows it.

NEEDLE DISPOSAL CONTAINERS

Once you have withdrawn the needle from the patient's arm, it must be handled with extreme care to avoid an accidental needle stick. A used needle is considered biohazardous waste and must be treated as such. Dispose of the needle and needle adapter immediately after activating the needle safety device. Needles must be placed in a clearly marked, puncture-resistant biohazard disposal container (Figure 8-11). Containers must be closable or sealable, puncture resistant, leakproof, and labeled with the correct biohazard symbol.

You must become familiar with the system in use at your workplace. Practice with a new system *before* you draw your first sample.

REVIEW FOR CERTIFICATION

The phlebotomist's tray includes tourniquets for locating veins; antiseptics and disinfectants for cleaning the puncture site; a variety of needles in different sizes, including multisample needles, syringe needles, and butterflies; needle adapters or tube holders; evacuated collection tubes; bandages; and a variety of other materials. The phlebotomist chooses the needle type and size to fit the characteristics of the patient and the test and uses tubes that contain additives appropriate for the tests that have been ordered. A prescribed order of draw is used to minimize the effects of contamination among tubes.

BIBLIOGRAPHY

2006 Medical Safety Product Directory: Advance for Medical Laboratory Professionals. March 13, 2006.

Calfee DP, Farr BM, Comparison of four antiseptic preparations for skin in the prevention of contamination of percutaneously drawn blood cultures: a randomized trial. J Clin Microbiol. 2002 May; 40(5): 1660-5.

Clinical and Laboratory Standards Institute: H3-A5: Procedures for the Collection of Diagnostic Blood Specimens by Venipuncture, ed 5. Villanova, PA, 2003.

Clinical and Laboratory Standards Institute: H1-A5: Tubes and Additives for Venous Blood Specimen Collection, ed 5. 2003.

Pallatroni L: The Price of Needle Safety. Medical Laboratory Observer. July 1998.

Winkelman J, Tanasijevic M: How RBCs Move through Thixotropic Gels. Laboratory Medicine. July 1999.

STUDY QUESTIONS

1. Explain the purpose of a tourniquet.
2. What does the gauge of a needle indicate?
3. Describe the consequences of using a needle with a large gauge number.
4. Explain the purpose of the rubber sleeve on the multisample needle.
5. Explain the advantages and disadvantages of the syringe method of drawing blood as opposed to the evacuated system.
6. Blood tubes are evacuated. Explain what this means.
7. Why must unused blood tubes be discarded when they expire?
8. Define SPS and what it is used for.
9. If a collection tube contains an anticoagulant, what must you do immediately after collection?
10. Explain the purpose of thixotropic gel in a collection tube.
11. Define glycolysis.
12. Name the three types of blood specimens used for analysis.

Match the collection tube stopper color to the type of test it is commonly used for.

13. tan	a. blood bank
14. red	b. lead analysis
15. light blue	c. glucose tolerance test
16. lavender	d. chemistry testing
17. gray	e. sedimentation rate
18. black	f. arterial blood gases
19. gold BD Hemogard™ Closure	g. CBC
20. green	h. trace metals
21. dark (royal) blue	i. coagulation

22. Number the following in the correct order of draw using the evacuated method.

_____ light blue
_____ lavender
_____ green
_____ red (plastic tube)
_____ yellow (sterile)
_____ gray
_____ gold BD Hemogard™ Closure

CERTIFICATION EXAM PREPARATION

1. Which of the following is not an anticoagulant?
   a. thixotropic gel
   b. sodium heparin
   c. sodium citrate
   d. EDTA

2. The most common antiseptic used in routine venipuncture is:
   a. povidone-iodine solution
   b. bleach
   c. isopropyl alcohol
   d. chlorhexidine gluconate

3. How many times may a needle be used before discarding it?
   a. 1
   b. 2
   c. 3
   d. no limit

4. Which of the following indicates the largest-sized needle?
   a. 20 gauge
   b. 23 gauge
   c. 16 gauge
   d. 21 gauge

5. Complete blood clotting takes _____ minutes.
   a. 10 to 20
   b. 25 to 45
   c. 30 to 60
   d. 30 to 40

6. Serum contains:
   a. fibrinogen
   b. clotting factors
   c. plasma
   d. none of the above

7. Which color-coded tube does not contain any additives?
   a. red (plastic tube)
   b. red (glass tube)
   c. gold BD Hemogard™
   d. dark blue

8. EDTA prevents coagulation in the blood tubes by:
   a. inactivating thrombin
   b. binding calcium
   c. inactivating thromboplastin
   d. inhibiting glycolysis

9. Tubes with gray stoppers are used for:
   a. sedimentation rate tests
   b. glucose tolerance tests
   c. coagulation studies
   d. CBC

10. Tubes with green stoppers may contain:
    a. sodium citrate
    b. sodium heparin
    c. sodium oxalate
    d. sodium phosphate

11. The smaller the gauge number, the:
    a. larger the lumen diameter
    b. longer the needle
    c. shorter the needle
    d. smaller the lumen diameter

12. The syringe method of draw is useful for patients:
    a. who are very young
    b. who are obese
    c. who have large veins
    d. who have fragile or small veins

13. The additive sodium citrate is used in blood collection to test for:
    a. blood alcohol
    b. sedimentation rate
    c. lactic acid
    d. lead

14. The most common gauge used for a *routine* venipuncture is:
    a. 16
    b. 20
    c. 25
    d. 23

CERTIFICATION EXAM PREPARATION—cont'd

15. Blood banks use a _____-gauge needle to collect blood from donors for transfusions.
    a. 16
    b. 20
    c. 25
    d. 23

16. Blood collection tubes containing an anticoagulant should be:
    a. inverted gently and repeatedly after blood collection
    b. shaken aggressively after blood collection
    c. allowed to sit for 30 minutes before centrifugation
    d. centrifuged immediately

17. Tubes containing the SPS anticoagulant are used for:
    a. antibody screen
    b. HLA studies
    c. nutritional analysis
    d. blood culture analysis

18. Blood collected in lavender-stoppered tubes is used for which test?
    a. FBS
    b. CBC
    c. stat potassium
    d. stat chemistry

19. Blood collected in gray-stoppered tubes is used for which test?
    a. FBS
    b. CBC
    c. stat potassium
    d. stat chemistry

20. Blood collected in light blue-stoppered tubes is used for which test?
    a. sedimentation rate
    b. glucose tolerance
    c. toxicology
    d. coagulation

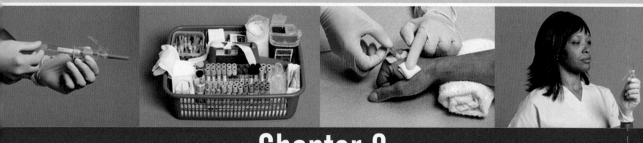

Chapter 9

Routine Venipuncture

OUTLINE

Requisitions
Routine Venipuncture Procedure

Routine Venipuncture with a Syringe
Review for Certification

OBJECTIVES

After completing this chapter, you should be able to:

1. List the information that is commonly found on a test requisition.
2. List in order the steps in a routine venipuncture.
3. Discuss the information that must be verified for inpatient identification before the blood collection procedure.
4. Explain how the identification of outpatients differs from that of inpatients.
5. Describe patient preparation and positioning.
6. Describe how to assemble the evacuated tube system.
7. Explain how to apply a tourniquet and list three consequences of improper application.

8. List the veins that may be used for blood collection, including the advantages and disadvantages of each.
9. Explain how to clean the venipuncture site.
10. Describe how to properly insert the needle into the vein.
11. Discuss how the needle should be removed when the last tube of blood has been collected.
12. List the information that must be included on the label of each tube.
13. Describe how venipuncture using a syringe differs from that using the evacuated tube system.

KEY TERMS

hematoma
hemoconcentration
informed consent

palpation
petechiae
requisition

ABBREVIATIONS
DOB: date of birth

ID: identification

Routine venipuncture is the most common procedure a phlebotomist performs. The single most important step in venipuncture is positive identification of the patient. This is done by matching the information on the requisition with, for inpatients, the information on the patient's identification band or, for outpatients, the information provided by the patient. Although most patients are suitable candidates for drawing blood with evacuated tubes, patients with fragile veins may be better candidates for syringe collection, with the blood being transferred to evacuated tubes after the draw.

REQUISITIONS

All blood collection procedures begin with a request for a test from the treating physician. The laboratory processes this request and generates a **requisition**. The requisition is the form the phlebotomist uses to determine what type of sample to collect from the patient (Figure 9-1).

Requisitions may be computer generated or handwritten. At a minimum, the requisition has the following information:

- Patient demographics—full name, date of birth (DOB), sex, and race.

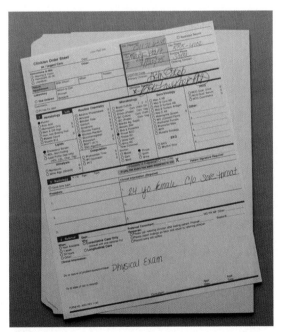

Figure 9-1
The phlebotomist uses the requisition form to determine what type of sample to collect from the patient. The requisition may be computer-generated or written by hand.

- If an inpatient, hospital identification (ID) number and room number and bed.
- Name or code of the physician making the request.
- Tests requested with the accompanying ICD-9 code.
- Test status (e.g., stat, timed, fasting).

The requisition may also contain information about the patient's status, such as potential bleeding complications or puncture sites to avoid. The number and type of tubes to collect may also be indicated. Test names may be abbreviated, so it is important to know the meaning of test abbreviations.

 FLASHBACK

Most common lab tests and their abbreviations were covered in Chapters 2, 6, and 7.

The information on the requisition serves several purposes. First, it allows you to identify the patient correctly and may provide some helpful information about the patient. Second, it tells you what specimen should be collected. And third, it allows you to gather the necessary equipment for the collection before you encounter the patient. Computer-generated requisitions may also have a set of labels used for the collection tubes. The requisition may not indicate any special handling procedures, and you may be required to consult the laboratory resources to ensure both correct collection and handling of samples. For instance, a sample for a bilirubin test must always be shielded from light after collection, even though the requisition does not state this.

FLASH FORWARD

Special collection procedures are covered in Chapter 14.

The requisition may arrive in one of several ways. Requisitions for inpatients are usually picked up at either the lab or the nursing station. Outpatients typically carry their own requisitions with them. Emergency requisitions may be telephoned in to the lab; in this case, the phlebotomist picks up the form at the unit where the patient is located.

There are several steps you should perform when you receive requisitions:

- Examine them to make sure that each has all the necessary information: Full name, DOB, ordering physician, and test ICD-9 codes.
- Check for duplicates. If there are several requisitions for one patient, group them together so

that all collections can be made with a single puncture.

- Prioritize the requisitions (stat, timed collections, routine).
- Collect all the equipment you will need for the collections you will be performing.

ROUTINE VENIPUNCTURE PROCEDURE

Procedure 9-1 describes the steps for a routine venipuncture using evacuated tubes, from the first encounter with the patient until the sample is complete and labeled, the puncture site has stopped bleeding, and the patient is discharged or the phlebotomist leaves the patient's room.

ROUTINE VENIPUNCTURE WITH A SYRINGE

Procedure 9-2 describes the steps for a routine venipuncture with a syringe. Patients with fragile veins may need to have blood drawn using a syringe, because the stronger vacuum of the evacuated tube may collapse the vein. A small needle is usually used for the draw. After the blood is drawn, the needle is removed from the syringe and disposed of. Blood is transferred to evacuated tubes using a needleless blood transfer device.

REVIEW FOR CERTIFICATION

The steps of routine venipuncture are designed to produce a blood sample quickly and efficiently while ensuring the safety of both the phlebotomist and the patient during the collection. Positive patient identification is the single most important step in the procedure. A tourniquet is used to locate a vein, but care must be taken to avoid applying it too tightly or leaving it on too long. Once the site is cleaned, the needle is inspected, and the first tube is prepared, the needle is inserted at an angle of 15 to 30 degrees in a single smooth, quick motion. Tubes are held at a slight downward angle while filling and are mixed immediately after filling. They are labeled after filling, once the needle has been withdrawn and gauze has been applied to the puncture site. Syringe collection is used for patients with fragile veins. Blood is transferred to evacuated tubes after drawing.

Procedure 9-1
Routine Venipuncture

1. Greet and identify the patient.

Knock gently before entering the room, even if the door is open. This alerts the patient to your presence.

Announce yourself if a curtain is closed around the bed.

Introduce yourself.

Explain that you are there to collect a blood sample. If the patient asks the purpose of the test, it is usually best to simply say that the doctor has ordered the test, without discussing specifics. Information about the purposes and results of the test should come from the patient's doctor.

Positive identification of the patient is the single most important aspect of any phlebotomy procedure. Identification errors can lead to incorrect diagnosis and treatment of the patient and may even cause death. Drawing blood from the wrong patient is grounds for dismissal and possibly a lawsuit.

Ask the patient to state his or her full name. Do not ask, "Are you Jane Doe?" because confused or hard-of-hearing patients may say yes without understanding the question.

Check the requisition against this patient-provided information *and* the patient's ID band. The ID band is usually on the patient's wrist, or it may be on the ankle.

The ID band contains the patient's name, DOB, and, most importantly, ID number. Although two patients in a hospital may have the same name and even the same birth date, they will not have the same ID number. The ID number must match the number on the requisition. If the wristband is not attached to the patient—even if it is on the bedside table—*do not draw blood*. Ask the patient's nurse to attach a new one before proceeding.

Outpatients do not have ID bands. Have the patient state his or her name and DOB, and compare this information with that on the requisition. You may also ask the patient to present a photo ID.

Ask the patient if he or she is taking any medications. Patients taking blood-thinning medications such as warfarin, heparin, or aspirin

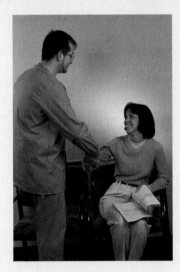

Procedure 9-1—cont'd
Routine Venipuncture

may require extra compression to stop bleeding after the draw.

Place your phlebotomy tray on a flat, stable surface nearby, but not on the patient's bed. Take the necessary safety precautions to avoid contamination of yourself and your equipment if the patient has an infection.

2. Position and prepare the patient.

The patient should be positioned for both safety and comfort. Never draw blood from a standing patient or from one sitting on a high stool. Outpatients can be seated in a special chair with arm support. For inpatients, you may lower the bed rail for better access, *but you must remember to raise it again after the procedure.*

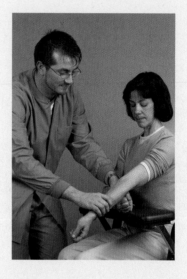

Support the arm for venipuncture under the elbow, either with the patient's fist or with a pillow.

Ask the patient to remove all foreign objects, such as gum, from his or her mouth.

Explain the procedure, and get a verbal *informed consent* from the patient. The patient must consent to the procedure before you proceed.

 FLASH FORWARD

The issue of informed consent is covered in Chapter 18.

As noted earlier, refer any specific questions to the doctor in charge. Explain to the patient that he or she will feel a small poke or pinch, and should remain still throughout the collection. If the patient seems nervous, try to calm him or her. Distracting the patient with small talk about the weather or other neutral subjects often relieves anxiety.

Verify any pretest preparation, such as fasting or abstaining from medications. If the sample requires pretest fasting, ask the patient, "When was the last time you had anything to eat or drink?"

 FLASH FORWARD

Special collections are discussed further in Chapter 14.

Procedure 9-1—cont'd

Routine Venipuncture

3. **Assemble your equipment.**
   Wash your hands and put on gloves.

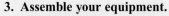
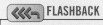

> See Procedures 4-1 and 4-2.

Collect antiseptic pads, sterile gauze, bandages, tourniquet, tubes, and needle disposal system.

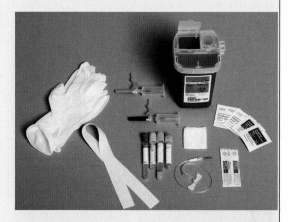

Attach the needle to the adapter.

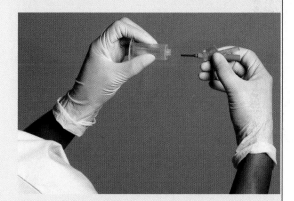

Insert the tube into the adapter up to the tube advancement mark.
Carry everything to the patient drawing area.

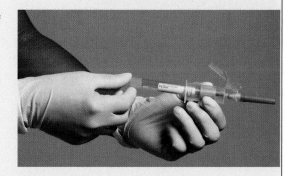

Procedure 9-1—cont'd
Routine Venipuncture

4. Apply the tourniquet.

Most venipunctures are in the arm. The tourniquet should be applied 3 to 4 inches above the puncture site. Direct skin contact may be uncomfortable for people with hairy arms; in this case, you can tie the tourniquet over a shirt sleeve. Do not place the tourniquet over an open sore.

To tie the tourniquet, follow these steps (these directions are for right-handed people; left-handers can adapt them as necessary):

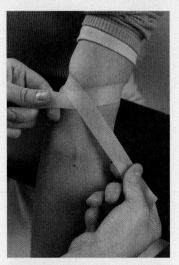

- Hold one free end of the tourniquet close to the patient's arm. Bring the other end around behind the arm, crossing it over the first end on top of the arm, forming an X.
- Pull the lower side of the tourniquet taut, and grasp the X between the thumb and forefinger of one hand.
- With the other hand, tuck in the upper strip close to the X by sliding it under the other side from above. Both free ends should be away from the puncture area.

The tourniquet should not be left on longer than 1 minute. The patient will notice some slight restriction, but it should not pinch or hurt. The arm should not turn red, the fingers should not tingle, and you should continue to be able to feel a radial pulse. In addition to discomfort for the patient, there are three consequences of improper tourniquet application:

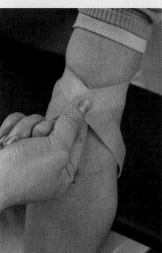

- **Hemoconcentration**—an increase in the ratio of formed elements to plasma caused by leaving the tourniquet on too long. Hemoconcentration can alter some test results.
- **Hemolysis**—this can occur if the tourniquet is too tight or left on too long. Destruction of red blood cells can alter test results.
- **Petechiae**—small red spots on the skin, caused by a tourniquet that is too tight.

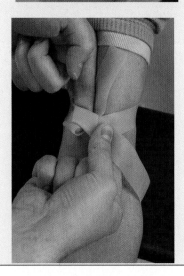

Procedure 9-1—cont'd

Routine Venipuncture

5. Select the site.

The best veins for venipuncture are located in the antecubital fossa, on the anterior surface of the arm just distal to the elbow. Refer back to Chapter 7 to review the anatomy of this area.

The median cubital vein is the first choice. It is located in the middle of the arm's surface, is large and well anchored, and does not move when the needle is inserted.

The cephalic vein, on the same side of the arm as the thumb, is the second choice. It can be hard to locate and is not well anchored, so it has a tendency to move. However, it is often the only vein that can be palpated (located by touch) in an obese patient.

The basilic vein, on the same side of the arm as the pinky finger, is the third choice. It is the least firmly anchored, and its location near the brachial artery means that if you insert the needle too deep, you may puncture the artery.

Blood can also be drawn from wrist and hand veins, but these require winged infusion sets with smaller needles and tubes, making the draw slower and increasing the risk of hemolysis.

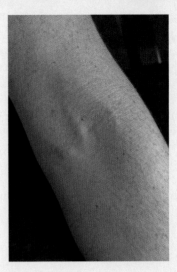

6. Palpate the vein.

Veins are best located by **palpation**, or feel, rather than by sight. Palpating is done with the tourniquet on. Gently push up and down with the index finger—this determines both the depth and the direction of the veins. Veins feel spongy, bouncy, and firm. Arteries pulsate, and tendons feel rigid.

If you have difficulty locating the vein, you can increase the circulation by gentle massage of the arm where the vein is located, or by asking the patient to make a fist. You can also gently warm the arm with a warm towel or hot pack, after removing the tourniquet. Beginners should remove the tourniquet once the vein is located.

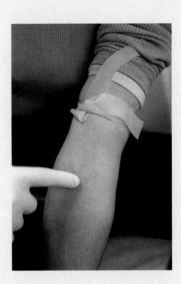

Procedure 9-1—cont'd

Routine Venipuncture

7. **Clean the site.**

   Using 70% isopropyl alcohol or other antiseptic, clean the area in concentric circles spiraling outward from the puncture site. (Other antiseptics may be used in special situations; see Chapters 8 and 14.)

   Allow the site to dry for 30 to 60 seconds. This provides maximum bacteriostatic action, avoids specimen hemolysis, and prevents stinging the patient. Do not blow on it. If you need to repalpate the vein, the area must be cleaned again prior to the puncture.

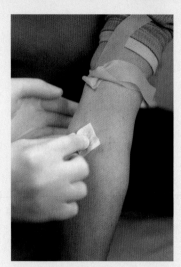

8. **Reapply the tourniquet.**

   If you removed the tourniquet during cleaning to prevent hemoconcentration or hemolysis, reapply it at this time. (As you become more proficient in routine venipuncture, removing and reapplying the tourniquet will become unnecessary, because you will be able to locate the vein, scrub and dry the site, inspect the needle, and insert the needle within 30 to 60 seconds.)

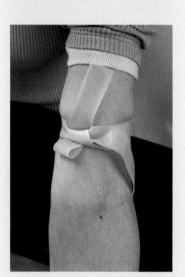

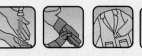

Procedure 9-1—cont'd
Routine Venipuncture

9. **Examine the needle.**
   Uncap the needle and examine it for defects, such as a blunted or barbed point, an obstructed lumen, or a bent shaft.

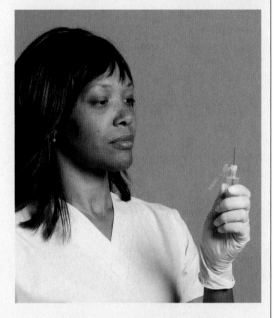

10. **Perform the venipuncture.**
   Anchor the vein 1-2 inches below the venipuncture site and brace the arm using the thumb of your nondominant hand (your left hand, if you are right-handed).

   Hold the needle assembly with your dominant hand, with the tube inserted up to the line on the adapter. Angle the needle at 15 to 30 degrees above the skin. The best way to grasp the assembly is with your thumb on top, your index finger close to the front of the holder, and your other fingers gently grasping the underside. Placing your fingers too far forward can elevate the tube holder beyond the ideal angle.

   Insert the needle, bevel up, in one smooth, quick motion. You will feel a slight give when the needle enters the vein.

   Hold the needle assembly very steady. Do not pull up or push down on the needle while it is in the vein. It helps to rest your hand on the patient's arm. Keep the assembly angled downward to prevent backflow of blood into the needle from the tube. This prevents additive from contaminating the needle, and hence the next tube. It also prevents additive from entering the patient's circulation, a potentially harmful event.

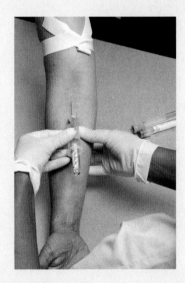

Procedure 9-1—cont'd

Routine Venipuncture

11. Fill the first tube.

Push in the tube with the hand that anchored the vein. Use your thumb to push the tube in, but be sure to pull back with your fingers on the flanges of the adapter to prevent pushing the needle in farther. (Some phlebotomists switch hands at this point, so that the dominant hand is pushing and switching tubes. This switch must be done carefully to avoid moving the needle.)

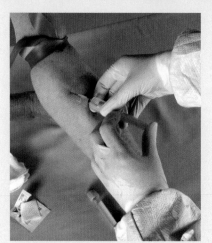

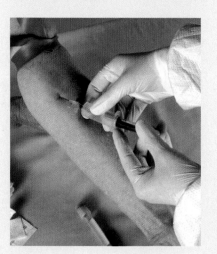

12. Remove the tourniquet.

To be sure the tourniquet stays on no longer than 1 minute, remove it as soon as blood flow is established. This is done while the first tube is filling.

The tourniquet must be removed prior to needle removal to prevent formation of a **hematoma**, which is a reddened, swollen area where blood collects under the skin. A hematoma forms when the extra pressure from the tourniquet forces blood out through the puncture.

To remove the tourniquet, pull on the free end to release it from the patient's arm.

Procedure 9-1—cont'd

Routine Venipuncture

13. Advance and change the tubes.

Remove a tube when blood stops flowing into it. This will occur before it is completely filled. Gently pull the tube to remove it, again ensuring that the needle remains still.

If the tube contains additives, mix it by gently inverting it the number of times specified by the manufacturer as soon as it is removed.

Insert another tube, if needed, being sure to keep the needle assembly still and angled downward.

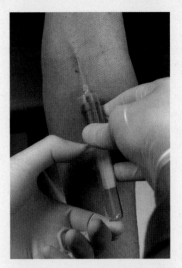

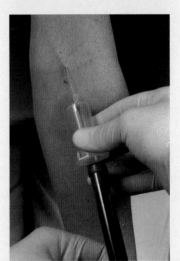

14. Prepare for needle removal.

Remove the last tube before removing the needle, to prevent blood from dripping out of the tube.

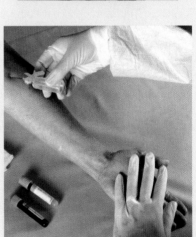

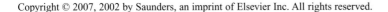

Procedure 9-1—cont'd

Routine Venipuncture

15. **Withdraw the needle.**

Pull the needle assembly straight out.

Activate the safety feature on the needle.

Apply a gauze square folded in quarters to the puncture site. Do not press down on the site until after withdrawal. The patient's arm should be straight or slightly bent, but not bent back up over the puncture site, which can cause a hematoma. The arm may be elevated. Apply pressure for up to 2 minutes for patients on anticoagulants, especially if the cephalic or basilic vein is used.

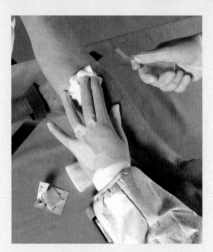

16. **Dispose of the used needle in the needle collection container.**

Use the disposal method and container designed for the type of needle you are using.

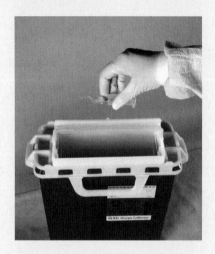

17. **Label the tubes.**

Label each tube at the patient's bedside. *Do not leave the room without first labeling the tubes.* If you are labeling by hand, use either a ballpoint pen or a permanent marker—never pencil or nonpermanent marker. The label must have the patient's name and ID number, the date and time of collection, and your initials or ID number. If you are using computer-generated labels, make sure that the label has all the required information, and then add your initials or ID number.

Never label a tube before collection. This can lead to serious errors if, for instance, another person makes the collection or tubes for different patients are mixed before collection. If possible, compare the information on the labeled tube to the patient's ID band, or ask the patient to confirm the information on the label.

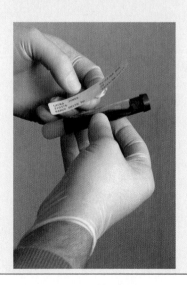

Procedure 9-1—cont'd
Routine Venipuncture

18. Attend to the patient.

Check the puncture site to be sure bleeding has stopped.

Apply a bandage, using a fresh adhesive bandage or placing adhesive tape over the gauze square.

Raise the bed rail, if you lowered it.

Dispose of all contaminated materials in a biohazard container.

Remove your gloves (follow Procedure 4-2), and wash your hands.

Thank the patient and smile.

In some inpatient situations, it is appropriate to report to the nursing station that you are finished with the patient. For instance, a fasting patient may be able to eat after the phlebotomist is finished.

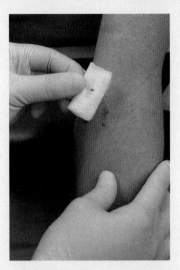

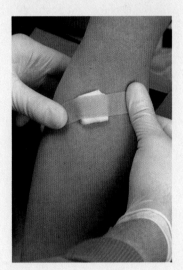

19. Deliver the specimen.

Deliver the specimen to the lab.

Follow the lab's policy about recording your work in the computer, logbook, or other tracking system.

Log in the specimen arrival time in the logbook.

Complete all your paperwork.

Procedure 9-2

Venipuncture with a Syringe

1. **Follow the beginning steps for a routine venipuncture.**

   Perform steps 1, 2, 4 to 7, and 9 of Procedure 9-1, including removing and inspecting the needle. The needle should be checked immediately before insertion, because its small size makes it susceptible to damage from improper handling during preparation.

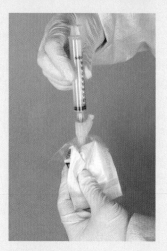

2. **Prepare the syringe and perform the venipuncture.**

   Twist the needle onto the tip of the syringe.

   Pull the plunger back to be sure it moves freely, then push it all the way back in to expel any air.

   Reapply the tourniquet and perform the venipuncture, as in steps 8 and 10 of Procedure 9-1. A flash of blood should appear in the syringe hub, indicating that the vein has been entered.

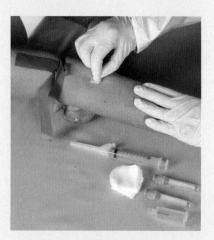

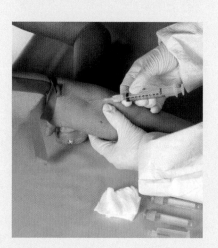

Procedure 9-2—cont'd

Venipuncture with a Syringe

3. **Fill the syringe.**

   Unlike the evacuated tube, the syringe does not automatically fill with blood. Pull back the plunger evenly, gently, and slowly to withdraw the blood.

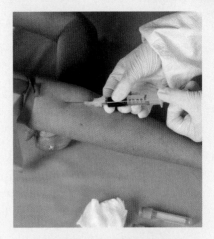

4. **Withdraw the needle, and transfer the blood to evacuated tubes.**

   Withdraw the needle and stop the bleeding as in steps 12 to 14 of Procedure 9-1. Activate the safety device.

   Transferring the blood to evacuated tubes is done in the same order as if the evacuated tube system were used (blood culture, light blue, and so on). Rubber stoppers should not be removed.

   Place the tubes in a tube holder.

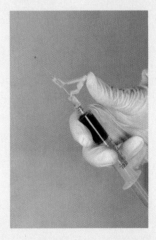

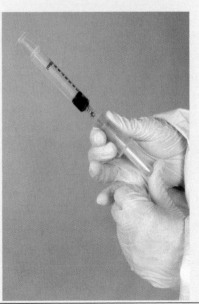

Procedure 9-2—cont'd
Venipuncture with a Syringe

Never transfer blood from a syringe with an exposed needle. Instead, activate the safety device on the needle, remove it from the syringe, and dispose of it according to your institution's procedures. Then, attach a needleless blood transfer device to the syringe.

Holding the syringe upright, push the first tube up into the transfer device. Allow the tube to fill without applying any pressure to the plunger. Pushing on the plunger causes hemolysis and increases the risk of causing an aerosol spray when the needle is removed. The evacuated tube will fill according to its vacuum capacity. If you need to fill a second tube, remove the first and insert the second tube just as you did the first.

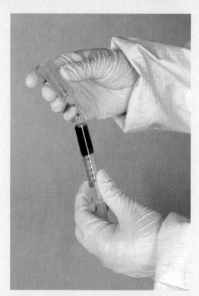

5. **Dispose of the syringe and transfer device together in the appropriate container.**

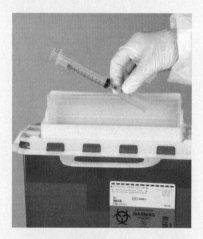

6. **Complete the procedure.**
   Finish the procedure as in steps 15-17 of Procedure 9-1.

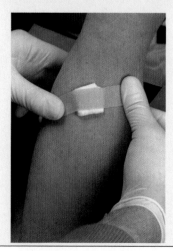

BIBLIOGRAPHY

College of American Pathologists: So You're Going to Collect a Blood Specimen: An Introduction to Phlebotomy, ed 6. Northfield, IL, College of American Pathologists, 1994.

Clinical and Laboratory Standards Institute (CLSI). Procedures for the Collection of Diagnostic Blood Specimens by Venipuncture; Approved Standard—Sixth Edition. CLSI Document H3-A6. November, 2007.

Ernst DJ: The Ten Commandments of Phlebotomy. Advance for Medical Laboratory Professionals. June 28, 1999.

Phelan S: Phlebotomy Techniques: A Laboratory Workbook. Chicago, College of American Pathologists, 1993.

Slockbower JM: Venipuncture Procedures. Laboratory Medicine. December 1979.

STUDY QUESTIONS

1. What is the single most important aspect of any phlebotomy procedure?
2. Describe how to properly identify a patient.
3. What information is typically on a requisition form?
4. List the steps you should perform when requisitions are received.
5. Define hemoconcentration.
6. Name three veins in the antecubital area suitable for venipuncture.
7. Explain why the median cubital vein is the first choice for venipuncture.
8. Describe how veins, arteries, and tendons feel when palpating them.
9. What techniques can you use to help locate a vein?
10. Define hematoma.
11. Describe the correct position of the patient's arm after withdrawing the venipuncture needle.
12. Explain the correct procedure for labeling blood tubes.
13. Describe the proper way blood should be transferred to collection tubes when using a syringe.
14. List the information a phlebotomist must look for on a requisition slip.
15. Explain the reasoning behind preparing the patient *before* you wash your hands and put on gloves.

CERTIFICATION EXAM PREPARATION

1. Which is not a purpose of the requisition?
   a. filing insurance claims
   b. identifying the patient
   c. determining the specimens to be collected
   d. allowing the equipment necessary for the collection to be gathered

2. Which vein is often the only one that can be palpated in an obese patient?
   a. median
   b. cephalic
   c. basilic
   d. iliac

3. Upon entering a patient's room, you should first:
   a. assemble your equipment
   b. put your gloves on
   c. introduce yourself
   d. identify the patient

4. Which vein lies close to the brachial artery?
   a. cephalic
   b. median cubital
   c. basilic
   d. iliac

5. At what angle should a venipuncture needle penetrate the skin?
   a. 10 to 15 degrees
   b. 15 to 30 degree
   c. 30 to 40 degrees
   d. 45 degrees

6. Which information must match on the patient's ID band and requisition?
   a. DOB
   b. physician's name
   c. ID number
   d. patient's name

7. When should the tourniquet be removed from the arm in a venipuncture procedure?
   a. After the needle is withdrawn.
   b. As the needle is withdrawn.
   c. Before the needle is withdrawn.
   d. The tourniquet should not be removed.

8. Tourniquets should be placed _____ inches above the venipuncture site.
   a. 1 to 2
   b. 2 to 3
   c. 3 to 4
   d. 4 to 5

9. The following can occur if the tourniquet is left on the patient too long:
   a. nerve damage
   b. petechiae
   c. occluded radial pulse
   d. hematoma

10. Hematomas can be caused by:
    a. Removing the tourniquet after removing the needle.
    b. Withdrawing the needle before removing the last tube.
    c. Withdrawing the needle too quickly.
    d. Removing the tourniquet before removing the needle.

11. An increase in the ratio of formed elements to plasma is called:
    a. hemolysis
    b. petechiae
    c. hemoconcentration
    d. hematoma

12. Small red spots on the skin are referred to as:
    a. hemolysis
    b. petechiae
    c. hemoconcentration
    d. hematoma

13. If you are asked to perform a venipuncture on an inpatient who is not wearing an ID band, you should:
    a. Identify the patient by asking his or her name, and perform the venipuncture.
    b. Ask the patient's nurse to attach a new ID before proceeding.
    c. Notify the physician.
    d. Refuse to perform the venipuncture.

14. Which vein is the first choice for venipuncture?
    a. basilic
    b. median
    c. cephalic
    d. iliac

15. During the venipuncture procedure, the tourniquet should stay on no longer than:
    a. 30 seconds
    b. 45 seconds
    c. 1 minute
    d. 2 minutes

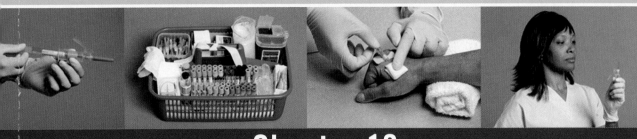

Chapter 10

Dermal Puncture

OUTLINE

Reasons for Performing Dermal
  Puncture
Differences between Venous and
  Capillary Blood
Equipment for Dermal Puncture
    Skin Puncture Devices
    Microsample Containers
    Additional Supplies

Site Selection
    General Considerations
    Puncture Depth and Width
    Dermal Puncture Sites in
      Adults and Older Children
    Dermal Puncture Sites in
      Infants

Dermal Puncture Procedure
Other Uses of Dermal Puncture
    Bleeding Time Test
    Ancillary Blood Glucose Test
Review for Certification

OBJECTIVES

After completing this chapter, you should be able to:

1. List situations in which a dermal puncture might
   be preferred.
2. Explain why it is necessary to inform the physician
   when capillary blood is collected.
3. Describe skin puncture devices, including safety
   features they may have.
4. Discuss containers that may be used to collect
   capillary blood.
5. List the steps in the BD Unopette™ dilution method.
6. Explain how circulation may be increased at the
   puncture site.
7. Discuss proper dermal puncture site selection.
8. Explain why it is important to control the depth of
   the puncture.

9. List in order the steps for dermal puncture.
10. Describe how the cut should be made when a
    finger is used.
11. Explain why the first drop of blood is discarded.
12. List precautions to be observed when collecting
    capillary blood.
13. State the order of the draw in collecting capillary
    blood.
14. Explain the use of the bleeding time test.
15. List the equipment required to perform a bleeding
    time test.
16. List in order the steps for performing a bleeding
    time test.
17. Explain the procedure for performing a bedside
    glucose test.

KEY TERMS

ancillary blood glucose test
bleeding time test
BURPP
calcaneus
capillary tubes (microhematocrit tubes)
diluent

microcollection tubes
micropipets (Caraway or Natelson pipets)
osteochondritis
osteomyelitis
venous thrombosis

ABBREVIATIONS

ABG: arterial blood gas
BT: bleeding time
BURPP: bilirubin, uric acid, phosphorus, and potassium

CBC: complete blood count
IV: intravenous
OSHA: Occupational Safety and Health Administration

Dermal puncture is an alternative collection procedure when minute amounts of blood are needed for testing, or for patients in whom venipuncture is inadvisable or impossible. It is the usual collection procedure for infants. In addition, it is the standard procedure for the bleeding time test and the ancillary blood glucose test. The depth of puncture must be carefully controlled to produce adequate flow while avoiding contact with underlying bone. Skin puncture devices deliver a precise incision, and microsample containers, sized to fit the desired sample, collect the blood from the puncture site.

REASONS FOR PERFORMING DERMAL PUNCTURE

Although venipuncture is the most common way to obtain a blood sample, there are times when it is impossible or inadvisable to do so. In these situations, dermal (skin) puncture offers a valuable alternative. Dermal puncture is also used for bleeding time determinations and bedside glucose testing and can be used as an alternative to arterial puncture for arterial blood gas (ABG) determination.

A requisition form generally does *not* state that a dermal puncture should be performed, and it is up to the phlebotomist to choose the best collection method for the tests ordered. For this reason, you must be familiar with the advantages, limitations, and appropriate uses of the dermal puncture. Knowing how and when to perform a dermal puncture is a vital skill for a phlebotomist.

Dermal puncture is preferred in several situations and for several types of patients (Box 10-1). Adult patients undergoing frequent glucose monitoring are excellent candidates for dermal puncture, because the test requires only a small amount of blood, which must be taken frequently. Patients requiring frequent blood tests are candidates for dermal puncture, as are those receiving intravenous (IV) therapy, because it spares the veins and keeps them available for the IV line. Access to venipuncture sites may be difficult in obese patients, whose veins are often hard to find, and in geriatric patients, who often have small or fragile veins that can make obtaining venous blood difficult. Venipuncture may be contraindicated in

---

BOX 10-1   Patients for Whom Dermal Puncture May Be Considered

Geriatric patients
Children, especially younger than age 2
Patients undergoing frequent glucose monitoring
Patients with burns or scars over venipuncture sites
Obese patients
Patients requiring frequent blood tests
Patients receiving IV therapy
Patients at risk for venous thrombosis
Patients at risk for serious complications associated with deep venous puncture
Patients at risk for injury from restraints that may be needed for successful venipuncture
Patients for whom only one blood test has been ordered, for which a dermal puncture is appropriate

---

patients with burns or scars over venipuncture sites or in those at risk for **venous thrombosis** (caused when clots form within the veins), because venipuncture increases the risk of venous thrombosis. Other patients may be at risk for serious complications associated with deep vein puncture, including anemia, hemorrhage, infection, organ or tissue damage, arteriospasm, or cardiac arrest. In some patients who require restraints, blood is more safely drawn by dermal puncture than by venipuncture. Finally, patients for whom only one blood test has been ordered may be good candidates for dermal puncture.

Dermal puncture is usually the preferred method of collection for newborns, infants, and children younger than 2 years old. Young children's smaller veins and lower blood volume make venipuncture both difficult and potentially dangerous. Reducing blood volume through venipuncture is a concern for all children. It may lead to anemia and even cardiac arrest and death.

⌐>>> FLASH FORWARD

Special considerations for collection in children and the elderly are discussed in Chapter 12.

However, there are some tests that cannot be performed on blood from a dermal puncture. These include blood cultures, erythrocyte sedimentation rate, and most routine coagulation tests. Dermal puncture may not be appropriate for severely dehydrated patients, because test results may not be accurate. (This may also be a concern with venipuncture in such patients.) Dermal puncture should not be used at sites that are swollen, or where circulation or lymphatic drainage is compromised (such as a mastectomy).

DIFFERENCES BETWEEN VENOUS AND CAPILLARY BLOOD

A dermal puncture collects blood from capillaries. Because capillaries are the bridges between arteries and veins, blood collected by dermal puncture is a mixture of venous blood and arterial blood. The arterial proportion in the sample is increased when the collection site is warmed, as may be done to help increase blood flow before collection. Small amounts of tissue fluid from the puncture site may also be in the sample, especially in the first drop.

The levels of many substances are the same in both capillary and venous blood, but this is not the case for all substances, as indicated in Table 10-1. For instance, the normal potassium reading obtained by dermal puncture is lower than the normal potassium reading obtained by venipuncture. Because of these differences, results obtained from the two techniques cannot be compared. For this reason as well, it is important to record that the sample was obtained by dermal puncture.

 Clinical Tip: If a patient needs repeated determinations of potassium, calcium, total protein, hemoglobin, or glucose, you must use the same collection technique each time.

EQUIPMENT FOR DERMAL PUNCTURE

Dermal puncture equipment allows the phlebotomist to puncture the skin safely and collect the sample quickly and efficiently, with a minimum of discomfort for the patient.

Skin Puncture Devices

There are many different types of skin puncture devices (Figure 10-1). The oldest and simplest is a hand-held lancet, a thin, flat piece of steel with a very sharp tip. These are no longer used due to new safety regulations that require a retractable blade on the puncture device; instead, automatic devices have largely replaced these simple lancets in the modern health care environment. Automatic puncture devices deliver a swift puncture to a predetermined depth, which can be a significant advantage in sites where the bone is close to the skin (see "Site Selection"). The dimensions of the puncture are controlled by the width and depth of the point. Some automatic puncture devices have a platform that is positioned over the puncture site, color-coded for different depths. (The automatic devices designed for home glucose testing make a cut that is too small for multiple tests or for filling several microcontainers and are not used in clinical practice.) Safety features may include retractable blades and locks that keep a blade from being used a second time and prevent accidental sticks to the phlebotomist.

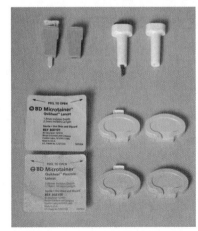

Figure 10-1
Skin puncture devices include simple lancets and automated devices that control the depth and width of the incision. (Courtesy of Zack Bent. From Garrels M, Oatis CS: Laboratory Testing for Ambulatory Settings: A Guide for Health Care Professionals. Philadelphia, Saunders, 2006.)

TABLE 10-1 Reference Values in Capillary and Venous Blood

Reference Values Higher in Capillary Blood	Reference Values Higher in Venous Blood
Hemoglobin	Potassium
Glucose	Calcium
	Total protein

The Lasette® laser lancing device is unique in that it uses a laser, rather than a sharp instrument, to pierce the skin, which causes less pain and bruising at the sample site. Cross-contamination between patients is avoided by disposing of the single-use lens cover between uses. The device is approved for patients 5 years and older.

Microsample Containers

Containers come in different sizes to accommodate different volumes of blood. From largest to smallest, they are microcollection tubes, micropipets (pronounced pie-PETS), and capillary tubes (Figure 10-2).

Microcollection tubes (also called "bullets") hold up to 750 μL (microliters) of blood. They are made of plastic and are available with a variety of anticoagulants and additives. The tubes are color-coded by additive to match the coding of evacuated containers. Microcollection tubes are used for all types of dermal puncture collections, and are the most common type of collection containers used for dermal puncture samples.

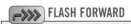 **FLASH FORWARD**

See Appendix A to review metric symbols.

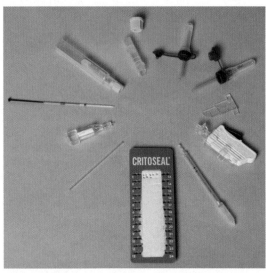

Figure 10-2
Microcollection tubes, micropipets, and capillary tubes are all used for dermal puncture collections. Microcollection tubes ("bullets") are increasingly used for all types of collection. (Courtesy of Zack Bent. From Garrels M, Oatis CS: Laboratory Testing for Ambulatory Settings: A Guide for Health Care Professionals. Philadelphia, Saunders, 2006.)

Micropipets, also called **Caraway** or **Natelson pipets**, are large plastic or glass capillary tubes with capacities up to about 470 μL. These tubes are used primarily for the collection of samples for ABG determinations. The use of these tubes has declined in recent years because of heightened attention to sharps injury prevention, and the Occupational Safety and Health Administration (OSHA) recommends against using glass tubes of this sort. They are available either plain, with a blue band, or heparin-coated, with a yellow or green band (colors may vary with the manufacturer). Once the sample is in the tube, one or both ends are sealed. Sealing used to be done by pushing the ends into soft clay. New, safer sealing methods are recommended that instead fit the ends with small plastic caps. Both ends must be sealed for an ABG determination. In the lab, the sample may be centrifuged to separate cells from plasma or serum. The sample can be removed with a syringe.

Capillary tubes, also called **microhematocrit tubes**, are small plastic tubes with a volume up to 75 μL. They are used primarily for hematocrit tests. Uncoated tubes have a blue band, and heparin-coated tubes have a red or green band. They are sealed in the same manner as micropipets. Although capillary tubes are not used routinely for dermal puncture collections, they are useful when only a serum sample is needed (although microcollection tubes are used even for this).

A micropipet and dilution system is useful for hematology or complete blood count (CBC) tests when a large sample is not needed for other tests. Called the BD Unopette™ system (BD, Franklin Lakes, NJ), it allows you to collect a very small blood sample, which is diluted to the correct volume for analysis in the Unopette reservoir. The system includes a capillary pipet in a holder, a pipet shield, and a sealed reservoir containing **diluent**, or liquid for dilution (Figure 10-3). In the lab, the sample is drawn into the analyzer directly.

Additional Supplies

As in venipuncture, alcohol pads are used to prepare the site, and gauze pads are used to help stop the bleeding. A sharps disposal container is needed for the lancet.

Warming devices increase circulation. Simple towels or washcloths may be soaked in warm water and applied to the site. Be sure that the site is completely dry before puncture, however, as residual water will cause hemolysis and dilution of the

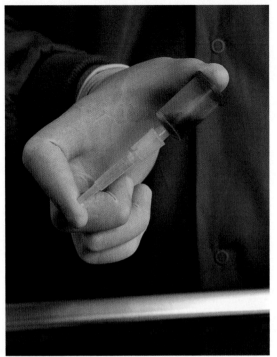

Figure 10-3
The BD Unopette™ system dilutes the sample to the proper concentration immediately after collection.

specimen. Commercial warming packs are also available. The pack is first wrapped in a dry towel and then activated by squeezing. Such "heel warmers" are often used when blood must be collected from infants. The temperature of the device should not exceed 42°C, and it should be applied for 3 to 5 minutes. *Glass slides* are used to prepare blood smears for microscopic examination of blood cells.

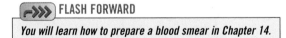 **FLASH FORWARD**
You will learn how to prepare a blood smear in Chapter 14.

SITE SELECTION
General Considerations
Dermal puncture should be performed on warm, healthy skin that is free of scars, cuts, bruises, and rashes. The site must be easily accessible and have good capillary flow near the skin surface, but there must be enough clearance above the underlying bone to prevent the lancet from accidentally contacting it. Bone puncture can lead to **osteochondritis**, a painful inflammation of the bone or cartilage, or **osteomyelitis**, a potentially serious, sometimes fatal, bone infection.

You should also avoid skin that has been damaged or compromised in any way. Specific areas to avoid include skin that is callused, scarred, burned, infected, bruised, edematous, or bluish. Also avoid previous puncture sites, and sites where circulation or lymphatic drainage is compromised.

Puncture Depth and Width
To minimize the risk of inflammation and infection, the lancet should never penetrate more than 3.0 mm. For a heel puncture, the maximum depth is 2.0 mm, because the **calcaneus**, or heel bone, can lie very close to the surface. In premature babies, the recommended depth is 0.65 to 0.85 mm.

Puncture width should not exceed 2.4 mm (Figure 10-4). In the right site, this achieves adequate blood flow but remains well above the bone. Puncture width is actually more important than depth in determining blood flow, because capillary beds may lie close to the skin, especially in newborns. A wider cut severs more capillaries and produces greater flow.

Dermal Puncture Sites in Adults and Older Children
For adults and for children older than 1 year, dermal punctures are almost always performed on the fingertips of the nondominant hand. The best sites are the palmar surface of the distal segments of the middle

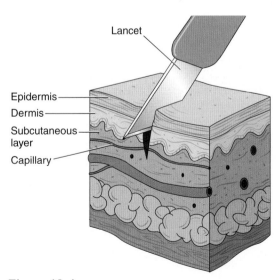

Labels: Lancet, Epidermis, Dermis, Subcutaneous layer, Capillary

Figure 10-4
The proper sites for dermal puncture are those that provide an adequate capillary bed and sufficient clearance from underlying bone.

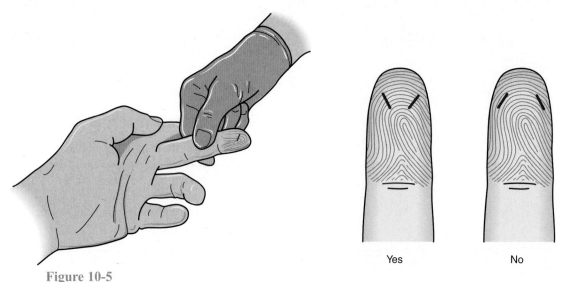

Yes   No

Figure 10-5
Dermal puncture in adults and children is performed on the middle or ring finger, on the palmar surface near the fleshy center of the distal segment.

and ring fingers (Figure 10-5). The thumb is likely to be callused, and the index finger's extra nerve endings make punctures more painful. The pinky has too little tissue for safe puncture. If the fingers cannot be used, the big toe may be an option—check the policy at your workplace. Earlobes are never used for dermal puncture.

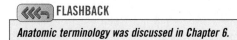 **FLASHBACK**

Anatomic terminology was discussed in Chapter 6.

The puncture should be made near the fleshy center of the chosen finger. Avoid the edge of the finger, as the underlying bone is too close to the surface. As indicated in Figure 10-5, the puncture should be made perpendicular to the ridges of the fingerprint, which lessens the flow of blood into the grooves.

Dermal Puncture Sites in Infants

For children younger than 1 year, there is too little tissue available in any of the fingers. For this reason, dermal puncture is performed in the heel. As shown in Figure 10-6, only the medial and lateral borders of the plantar (bottom) surface can be used. The center of the plantar surface is too close to the calcaneus, as is the posterior (back) surface. The arch is too close to nerves and tendons. In older infants, the big toe may be used if the heel is unacceptable.

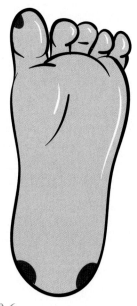

Figure 10-6
Dermal puncture in infants is performed on the heel, on the medial and lateral borders only.

DERMAL PUNCTURE PROCEDURE

Procedure 10-1 outlines the steps for a dermal puncture. In addition to these specific steps, you should always greet the patient, obtain consent, and identify the patient, as you would for a routine venipuncture.

Procedure 10-1
Dermal Puncture

1. **After documenting on the requisition that you are performing a dermal puncture, sanitize your hands and put on gloves.**

   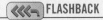 **FLASHBACK**

   Proper hand sanitation and gloving techniques were covered in Procedures 4-1 and 4-2.

   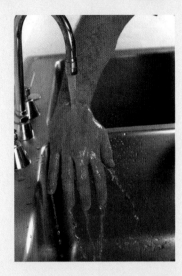

2. **Assemble your equipment.**

   Use the patient's age and the tests ordered to determine which type of collection tube you will need, what type of skin puncture device to use, and whether to use a warming device.

   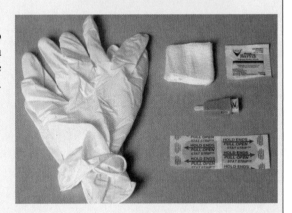

3. **Select and clean the site.**

   Warm the area first, if necessary. If the site feels cold, it should be warmed for at least 3 minutes with a temperature no greater than 42°C. If a wet washcloth is used, be sure to remove any residual water, as residual water will cause hemolysis and dilution of the specimen.

   Use 70% isopropyl alcohol to clean the site. Allow the site to dry completely. In addition to causing stinging, contamination, and hemolysis, residual alcohol interferes with the formation of rounded drops of blood on the skin surface. (Use of povidone-iodine is not recommended for dermal punctures, because it may elevate test results for bilirubin, uric acid, phosphorus, and potassium. Remember

Procedure 10-1—cont'd

Dermal Puncture

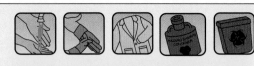

the acronym **BURPP** to help you learn this group of tests.)

Massaging the finger proximal to the puncture site (closer to the palm) can help increase blood flow. To avoid hemolysis, massage gently, and do not squeeze.

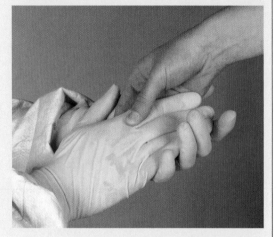

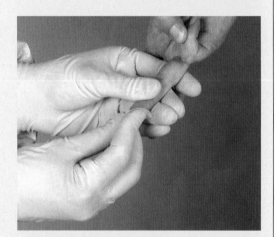

4. **Position and hold the area.**

   Hold the finger or heel firmly. This prevents it from moving during the puncture and also reassures the patient.

   Grasp the patient's finger with its palmar surface up, holding it between your thumb and index finger.

   To hold the patient's heel, place your thumb in the arch, wrap your hand over the top of the foot, and place your index finger behind the heel.

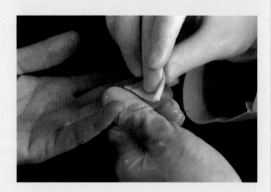

Procedure 10-1—cont'd

Dermal Puncture

5. **Make the puncture.**

Align the device so the cut is made across the fingerprint ridges or heel lines. This allows the blood to flow out and make a rounded drop, rather than run into the grooves. Do not lift the device immediately after the puncture is complete. Count to two before lifting the device to ensure that the blade has made the puncture to the full depth and then fully retracted. Scraping of the skin may occur if the blade is not retracted.

Dispose of the used blade immediately in an appropriate collection container.

Failure to obtain blood: If you are unable to obtain sufficient blood with the first puncture, the policy at most institutions is to attempt one more puncture. You must use a sterile lancet to make the new puncture. After two unsuccessful punctures, notify the nursing station and contact a different phlebotomist to complete the procedure.

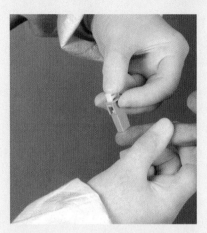

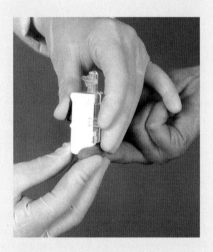

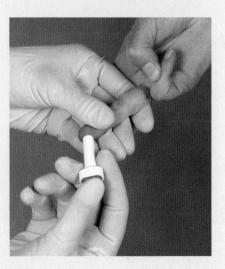

Procedure 10-1—cont'd
Dermal Puncture

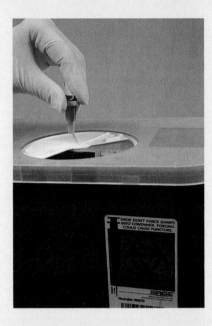

6. Prepare to collect the sample.

Wipe away the first drop of blood with a clean gauze pad, to prevent contaminating the sample with tissue fluid.

Keep the finger in a downward position to help encourage flow.

You can alternate applying and releasing firm pressure below the site to increase flow, but avoid *constant massaging*, as this will cut off flow, cause hemolysis, and introduce tissue fluid back into the sample.

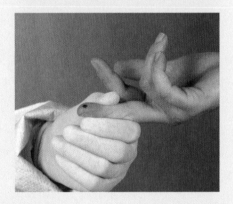

7. Collect the sample.

Once blood is flowing freely, position the container for collection.

Microcollection tubes should be slanted downward. Lightly touch the scoop of the tube to the blood drop, and allow the blood to run into the tube. Tap the container lightly to move blood to the bottom. Close the lid after the sample has been collected. Invert the tube 8 to 10 times after filling if additives are present.

Capillary tubes are held *horizontally* to prevent trapping air bubbles. Lightly touch the tube to the blood drop, and allow the tube to fill by capillary action. Do not allow the capillary

Procedure 10-1—cont'd
Dermal Puncture

tube to touch the skin. This allows tissue fluids to enter into the tube.

With either type of container, do not scrape the skin with the container. This causes hemolysis, activates platelets, and contaminates the sample with epithelial skin cells.

Order of collection: Blood smears are collected first, to minimize the effect of ongoing platelet aggregation at the puncture site. Platelet counts, CBCs, and other hematology tests are collected next, followed by other tests.

Seal the dry end using a small cap or other sealant.

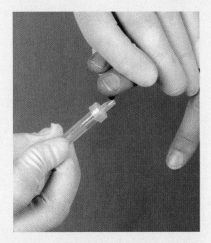

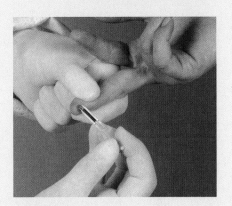

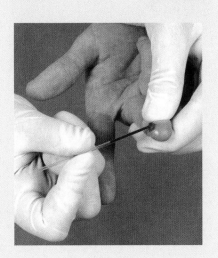

Procedure 10-1—cont'd
Dermal Puncture

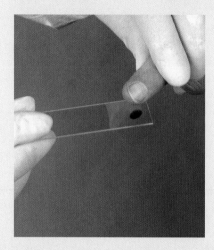

8. Complete the procedure.

Apply pressure to the puncture site using a clean gauze square. Once bleeding has stopped, you can bandage the site for older children and adults. Do not use a bandage on children younger than age 2, as they may remove the bandage and choke on it. When drawing blood from children and infants, be especially careful that all equipment has been picked up and bed rails have been placed back in position.

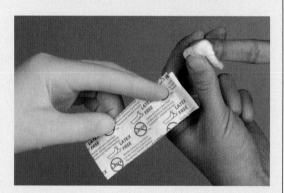

Place capillary tubes in a larger tube, and label the tube.

As always, thank the patient.

OTHER USES OF DERMAL PUNCTURE

In addition to serving as a substitute for venipuncture, dermal puncture is commonly used for bleeding time tests and bedside glucose testing (also called ancillary glucose testing). It can also be used as an alternative to arterial puncture for ABG determination, covered in Chapter 13.

Bleeding Time Test

A **bleeding time** (BT) **test** measures the length of time required for bleeding to stop after an incision is made. A BT test is a screening test that helps assess the overall integrity of primary hemostasis, involving the vascular system and platelet function. A BT test may be ordered before surgery. Abnormal results may be due to a number of different factors, including vascular disorders, platelet disorders, skin conditions, or medications that interfere with clotting, such as aspirin, streptokinase, or ethanol. An abnormal BT test result may be followed by further testing to determine the cause of the problem.

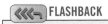 **FLASHBACK**

Hemostasis was discussed in Chapter 7.

The original BT test, developed in 1910 by Duke, was an earlobe puncture. This test is rarely performed today. In 1941, Ivy modified the test by performing it on the volar surface of the forearm, with constant pressure applied by a blood pressure cuff. Mielke improved the test further in 1969 by introducing a template that standardized the depth of the incision. The template has since been replaced by puncture devices that deliver the correct incision automatically. Incision depth is set at 1 mm, and length at 5 mm. Some devices make one incision; others make two incisions at the same time. The steps of the bleeding time test are shown in Procedure 10-2.

Results and Complications

Normal bleeding time is 2 to 10 minutes and depends somewhat on the device used. Bleeding that does not stop within 15 to 20 minutes means one of two things: Either the patient has a condition that is interfering with normal platelet plug formation, or the test was performed incorrectly—a capillary was scratched, the incision was too deep, or some technical error was made. If only one incision was made, the test may have to be repeated on the other arm. If two incisions were made and the two bleeding times are within several minutes of each other, it is unnecessary to repeat the test. Be sure to learn the exact protocol for your lab *before* this situation occurs. Abnormally short bleeding times are probably due to a test error—for instance, the incision may have been too shallow, the device may have been lifted too soon, or there may have been hair at the incision site.

Ancillary Blood Glucose Test

The **ancillary blood glucose test** is performed at the bedside, most often for patients with diabetes mellitus. Steps for this test are shown in Procedure 10-3. Blood collected by dermal puncture is applied to a paper reagent strip. Because different manufacturers have somewhat different procedures for their machines and test strips, be sure to read and understand the directions for the one you are using. Before any patient sample can be tested, the machine must be calibrated with materials provided by the manufacturer. This is usually performed by lab personnel at scheduled times. Control solutions must also be run using the same procedure as for the patient's test. These results are recorded as well. If any values fall outside the ranges provided by the manufacturer, troubleshooting must be performed until the values are correct. Proper calibration and control are critical for accurate results. Be sure to follow your institution's instructions exactly regarding performance and frequency.

REVIEW FOR CERTIFICATION

Dermal puncture is used in a variety of patients with compromised or otherwise inaccessible veins, including infants, or when only a small sample is needed. A calibrated puncture device delivers a precise, carefully controlled puncture, avoiding contact with the bone and reducing the risk of osteomyelitis or osteochondritis. The size and purpose of the sample dictate the collection container used, although microcollection tubes are increasingly used for most collections. The bleeding time test assesses the integrity of primary hemostasis by measuring the time required to stop bleeding after a standard incision is made. The ancillary blood glucose test uses blood from a standard dermal puncture to measure blood glucose levels on a paper strip.

Procedure 10-2

Bleeding Time Test

1. Assemble your equipment.
You will need:

- Antiseptic materials (alcohol pads)
- Blood pressure cuff
- Automated bleeding time device
- Stopwatch or timer with a second hand
- Filter paper
- Bandages

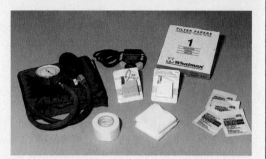

2. Prepare the patient.
Explain the procedure to the patient. Be sure to explain that scarring may occur, especially in dark-skinned patients.

Ask the patient about any medications he or she is taking or has taken recently, especially aspirin or other drugs that interfere with clotting. Salicylates, including aspirin, inhibit platelet function for 7 to 10 days after the last dose. Ibuprofen inhibits function for 24 hours. If the patient has taken such medications recently, follow the policy of your institution or consult with your supervisor about proceeding with the test.

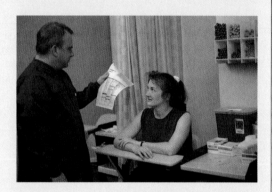

3. Position the arm, select the site, and clean the site.
Place the arm on a flat, steady surface, with the volar surface facing up. Select a site 5 cm below the antecubital crease. The area must be free of veins, scars, hair, and bruises. For patients with very hairy arms, you may need to shave the site before cleaning it. Clean the site and allow it to dry, as you would for other dermal procedures.

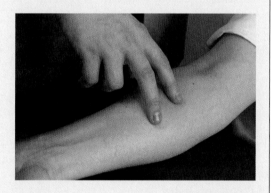

Procedure 10-2—cont'd

Bleeding Time Test

4. Apply the blood pressure cuff.

Place the cuff on the upper arm. Inflate it to 40 mm Hg. This pressure must be maintained throughout the procedure.

Wait 30 to 60 seconds to ensure that the pressure is stable before making the incision.

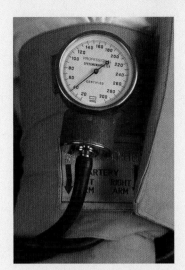

5. Position the device.

The blade may be placed either parallel or perpendicular to the antecubital crease. Although orienting the blade perpendicular to the crease produces less scarring, the results are not as accurate. Follow the policy set by your institution.

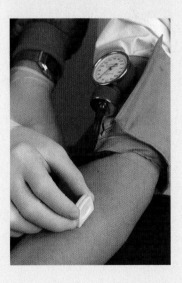

Procedure 10-2—cont'd

Bleeding Time Test

6. **Make the incision, and start timing.**
   Press the device on the arm without making an indentation.
   Press the trigger.
   Start timing as soon as the cut is made.
   Remove the device only after the blade has retracted.

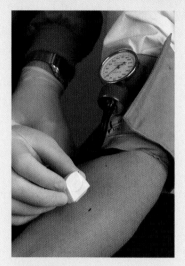

7. **Wick the blood away every 30 seconds.**
   Use filter paper to absorb blood from the cut without touching the incision. Touch the edge of the filter paper to the surface of the blood drop without touching the skin or the incision. Wick until the drop disappears.
   Repeat every 30 seconds.
   If two incisions are made, follow this procedure for each incision independently.

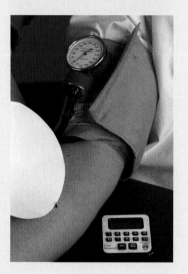

Procedure 10-2—cont'd
Bleeding Time Test

8. Complete the test.

When blood is no longer absorbed by the filter paper, bleeding has stopped.

Record the time.

Remove the pressure cuff.

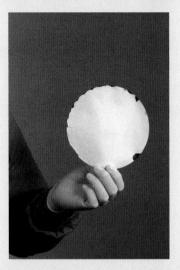

9. Attend to the patient.

Clean the arm and apply a butterfly bandage. Be sure to pull the edges of the incision together when applying the butterfly bandage. Instruct the patient to keep the bandage in place for 24 hours to minimize scarring.

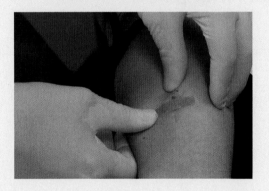

Procedure 10-3

Ancillary Blood Glucose Test

1. **Perform a routine dermal puncture (presented in Procedure 10-1).**

   Some manufacturers do not recommend wiping away the first drop of blood. Check the insert for the product you are using.

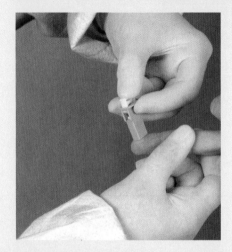

2. **Collect the sample.**

   You can either collect the blood drop directly on the strip or use a glass capillary tube to transfer blood to the strip.

   Cover the appropriate area on the stick with a free-falling drop of blood. Be careful not to touch the strip yourself or allow the patient's skin to touch it, because this can contaminate the strip.

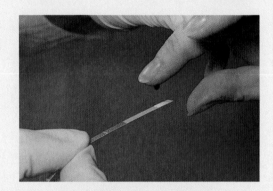

3. **Read and record the result.**

   Values that are well outside the range of normal (called "panic values") should be reported immediately to the nursing staff or the physician in charge. Your lab should have a policy regarding the exact values that trigger such notification.

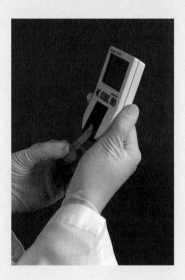

BIBLIOGRAPHY

Blumenfeld TA, Turi GK, Blanc WA: Recommended Site and Depth of Newborn Heel Skin Punctures Based on Anatomical Measurements and Histopathology. Lancet. February 1979.

Clinical and Laboratory Standards Institute: H45-A2: Performance of the Bleeding Time Test, ed 2. Villanova, PA. 2004.

Clinical and Laboratory Standards Institute: H4-A5: Procedures for the Collection of Diagnostic Blood Specimens by Skin Puncture, ed 5. Villanova, PA. 2004.

Hammond KB: Blood Specimen Collection from Infants by Skin Puncture. Laboratory Medicine ASCP 11, no 1. January 1980.

Smith B, Hill J: Performing a Capillary Puncture: SIP. Kettering Medical Center, School of Medical Technology, Kettering, OH, 1976. NIH Grant AH 00721.

STUDY QUESTIONS

1. Name two sites commonly used for adult capillary collection.
2. Explain why it is best to perform a dermal puncture rather than a venipuncture on children.
3. List six types of patients, other than infants, in whom dermal puncture may be advisable.
4. Explain why, in a dermal puncture, the first drop of blood is wiped away with clean gauze.
5. Describe what micropipets are used for.
6. Describe the Unopette system and what it is used for.
7. What can be used to stimulate blood flow to the capillaries?
8. List six specific areas of the skin to avoid when performing a capillary stick.
9. At what age are heel sticks preferred to finger sticks?
10. List four reasons why alcohol must air-dry before a capillary stick.
11. Explain why povidone-iodine should not be used for capillary collection procedures.
12. Which fingers are acceptable to use for dermal puncture?
13. Describe the order of collection for a dermal puncture.
14. Explain the purpose of the bleeding time test.
15. Why should bandages not be placed on young children following a dermal puncture?

CERTIFICATION EXAM PREPARATION

1. Dermal punctures are performed on:
   a. capillaries
   b. veins
   c. arteries
   d. arterioles

2. Which of the following has a higher value in capillary blood as opposed to venous blood?
   a. potassium
   b. calcium
   c. total protein
   d. hemoglobin

3. A red-banded microhematocrit tube contains which anticoagulant?
   a. sodium citrate
   b. potassium oxalate
   c. heparin
   d. EDTA

4. The Unopette system can be used for which kind of tests?
   a. chemistry
   b. blood banking
   c. hematology
   d. coagulation

5. An infant heel-warming device should be applied for approximately:
   a. 1 to 2 minutes
   b. 8 to 10 minutes
   c. 30 seconds
   d. 3 to 5 minutes

6. The depth of a heel puncture should not be more than:
   a. 3.0 mm
   b. 2.0 mm
   c. 2.0 cm
   d. 1.5 cm

7. Which finger is most widely used for capillary collection?
   a. thumb
   b. index
   c. ring
   d. pinky

8. In performing a dermal puncture, the puncture should be:
   a. aligned with the whorls of the fingerprint
   b. perpendicular to the whorls of the fingerprint

   c. on the edge of the finger
   d. on the tip of the finger

9. The location for heel sticks is the:
   a. center of the plantar surface
   b. medial or lateral borders of the plantar surface
   c. posterior surface
   d. arch

10. In a dermal puncture, which test is collected first?
    a. electrolytes
    b. blood smear
    c. platelet counts
    d. CBC

11. Which test cannot be collected by dermal puncture?
    a. glucose
    b. blood cultures
    c. CBC
    d. platelet counts

12. Which medication does not interfere with the bleeding time test?
    a. ethanol
    b. ibuprofen
    c. aspirin
    d. acetaminophen

13. At what level does the blood pressure cuff remain during a bleeding time test?
    a. 20 mm Hg
    b. 10 mm Hg
    c. 50 mm Hg
    d. 40 mm Hg

14. A normal bleeding time result is:
    a. 30 to 45 seconds
    b. 2 to 10 minutes
    c. 15 to 20 minutes
    d. 1 to 2 minutes

15. How frequently is the blood wicked during a bleeding time test?
    a. every 5 seconds
    b. every 10 seconds
    c. every 30 seconds
    d. every 45 seconds

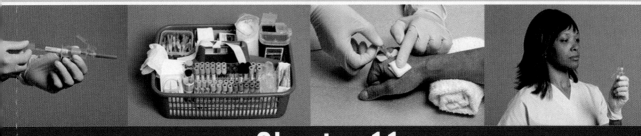

Chapter 11
Venipuncture Complications

OUTLINE

OBJECTIVES

After completing this chapter, you should be able to:

1. Explain the procedure to be followed
   in these situations:
   a. The patient is not in his or her room.
   b. The patient has no identification band.
   c. The patient is sleeping, unconscious,
      or apprehensive.
   d. Clergy or a physician is with the patient.
   e. Visitors are present.
   f. The patient cannot understand you.
   g. The patient refuses to have blood drawn.

2. List at least four sites that must be avoided when
   collecting blood, and explain why.
3. Describe techniques that can be used to help
   locate a vein.
4. Discuss limitations and precautions to be followed
   if a leg or hand vein is considered for
   venipuncture.
5. List at least two situations in which alcohol should
   not be used to clean the venipuncture site, and
   state at least one alternative.

Continued

OBJECTIVES—cont'd

6. Describe four potential problems associated with tourniquet application.
7. Define syncope, and explain what to do when a patient experiences this condition during the collection of blood.
8. Describe the actions to be taken if a patient has a seizure, complains of nausea, or vomits.
9. List three reasons why blood may not flow into a tube, and explain how to prevent or correct the problem.
10. Explain what should be done in the following situations:
    a. An artery is inadvertently punctured.
    b. No blood is collected on the first try.
    c. The patient requests something.
    d. There is prolonged bleeding from the puncture site.
11. List the causes of a hemolyzed sample, and name the test results that may be affected.
12. List tests that may be affected by a patient's position.
13. Describe five long-term complications associated with venipuncture, and explain how they can be avoided.
14. State reasons why a sample may be rejected by the laboratory.

KEY TERMS

compartment syndrome
emesis
hemolysis

lymphostasis
occluded
petechiae

reflux
sclerosed
syncope

ABBREVIATIONS

BURPP: bilirubin, uric acid, phosphorus, and potassium
CBC: complete blood count
ER: emergency room

ICU: intensive care unit
ID: identification
WIS: winged infusion set

Although most venipuncture collections are routine and without problems, complications can arise. Many factors can interfere with the collection of blood, but most complications can be dealt with by knowing what to expect and planning ahead. Complications include problems with access to the patient, site selection, site cleaning, tourniquet application, sample collection, completion of the procedure, and sample integrity. In addition, patients may experience long-term health-related complications from venipuncture. Specimens may be rejected for a variety of reasons, requiring a redraw. By learning the most common complications and the best approaches for avoiding or overcoming them, you will be better prepared in your work as a phlebotomist.

FACTORS THAT PREVENT ACCESS TO THE PATIENT

Locating the Patient

If the patient is not in his or her room, make every effort to locate the patient by checking with the nursing station. If the patient is in another department

and the test is a stat or timed request, proceed to that area and draw the blood there.

Always let the nurse know if the request needs to be rescheduled.

Identifying the Patient

As you learned earlier, positive identification of the patient is the most important procedure in phlebotomy.

Several situations can make identification difficult, including:

- Emergency requisitions
- Emergency room (ER) collections
- Orders telephoned in to the lab
- Requisitions picked up at the site

Despite the difficulties these situations may present, the information on the requisition *must* match exactly the information on the patient's identification (ID) band. *Any discrepancies must be resolved before collecting the specimen.* When the ID band is missing, contact the nursing station so that one can be attached by the nurse on duty. Even if an ID band is in the room, unless it is on the patient, you must not draw blood. Specific policies regarding the resolution of patient identification problems may vary from institution to institution. Be sure to follow the policy of your institution.

The American Association of Blood Banks requires special ID for patients receiving blood transfusions. Most institutions use a commercial ID system, in which the ID band comes with matching labels for the specimens. If you are collecting a blood bank specimen and your institution uses this system, be sure to have the appropriate labels.

BARRIERS TO COMMUNICATING WITH THE PATIENT

Sleeping or Unconscious Patients

Never draw blood from a sleeping patient. Instead, gently wake the patient before proceeding. Unconscious patients are often encountered in the ER and intensive care unit (ICU). If you know the patient to be unconscious, you may proceed with the collection. However, treat an unconscious patient just as you would a conscious one, including identifying yourself and describing the procedure. Unconscious patients may be able to hear you, even if they cannot respond.

Presence of Physicians or Clergy

If a physician or clergy member is in the room, return at another time for the procedure, unless it is a stat or timed collection. In that case, you should respectfully interrupt and explain the reason for the interruption.

Presence of Visitors

When you enter a room with visitors, greet them as you would the patient. Explain the purpose of your visit to the patient, and ask the visitors to step outside. If the patient is a child, the presence of visitors or family members during the collection may be helpful.

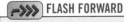 **FLASH FORWARD**

Collecting blood from children is covered in Chapter 12.

Apprehensive Patients

Many patients have some apprehension about being stuck with a needle or having their blood drawn. Most patients can be easily calmed by engaging them in a little distracting conversation on neutral topics such as the weather, traffic, or local news. If a patient is very nervous or you expect difficulty keeping the patient still or calm during the collection, it is helpful to request a nurse's assistance. This is especially true if the patient is a child.

Language Problems

When the patient cannot understand you, he or she cannot give informed consent. In this situation, you may need a translator. Alternatively, if you can effectively communicate with the patient by showing him or her what you will do, you may be able to obtain consent without a translator.

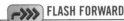 **FLASH FORWARD**

See Appendix B for useful Spanish phrases and vocabulary.

Patient Refusal

The patient always retains the right to refuse a blood collection. When a patient refuses to have his or her blood drawn, stress in a calm, professional way that the results are needed for treatment. If the patient still refuses, document this on the request, and notify the health care provider. Remember: Never force a patient to have blood drawn.

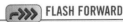 **FLASH FORWARD**

Informed consent and legal issues are discussed further in Chapter 18.

PROBLEMS IN SITE SELECTION

The antecubital fossa is the most common site for routine venipuncture. However, the presence of certain conditions at the chosen site may alter the quality of a specimen or cause harm to the patient. In that case, another site must be chosen.

Occluded Veins

Veins that are **occluded** (blocked) or **sclerosed** (hardened) feel hard or cordlike and lack resiliency. Occlusion and sclerosis can be caused by inflammation, disease, chemotherapy, or repeated venipunctures. Such veins are susceptible to infection, and because the blood flow is impaired, the sample may produce erroneous test results.

Hematomas

Hematomas may be caused by the needle going through the vein, by having the bevel opening only partially in the vein, or by failing to apply enough pressure after withdrawal. Blood from a hematoma is no longer fresh from the vein, and the hematoma can also obstruct the vein, slowing blood flow. Each of these factors can alter test results.

Edematous Tissue

The arm may appear swollen due to the accumulation of tissue fluid. Collection from edematous tissue alters tests results.

Burns and Scars

Areas with burns or scars are susceptible to infection and may be painful or difficult to penetrate.

Mastectomies

The removal of lymph tissue on the side of the mastectomy causes **lymphostasis**, or lack of lymph fluid movement. This can affect test results. The collection also may be painful to the patient, and the risk of infection may be increased.

Other Situations

Any condition resulting in disruption of skin integrity means that the site should be avoided. Open or weeping lesions, skin rashes, recent tattoos, or incompletely healed stitches are examples of sites that should be avoided because of the increased risk of infection.

Difficulty Finding a Vein

When you cannot find a vein, several techniques can help.

Check the Other Arm

Examine the other arm for a suitable site. Ask the patient about sites of previous successful phlebotomy.

Enhance Vein Prominence

- Massage gently upward from the wrist to the elbow.
- Dangle the arm in a downward position to increase blood in the arm.

- Apply heat. Moist heat should be avoided if possible.
- Rotate the wrist to increase the prominence of the cephalic vein.
- Tapping the antecubital area with the index and middle finger may help, but it increases the risk of damage to fragile skin.

Use a Blood Pressure Cuff

A blood pressure cuff can be used instead of a tourniquet for hard-to-find veins. Inflate the cuff halfway between the diastolic and systolic readings. The phlebotomist needs special training to use the blood pressure cuff in this way.

> **◀◀◀ FLASHBACK**
>
> *You learned about diastole and systole in Chapter 7.*

Use an Alternative Site

When a suitable vein cannot be found in the antecubital fossa, you will have to collect the blood from somewhere else—the hand, foot, or leg. The leg and foot are more susceptible to infections and clots, and they are not recommended sites for patients with diabetes or those on anticoagulant therapy (heparin or warfarin). Collection from the leg and foot usually requires the physician's permission.

The veins of the back of the hand (Figure 11-1) are small and fragile. For this reason, you should use a smaller gauge needle and tube, or a syringe.

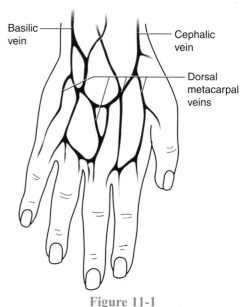

Figure 11-1
The veins of the back of the hand.

The steps in collecting blood from the back of the hand are similar to those for routine venipuncture, as described in Chapter 9. A winged infusion set (WIS), or butterfly, is ideal for a hand draw, because the tubing allows for a lower angle of insertion than a standard needle and tube holder. A syringe allows you to control the suction to protect the veins, which is particularly important for elderly and pediatric patients. Procedure 11-1 outlines hand collection using a WIS.

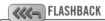 **FLASHBACK**

Butterflies were discussed in Chapter 8.

 FLASHBACK

Syringe collection was discussed in Chapter 9.

PROBLEMS ASSOCIATED WITH CLEANING THE SITE

Alcohol cannot be used for site cleaning when drawing a blood alcohol test. It is also not a strong enough disinfectant for drawing blood cultures and blood gases. In these cases, povidone-iodine is used instead. For patients allergic to iodine, chlorhexidine gluconate is available.

Povidone-iodine is not recommended for dermal punctures, because it may elevate test results for bilirubin, uric acid, phosphorus, and potassium (BURPP).

PROBLEMS ASSOCIATED WITH TOURNIQUET APPLICATION

Hemoconcentration

In Chapter 9, you learned that a tourniquet should not remain in place for more than 1 minute at a time. This is to prevent hemoconcentration, or alteration in the ratio of elements in the blood. When a tourniquet remains in place too long, the plasma portion of the blood filters into the tissue, causing an increase in the proportion of cells remaining in the vein. Primarily, this affects determinations of the large molecules, such as plasma proteins, enzymes, and lipids. It also increases red blood cell counts and iron and calcium levels. Prolonged tourniquet application can also alter potassium and lactic acid levels, by a different mechanism. These problems can be avoided by releasing the tourniquet as soon as blood flow begins in the first tube. Hemoconcentration can also be caused by pumping of the fist,

sclerosed or occluded veins, long-term intravenous therapy, or dehydration.

Formation of Petechiae

Petechiae are small, non-raised red spots that appear on the skin when the tourniquet is applied to a patient with a capillary wall or platelet disorder. The appearance of petechiae indicates that the site may bleed excessively after the procedure.

Tourniquet Applied Too Tightly

If there is no arterial pulse or the patient complains of pinching or numbing of the arm, the tourniquet is too tight. Loosen it slightly before proceeding.

Latex Allergy

Latex allergy is becoming increasingly common, and all patients *must* be asked whether they have a latex allergy. Nonlatex tourniquets and gloves are available. Latex bandages should also be avoided in these patients.

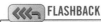 **FLASHBACK**

You learned about latex allergy in Chapter 3.

COMPLICATIONS DURING COLLECTION

Changes in Patient Status

Syncope

Syncope (pronounced SIN-co-pee) is the medical term for fainting. The patient's skin often feels cold, damp, and clammy before syncope. If syncope occurs during the procedure, remove the tourniquet and needle immediately, and apply pressure to the site. All incidents of syncope must be documented.

Seizures

If a patient has a seizure during the procedure, remove the tourniquet and needle immediately, and apply pressure to the site. *Do not* put anything in the patient's mouth; this is of no use during a seizure and can cause injury.

Nausea and Vomiting (Emesis)

When **emesis** occurs, reassure the patient and make him or her comfortable. Give the patient an emesis basin, and instruct him or her to breathe slowly and deeply. A wet washcloth for the head is often helpful.

Procedure 11-1

Hand Collection Using a Winged Infusion Set

1. **Assemble your equipment.**

Remove the WIS from the package. Straighten out the coiled tubing. Attach the WIS to the evacuated tube holder or the syringe.

Insert the first tube. Lay this assembly next to the patient's hand. If using a syringe, loosen the plunger by pulling the barrel in and out.

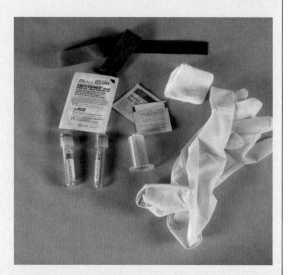

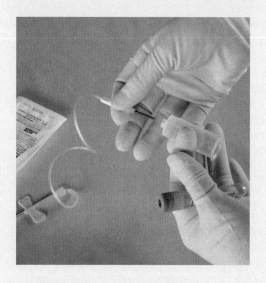

Procedure 11-1—cont'd

Hand Collection Using a Winged Infusion Set

2. Position the patient's hand, and apply the tourniquet.

Place the hand in an accessible position. Place a support (e.g., a towel) under the wrist, and ask the patient to gently curl his or her fingers under the hand. Tie the tourniquet in the usual manner around the wrist below the antecubital fossa.

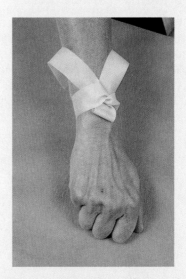

3. Insert the needle.

Choose the largest and straightest vein, and clean the site in the usual manner.

Anchor the vein firmly with your nondominant hand.

Grasp the needle between the thumb and index finger by folding the wings together in the middle.

Insert the needle into the vein, bevel side up and lined up in the direction of the vein. The angle of insertion should be 10 to 15 degrees.

Once the needle has entered the vein, a flash of blood should appear in the tubing. When using the syringe system, never pull the syringe plunger back if you do not see blood flash in the top of the syringe.

Gently thread the needle up the lumen of the vein until the bevel is not visible, keeping the angle shallow.

Hold the needle in place by one wing with the thumb of the opposite hand.

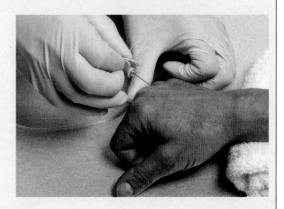

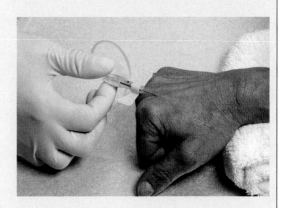

Procedure 11-1—cont'd

Hand Collection Using a Winged Infusion Set

4. Collect the sample.

If you are using evacuated tubes, push the collection tube into the adapter. Blood should appear in the tube. If you are using a syringe, pull the plunger back slowly, only matching the rate at which the blood is flowing into the syringe.

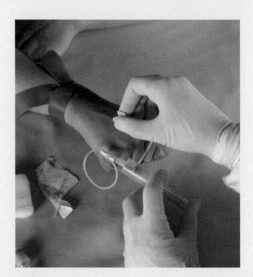

5. Finish the collection.

When the tube is completely filled, release the tourniquet and remove the needle. Activate the needle safety device.

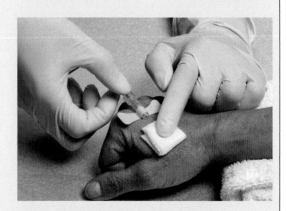

6. Attend to the patient.

Apply pressure to the site, as you would for routine venipuncture.

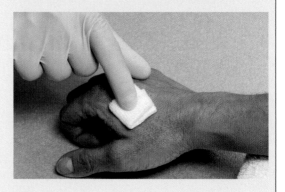

Procedure 11-1—cont'd

Hand Collection Using a Winged Infusion Set

7. **Dispose of the WIS.**

Special safety precautions must be observed when disposing of the WIS. The entire system should be gathered up in one hand. Leave nothing dangling that could get caught on something or cause an accidental needle-stick injury. Remove the tube from the adapter. Drop the tubing, needle, and the attached adaptor into the sharps container.

If using a syringe, discard the tubing and needle as above. Attach a needleless blood transfer device to the syringe in order to transfer the sample to the appropriate evacuated tubes, as outlined in Chapter 9.

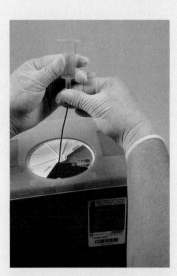

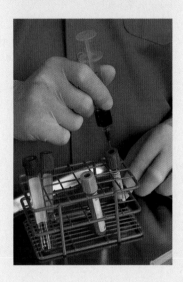

Pain

Warn the patient before the needle stick that there will be a little poke, pinch, or sting, to prevent the startle reflex.

Hematoma

When blood oozes from the vein into the surrounding tissue, a hematoma is formed. You can see the skin surrounding the puncture swell up and fill with blood. If this occurs during the procedure, remove the tourniquet and needle immediately, and apply pressure to the site. A cool cloth or cold pack can slow swelling from blood and ease pain.

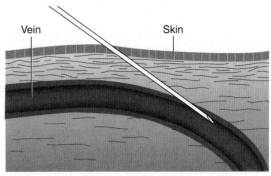

Figure 11-2
The bevel is stuck to the vein wall. Slightly rotate the needle.

Lack of Blood Flow

Lack of blood flow can be caused by a defective tube, an improperly positioned needle, or missing the vein. Intermittent or slow blood flow indicates improper needle position or a collapsed vein.

Defective Evacuated Tubes

Occasionally, blood will not flow into a tube because the vacuum in the tube has been depleted. This may occur from a manufacturing defect, use of an expired tube, or a very fine crack (which may occur if the tube is dropped). If the tube has been pushed past the indicator line on the holder before insertion in the vein, the vacuum has been depleted. Always take extra tubes to the bedside to be prepared for defects or errors.

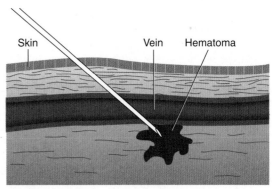

Figure 11-3
The needle has passed through both sides of the vein ("blowing" the vein). Slowly pull back on the needle.

 Clinical Tip: Be careful not to push the tube past the tube advancement mark.

Improperly Positioned Needle

If the tube is not the problem, the needle may not be properly positioned in the vein, and you may need to adjust it. When the needle is not in the correct position with respect to the vein, blood flow may stop or may be intermittent. Any one of the following may have occurred:

- The bevel is stuck to the vein wall. Slightly rotate the needle (Figure 11-2).
- The needle has passed through both sides of the vein ("blowing" the vein). Slowly pull back on the needle (Figure 11-3).
- The needle is not advanced far enough into the vein. Slowly advance the needle (Figure 11-4).

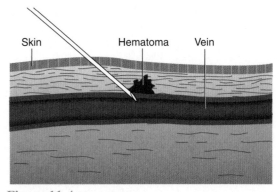

Figure 11-4
The needle is not advanced far enough into the vein. Slowly advance the needle.

- The vein was missed completely. Pull the needle out slightly, palpate to relocate the vein, and redirect the needle (Figure 11-5).

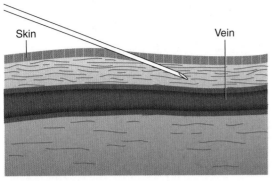

Figure 11-5
The vein was missed completely. Remove the tourniquet, pull the needle out slightly, palpate to relocate the vein, and redirect the needle.

- The tube is too large for the vein, causing the excessive vacuum to pull the vein onto the bevel and block blood flow. Remove the tube, wait a few seconds, and then switch to a smaller volume tube.

 Clinical Tip: Probing causes pain and hematoma. Do not probe if the needle is positioned incorrectly or if the vein cannot be located by palpation. Instead, repeat the puncture with a new tube and needle.

Collapsed Vein

A collapsed vein is caused by too much vacuum on a small vein. When using the evacuated tube system, a collapsed vein becomes evident when the tube is pushed onto the inner needle. During a syringe collection, it may occur when the plunger is pulled too quickly. Using smaller tubes or pulling the syringe plunger more gently can help prevent collapsed veins. Once a vein collapses, remove the tourniquet, pull out the needle, and select a different vein.

 Clinical Tip: Threading the needle up the vein minimizes collapsed veins and the likelihood of blowing the vein.

Inadvertent Puncture of the Artery

Puncture of the artery produces bright red blood and may also cause spurting or pulsing of blood into the tube. After sample collection and needle withdrawal, apply pressure for 5 minutes. The sample does not

have to be redrawn, but because some values are different for arterial versus venous blood, label the specimen as an arterial sample.

Failure to Collect on the First Try

The policy at most institutions is that a second try is acceptable. A new needle and tube must be used. For second tries, go below the previous site or use the other arm. After a second unsuccessful try, another phlebotomist should be found to draw blood from the patient.

PROBLEMS IN COMPLETING THE PROCEDURE
Patient Requests
Sometimes a patient may ask you for water or a change in bed position. Always check with the nurse on duty before you comply with any request.

Prolonged Bleeding

Normally, the site should stop bleeding within 5 minutes. However, aspirin or anticoagulant therapy can prolong bleeding times after the venipuncture procedure. In all cases, you must continue to apply pressure until the bleeding has stopped. Inform the nurse if the patient has a prolonged bleeding time. Failure to apply adequate pressure, particularly with patients on excessive doses of Coumadin or with a coagulation disorder, can cause compartment syndrome (see the following). In these patients, it is very important to apply pressure to the site beyond 5 minutes and ask the patient about any symptoms of significant pain.

FACTORS THAT AFFECT SAMPLE INTEGRITY
Hemolysis
Hemolysis is the destruction of blood cells, resulting in the release of hemoglobin and cellular contents into the plasma. Hemolysis can be caused by a range of factors, as indicated in Box 11-1. The serum or plasma is red in a hemolyzed sample, due to rupture of red blood cells. Hemolysis interferes with many test results, as shown in Box 11-2. The lab may request a redraw if the sample cannot give accurate results for the requested test.

Blood Drawn from a Hematoma

The blood in a hematoma is older than fresh venous blood, and use of such a sample can alter the results of some tests. The most frequent cause of hematoma

---

BOX 11-1 Causes of Hemolysis

Using too small a needle with respect to vein size
Using a needle smaller than 23 gauge (Usually any needle smaller than 23 gauge causes hemolysis)
Using a small needle with a large vacuum tube
Using a small needle to transfer blood from syringe to tube
Too much agitation of the blood
Vigorously mixing or shaking of tubes
Blood frothing, from a needle improperly attached to a syringe
Drawing blood too quickly into a syringe
Failing to allow the blood to run down the side of the tube when using a syringe to fill the tube
Forcing blood from a syringe into a vacuum tube

BOX 11-2 Tests Affected by Hemolysis

Seriously Affected
Potassium
Lactate dehydrogenase
Aspartate aminotransferase

Moderately Affected
Complete blood count (CBC)
Serum iron
Alanine aminotransferase
Thyroxine

Slightly Affected
Phosphorus
Total protein
Albumin
Magnesium
Calcium
Acid phosphatase

---

is improper insertion or removal of the needle, causing blood to leak or be forced into the surrounding tissue.

Patient Position

The position of the patient during collection can affect some test results (Box 11-3). The physician may request that an outpatient lie down before specimen collection.

Reflux of Anticoagulant

Reflux is the flow of blood from the collection tube back into the needle and then into the patient's vein. This is rare, but it can occur when the tube contents

---

BOX 11-3 Tests Affected by Patient Position

Cell counts
Hemoglobin or hematocrit
Protein
Albumin
Bilirubin
Calcium
Enzymes
Triglycerides
Cholesterol

---

come in contact with the stopper during the draw. Anticoagulant, as well as blood, may be drawn back into the patient's vein. This is a problem, because some patients have adverse reactions to anticoagulants (e.g., EDTA), and loss of additive from the tube can alter test results. It may also result in the contamination of the next tube with additive from the previous tube. To prevent reflux, keep the patient's arm angled downward, so that the tube is always below the site, allowing it to fill from the bottom up. Also, remove the last tube from the needle before removing the tourniquet or needle.

LONG-TERM COMPLICATIONS ASSOCIATED WITH VENIPUNCTURE

Anemia

Removal of as little as 3 or 4 mL of blood per day may result in the development of iron deficiency anemia in some patients. For this reason, it is important to minimize the amount of blood drawn and the frequency of collection. Your institution should have a procedure in place for documenting the total volume of blood drawn from a patient. If a single test is required, it may be appropriate to acquire blood with a dermal puncture instead of venipuncture.

Hematoma

The most common causes of hematoma are:

- Excessive probing to obtain blood.
- Failure to insert the needle far enough into the vein.
- The needle going through the vein.
- Failure to remove the tourniquet before removing the needle.
- Inadequate pressure on the site after removal of the needle.
- Bending the elbow while applying pressure.

Compartment Syndrome

In patients receiving excessive doses of anticoagulants such as Coumadin, or who have a coagulation disorder, such as hemophilia, routine venipuncture may cause bleeding into the tissue surrounding the puncture site. A small amount of blood leads to a hematoma. Larger amounts may cause **compartment syndrome**, a condition in which pressure within the tissue prevents blood from flowing freely in the blood vessels. This causes swelling and pain, and carries the risk for permanent damage to nerves and other tissues. Severe pain, burning, and numbness may be followed by paralysis distal to the puncture site. The patient should seek immediate medical attention if compartment syndrome is suspected.

Nerve Damage

Nerves in the antecubital area can be damaged if they are contacted with the needle during collection. The patient will experience a shooting pain or "electric shock" sensation down the arm, numbness, or tingling in the fingers. If the patient experiences this type of sensation, immediately remove the needle. The procedure should be performed at another site, preferably in the other arm. This incident should be documented according to your institution's protocol. To prevent nerve damage, avoid excessive or blind probing during venipuncture. *Avoid using the basilic vein whenever possible.*

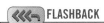 FLASHBACK

You learned about nerves in the antecubital area in Chapter 7.

BOX 11-4

Reasons for Specimen Rejection
No requisition form
Unlabeled or mislabeled specimens
Incompletely filled tube
Defective tube
Collection in the wrong tube
Hemolysis
Clotted blood in an anticoagulated specimen
Contaminated specimens and containers
Improper special handling

Infection

Infection can be prevented by proper aseptic technique before and during collection and by keeping the bandage on for at least 15 minutes afterward. Outpatients should be instructed to leave the bandage in place for at least that long.

SPECIMEN REJECTION

Specimens may be rejected by the lab for a variety of reasons (Box 11-4). Almost all of these can be avoided by proper care before, during, and after the procedure.

SPECIMEN RECOLLECTION

Sometimes, problems with the sample cannot be identified until after testing. In this case, another sample will have to be collected. Some of the reasons for recollection are shown in Box 11-5.

BOX 11-5 Reasons for Specimen Recollection

Site not properly cleaned
Use of the wrong antiseptic
Incomplete drying of antiseptic
Powder from gloves
Microscopic clots in an anticoagulated specimen
Contaminated specimens and containers
Improper special handling

REVIEW FOR CERTIFICATION

Complications of routine venipuncture may occur from a variety of causes. If the patient is not in the room, locate him or her if possible, especially if the collection is a stat request or for a timed test. Contact the nursing station for missing or improper ID bands. Apprehensive patients may need calming.

If the antecubital fossa is not appropriate due to scarring, burning, or other skin disruptions, use an alternative site such as the dorsal hand. Be aware of the potential for complications from improper tourniquet application. During the collection, remain aware of the patient's status, and be ready to cope with syncope, seizures, nausea, pain, and other responses to the procedure. Keep extra supplies handy in the event of defective tubes or needles. Specimen rejection, or redrawing and retesting, may be necessary due to improper collection, labeling, transport, or other errors.

BIBLIOGRAPHY

Clinical and Laboratory Standards Institute (CLSI). Procedures for the Collection of Diagnostic Blood Specimens by Venipuncture; Approved Standard—Sixth Edition. CLSI Document H3-A6. November, 2007.

Faber V: Lymph System's Intricacies Must Direct Phlebotomy. Advance for Medical Laboratory Professionals. February 8, 1999.

Flynn JC: What if the Patient Faints? (and Other Complications of Phlebotomy). Advance for Medical Laboratory Professionals. September 20, 1999.

Lindsay RL: Minimizing the Trauma of Phlebotomy. Laboratory Medicine. 1996.

Masoorli S. Caution: Nerve Injuries during Venipuncture. Nursing Spectrum. Retrieved 17 March 2006 from the world wide web: http://community.nursingspectrum.com/MagazineArticles/article.cfm?AID=13991

National Committee for Clinical Laboratory Standards: H 18-A: Procedures for the Handling and Processing of Blood Specimens. Villanova, PA, NCCLS, June 1984.

National Committee for Clinical Laboratory Standards: H3-A3: Procedures for the Collection of Diagnostic Blood Specimens by Venipuncture, ed 3. Villanova, PA, NCCLS, July 1996.

Roberge RJ, McLane M: Compartment Syndrome after Simple Venipuncture in an Anticoagulated Patient. Journal of Emergency Medicine. Jul–Aug 1999.

STUDY QUESTIONS

1. What must be done if the patient is not in the room when you come to collect a specimen?
2. What hospital protocol is followed when you are supposed to draw blood from a patient who is not wearing an ID bracelet?
3. How is an unconscious patient approached for blood collection?
4. Name six potential barriers to communicating with a patient.
5. Define hemolysis.
6. Define occluded, and describe what occluded veins feel like.
7. Describe where the tourniquet is applied when performing a dorsal hand stick.
8. What antiseptic must be used when collecting for a blood alcohol test?
9. List four things that can cause hemoconcentration.
10. What symptoms might a patient exhibit immediately before syncope?
11. How can you correct the position of a needle whose bevel has stuck to the vein wall?
12. What can cause a vein to collapse during a blood draw?
13. How many venipuncture attempts by a phlebotomist are usually considered acceptable?
14. How can a phlebotomist prevent reflux of an additive during collection?
15. List five reasons why specimens may be rejected.

CERTIFICATION EXAM PREPARATION

1. If a stat test is ordered and the patient is not in his or her room, you should:
   a. Wait in the patient's room until he or she returns.
   b. Leave the request at the nurse's station for the nurse to perform the draw.
   c. Locate the patient.
   d. Postpone the collection.

2. Which lab department may require special patient identification?
   a. microbiology
   b. chemistry
   c. hematology
   d. blood bank

3. Collapsed veins can be caused by:
   a. too large a needle for the vein
   b. too much vacuum asserted on the vessel
   c. the plunger being pulled too quickly
   d. all of the above

4. When an artery is inadvertently stuck during collection, all of the following are true *except:*
   a. The sample should be discarded.
   b. The blood will be bright red.
   c. The blood may spurt or pulse into the tube.
   d. Pressure should be applied for 5 minutes.

5. Which of the following could be a cause of hemolysis?
   a. vigorously mixing the tubes
   b. allowing the blood to run down the side of a tube when using a syringe to fill the tube
   c. drawing blood too slowly into a syringe
   d. using a needle larger than 23 gauge

6. Reasons for specimen recollection include all of the following *except:*
   a. incomplete drying of the antiseptic
   b. using the wrong antiseptic
   c. inadvertent puncture of an artery
   d. contamination by powder from gloves

7. To avoid reflux of an anticoagulant, you should do all of the following *except:*
   a. Keep the patient's arm elevated above the heart.
   b. Allow the tube to fill from the bottom up.

   c. Remove the last tube from the needle before removing the tourniquet.
   d. Remove the last tube from the needle before removing the needle.

8. Conditions that may alter the quality of a specimen or cause harm to the patient during a blood draw include:
   a. edematous tissue
   b. mastectomies
   c. hematomas
   d. all of the above

9. When performing a butterfly draw using a hand vein, place the tourniquet:
   a. on the patient's arm above the antecubital fossa
   b. on the patient's arm below the antecubital fossa
   c. on the patient's wrist
   d. A tourniquet is not required for a butterfly draw.

10. Povidone-iodine is not recommended for:
    a. blood alcohol draws
    b. dermal punctures
    c. blood gas draws
    d. blood cultures

11. Hemolysis is:
    a. the flow of blood from the collection tube back into the needle and the patient's vein
    b. alteration in the ratio of elements in the blood
    c. lack of lymph fluid movement
    d. destruction of blood cells

12. Test results affected by patient position include all of the following *except:*
    a. albumin
    b. blood alcohol
    c. cholesterol
    d. enzymes

13. Lymphostasis is:
    a. the flow of blood from the collection tube back into the needle and the patient's vein
    b. alteration in the ratio of elements in the blood
    c. lack of lymph fluid movement
    d. destruction of blood cells

14. To enhance vein prominence, you can:
    a. Elevate the arm in an upward position.
    b. Tap the antecubital area with your index and middle finger.
    c. Squeeze the patient's wrist.
    d. Apply a cold pack.

15. Hemoconcentration is:
    a. the flow of blood from the collection tube back into the needle and the patient's vein
    b. alteration in the ratio of elements in the blood
    c. lack of lymph fluid movement
    d. destruction of blood cells

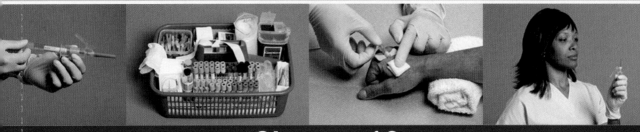

Chapter 12

Blood Collection in Special Populations

OUTLINE

OBJECTIVES

After completing this chapter, you should be able to:

1. Describe two physiologic differences between children and adults that should be considered when collecting blood from infants and children.
2. Describe steps that can be taken to help reduce a child's anxiety and make the venipuncture experience more pleasant.
3. Explain how blood collection supplies and the venipuncture procedure are modified for infants and children.
4. List the steps in dorsal hand vein puncture in children.
5. Define bilirubin, explain its significance, and describe precautions that must be observed when collecting blood for bilirubin testing.
6. Explain the usual procedure for collecting blood for neonatal screening tests, and list five tests that may be done.
7. Explain physical changes that may occur with aging that should be considered when collecting blood.
8. List conditions that may require blood draws for an extended period of time, and alternative collection sites for these patients.
9. Define vascular access device, and describe eight types.
10. Describe how blood should be collected from a vascular access device.
11. List steps to be followed when collecting blood from a patient with an intravenous line in place.

KEY TERMS

arterial line	fistula	maple syrup disease
arteriovenous shunt	galactosemia	peripherally inserted central
Bili light	Groshong	catheter
bilirubin	heparin lock	phenylketonuria
biotinidase deficiency	Hickman	saline lock
Broviac	homocystinuria	sickle cell anemia
central venous catheter	hypothyroidism	triple lumen
central venous line	implanted port	vascular access device
EMLA	internal arteriovenous shunt	
external arteriovenous shunt	jaundice	

ABBREVIATIONS

AV: arteriovenous
CBC: complete blood count
CVC: central venous catheter
ER: emergency room
ICU: intensive care unit
ID: identification

IV: intravenous
PICC: peripherally inserted central catheter
PKU: phenylketonuria
TLC: tender loving care
VAD: vascular access device

Four special populations—pediatric patients, geriatric patients, patients requiring chronic blood draws, and patients in the emergency room or intensive care unit—have special needs and require special knowledge and procedures to collect blood safely and considerately. In young children, loss of blood volume and the child's fear of the procedure are paramount concerns; in geriatric patients, skin changes and the possible presence of hearing loss or mental impairment are important considerations. Patients with certain diseases require regular blood tests for an extended or indefinite period, and the sites commonly used for drawing blood may become damaged from overuse. Patients in the emergency room or intensive care unit may have vascular access devices or intravenous lines in place. Only specially trained personnel can draw blood from these devices on a physician's order, but the phlebotomist may be called on to assist in the draw or handle the samples during and after collection. Each of these special populations requires approaches and equipment beyond those needed for routine blood collection. By understanding these special requirements, you will gain the skills you need to collect blood from the widest possible patient population.

perform phlebotomy on children than on adults, you should master your collection methods on adult patients first. Similarly, you should master collection in older children before moving on to young children and infants.

Special Physiologic Considerations

Children have a lower total blood volume than adults do. The younger (and smaller) the child, the lower the volume that can be safely withdrawn. For example, a 150-pound adult has about 5 liters of blood, so a 10-mL sample represents about 0.2% of total blood volume. In contrast, that same sample from a 1-year-old child represents 1% of total blood volume, and in a newborn about 3%. Removal of more than 10% can cause cardiac arrest. Repeated withdrawal of even smaller amounts may cause anemia. Infants and children should not have more than 5% of their blood volume removed within a 24-hour period unless medically necessary. Removal of 3% or less is the preferred maximum. No more than 10% should be removed over a 1-month period unless medically necessary. Table 12-1 provides guidelines for determining safe volumes that may be withdrawn.

PEDIATRIC PATIENTS

Collecting blood from pediatric patients presents both technical and psychological challenges. Because greater technical expertise is required to

 Clinical Tip: When collecting blood from a child, log the time and the volume of blood taken to avoid blood depletion.

TABLE 12-1 Blood Volume and Safe Withdrawal Calculations in Newborns and Infants

Age	Approximate Blood Volume/kg Body Weight	Patient Weight	× 0.03, Maximum Safe Withdrawal of 3%		Safe Volume for Withdrawal in 24 Hours
Premature neonate	95 mL/kg		× 0.03	=	
Full-term neonate	85 mL/kg		× 0.03	=	
Newborn	80 mL/kg		× 0.03	=	
1–12 Months	75 mL/kg		× 0.03	=	
Example: 7 lb Newborn	80 mL/kg	3.2 kg	× 0.03	=	7.68 mL

Dermal puncture requires a very small amount of blood and is the most common pediatric collection procedure. However, it cannot be used when a larger volume of blood is required, such as for blood culture or crossmatch testing. For blood culture in infants and small children, a sample of 1 to 5 mL is required. Consult with the laboratory's procedures manual for specific information on minimum draw volumes in infants.

Newborns also have a higher proportion of red blood cells than adults do (60% vs. 45%) and a lower proportion of plasma (40% vs. 55%), so more blood may be needed to obtain enough serum or plasma for testing.

Newborns and infants are also more susceptible to infection, because of the immaturity of their immune systems. Extra precautions should be taken to avoid exposing this group to potential sources of infection. Protective isolation procedures discussed in Chapter 4, are often used.

Special Psychological Considerations

Children differ in their levels of understanding, ability to cooperate, and anxiety about medical procedures. For many children, needles represent pain, and their fear of pain often makes the collection procedure challenging for the phlebotomist. In addition to the fear of pain, children may be anxious about being in a hospital and away from home. Some children associate a white coat with all these fears, and seeing a strange person in a white coat enter the room can increase their anxiety level even before they see a needle.

As a phlebotomist, your goal is to make the collection as calm, comfortable, and painless as possible for the child (Figure 12-1). Keeping the child calm not only helps the child, but also helps you carry out the procedure. Prolonged crying also affects the white

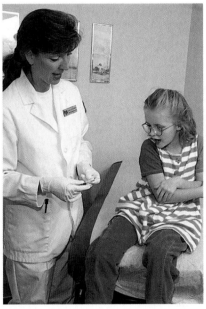

Figure 12-1
It is important that a phlebotomist use a calming approach with children. (From Chester GA: Modern Medical Assisting. Philadelphia, WB Saunders, 1998.)

blood cell count and the pH level of the blood; therefore, a calm experience ensures accurate test results.

Several strategies can be used to reduce the child's anxiety. Not all of them work for every child, and some are more appropriate for children of certain ages or dispositions. As you gain experience, you will be able to gauge how to best approach each child. To minimize the child's anxiety:

- Prepare your material ahead of time, before you encounter the child. This means less time for the child's anxiety to build before the stick.
- If possible, perform the procedure in a room that is not the child's hospital room. This allows the child to feel safe in his or her bed.

- Be friendly, cheerful, and empathetic. Use a soothing tone of voice.
- Explain what you will be doing in terms that are appropriate for the child's age. Even if the child will not or cannot respond, your explanation helps the child understand what is about to happen, lessening the fear of the unknown. Demonstrating on a toy can be helpful.
- *Do not say* that it will not hurt. Rather, explain that it will hurt a little bit and that it is okay to say "ouch" or even to yell or cry, but emphasize the need to keep the arm still.
- Give the child choices whenever possible, to increase his or her feeling of control. You can ask the child which arm or finger to use or which type of bandage he or she prefers. This also keeps the child occupied, lessening anxiety.
- Use the shortest possible needle for the procedure, and keep it out of sight for as long as possible.
- Distract the child just before the actual stick, so that he or she is looking away. If parents or siblings are in the room, they can be helpful here.
- During the draw, tell the child how much longer it will be ("just one more tube" or "a few more seconds"). This can help keep the child's anxiety from building during the procedure.
- Afterward, praise the child (even if he or she did not cooperate as well as you had hoped) and offer him or her a small reward, such as a sticker (for younger children) or a pencil (for older children).

Involvement of Parents and Siblings

Parents who are present during the procedure can help in several ways. Ask the parent whether the child has had blood drawn previously and, if so, what techniques helped ease the child's anxiety. Parents or siblings can help distract and comfort the child. Siblings should be offered small rewards as well.

Some parents may prefer not to remain with the child during the procedure because they are reluctant to see the child in pain or become queasy at the sight of blood. Respect their wishes. In some cases, parents can make the child more anxious through their words or reactions. If you feel that the parents cannot help the child, you can politely suggest that they might be more comfortable waiting outside.

Identification of Newborns

On their identification (ID) bracelets, newborns may be identified only by their last names, such as "Baby Boy (or Girl) Smith." As always, use the hospital ID number, not the name, as the ultimate proof of identification. Be especially careful with twins, who are likely to have similar names and ID numbers.

Supplies

When performing venipuncture, use shorter needles, if possible, and use the smallest gauge consistent with the requirements of the tests. Butterfly needles and smaller pediatric tubes should be used.

You may need additional protective equipment in the premature nursery (and possibly in the full-term nursery, as well) to reduce the risk of spreading infection. Check with the nursery supervisor regarding policy.

Take along a selection of rewards, such as stickers or small toys. Keep a stock of cartoon bandages as well. In a pinch, you can draw a smiley face on a regular bandage. Remember not to use these on infants younger than 2 years, due to the danger of choking.

Anesthetics

Topical anesthetic cream may be useful for venipuncture procedures in pediatric patients. The most commonly used agent is EMLA. It must be applied 60 minutes before the draw, however, which means that the site must be chosen at that time. It is possible to numb more than one area if it is not practical to choose the site ahead of time. Anesthetic is not recommended for phenylketonuria (PKU) testing (see later).

Immobilization of Infants and Children

Immobilizing pediatric patients may be necessary to ensure their safety during the draw. Wrapping newborns or very young infants in a receiving blanket is usually sufficient, as they are not strong enough to work themselves loose during the procedure. Older babies, toddlers, and young children need to be restrained. Older children may have the self-control to keep from moving, but a parent's care and attention can still be beneficial during the draw.

Pediatric draws are done with the patient either seated in the lap of a parent or other assistant or lying down, with the parent or assistant leaning over the child. For a seated child, the parent hugs the child's body and holds the arm not being used in the draw (Figure 12-2*A*). For a child lying down, the parent or assistant leans over the child, holding the unused arm securely (see Figure 12-2*B*). The assistant may

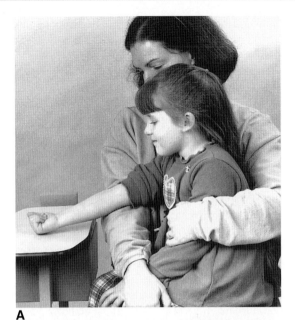

A

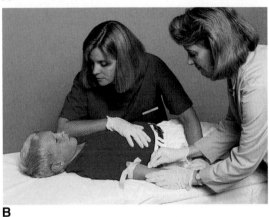

B

Figure 12-2
Suggested ways to restrain a child for phlebotomy. **A,** The parent hugs the child's body and holds the arm not being used in the draw. **B,** Obtaining a draw from a restrained child in a lying-down position. (*A* from Flynn JC: Procedures in Phlebotomy, ed 2. Philadelphia, WB Saunders, 1999, p 137; *B* from Wong D: Whaley and Wong's Nursing Care of Infants and Children, ed 6. St. Louis, Mosby, 1999.)

support the arm from behind, at the bend in the elbow, which helps immobilize the arm.

Pediatric Dermal Puncture

The procedures for dermal puncture were discussed in Chapter 10. As you learned in that chapter, heel puncture is preferred for children younger than age 1 year, because the tissue overlying the finger bones is not thick enough for safe collection there. Safe areas for heel collection were diagrammed in Figure 10-6.

Special Considerations

Several special considerations apply when performing dermal punctures in newborns and young children:

- The ID band must be present on the infant. Be sure to match the ID number to the number on the requisition.
- Keep your equipment out of the patient's reach.
- Warm the heel for 3 to 5 minutes, using a heel-warmer packet. The packet contains sodium thiosulfate and glycerin, which undergo a chemical reaction when activated by squeezing. Wrap the packet in a towel before placing it against the skin.
- At the end of the procedure, be sure to remove all equipment from the crib and secure all bed rails in the up position.
- Avoid using adhesive bandages.
- Document the collection in the nursery log sheet. Record the date, time, and volume of blood collected.

Special Dermal Puncture Procedures

Neonatal Bilirubin

Bilirubin is a substance produced by the normal breakdown of red blood cells. The liver is responsible for further processing of bilirubin so it does not reach excessive levels in the blood. In newborns the liver may not be developed enough to prevent bilirubin from accumulating in the blood. When this occurs, blood must be collected to assess the patient's clinical response to treatment to decrease bilirubin blood levels.

Excess bilirubin levels commonly occur when mother and child have mismatched blood groups, and antibodies from the mother break down the infant's red blood cells, increasing bilirubin levels beyond the infant's capacity to process it. Build-up of bilirubin causes **jaundice,** or yellowing of the skin, and can lead to brain damage if it is untreated.

When bilirubin is slightly above normal in a newborn, a **"Bili light,"** or ultraviolet light treatment, can be used. Higher levels, or levels that are rising rapidly, require blood transfusion.

Collection Precautions. Keep the following points in mind when collecting blood for bilirubin testing:

- Bilirubin is light sensitive. Bili lights should be turned off during collection. The specimen should be shielded from light using an amber-colored container, foil, or heavy paper to cover the container.

- Hemolysis of the specimen falsely lowers the results, so precautions against hemolysis must be taken.
- Collection times must be recorded exactly to track the rate of bilirubin increase. Samples for bilirubin testing are frequently collected as timed or STAT specimens.

Neonatal Screening

Neonatal screening tests are used to detect inherited metabolic disorders that cause severe brain damage. U.S. law mandates screening for **hypothyroidism** and **PKU.** Other diseases that are screened include **galactosemia, homocystinuria, maple syrup disease,** and **biotinidase deficiency. Sickle cell anemia** is an inherited disorder of the hemoglobin molecule that may also be screened for in newborns from ethnic groups with the highest risk.

Specimen Collection. Blood for neonatal screening is collected by capillary heel stick on special filter paper. Dorsal hand vein collection is not recommended. Recent studies have shown that the levels of phenylalanine are significantly different between capillary and venous samples. Reference values are based on capillary values.

The filter paper is supplied in a kit provided by the state agency responsible for screening tests (Figure 12-3). Both the ink and the paper are biologically inactive. When using the paper, you must be careful not to touch or contaminate the area inside the circles, as this will alter the results.

To collect a sample for neonatal screening, first perform a routine heel stick. Wipe away the first drop of blood, and then apply one large drop of blood directly to the circle. The drop must be evenly spread (see Figure 12-3*B*). Although applied to only one side of the filter paper, the blood should be visible from both sides. Air-dry the specimen in a suspended horizontal position. Keep it at room temperature and away from direct sunlight until it is delivered to the lab.

Screening samples also can be collected in a heparinized capillary tube and then transferred to the filter paper. However, direct application of the blood to the circle is the preferred method.

Venipuncture in Newborns

When a larger volume of blood is required, blood can be collected from newborns or children younger than age 2 years by venipuncture of the dorsal hand veins. A 23-gauge butterfly needle is used to puncture the vein, and blood is dripped from the hub

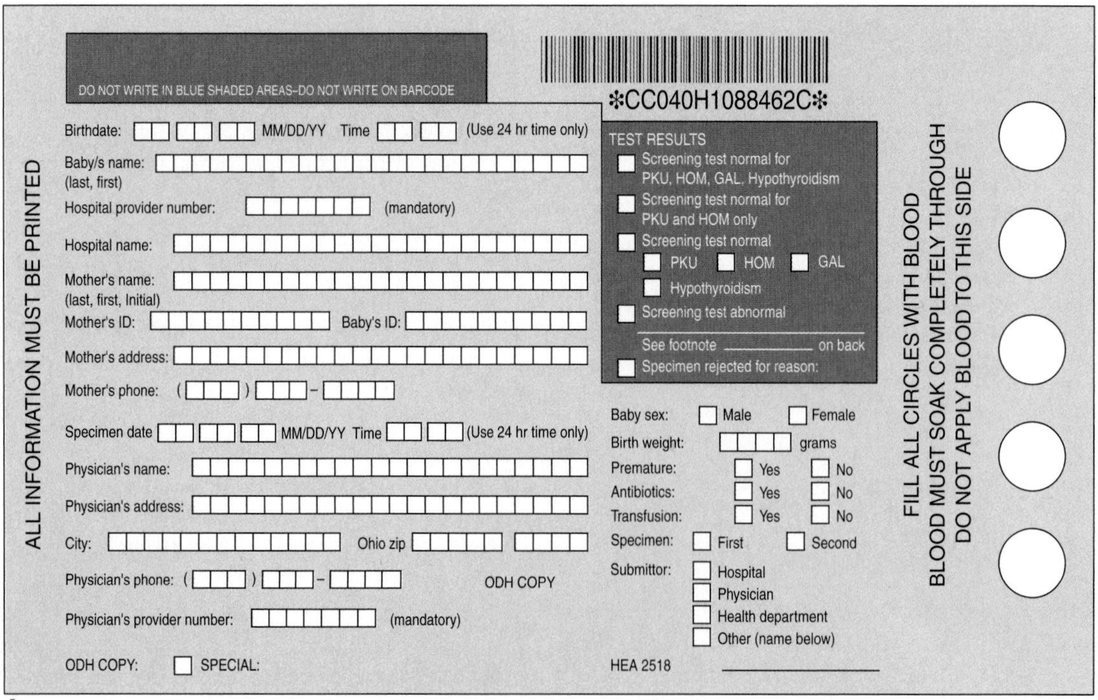
DO NOT WRITE IN BLUE SHADED AREAS-DO NOT WRITE ON BARCODE
CC040H1088462C
ALL INFORMATION MUST BE PRINTED
Birthdate: MM/DD/YY Time (Use 24 hr time only)
Baby/s name: (last, first)
Hospital provider number: (mandatory)
Hospital name:
Mother's name: (last, first, Initial)
Mother's ID: Baby's ID:
Mother's address:
Mother's phone: ( ) -
Specimen date MM/DD/YY Time (Use 24 hr time only)
Physician's name:
Physician's address:
City: Ohio zip
Physician's phone: ( ) - ODH COPY
Physician's provider number: (mandatory)
ODH COPY: SPECIAL:
TEST RESULTS
Screening test normal for PKU, HOM, GAL, Hypothyroidism
Screening test normal for PKU and HOM only
Screening test normal
PKU HOM GAL
Hypothyroidism
Screening test abnormal
See footnote on back
Specimen rejected for reason:
Baby sex: Male Female
Birth weight: grams
Premature: Yes No
Antibiotics: Yes No
Transfusion: Yes No
Specimen: First Second
Submittor: Hospital Physician Health department Other (name below)
HEA 2518
FILL ALL CIRCLES WITH BLOOD
BLOOD MUST SOAK COMPLETELY THROUGH
DO NOT APPLY BLOOD TO THIS SIDE

A

Figure 12-3
A, An example of filter paper used in neonatal screening.

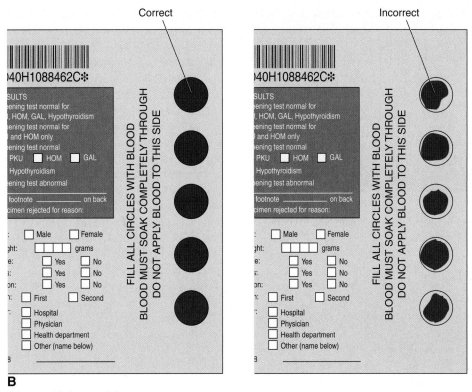

Figure 12-3, cont'd

B, Correct and incorrect ways to fill in the circles. (Modified from Bonewit-West K: Clinical Procedures for Medical Assistants, ed 5. Philadelphia, WB Saunders, 2000.)

directly into a microcollection container. A 3-mL syringe may be used for collection instead, followed by transfer to the microcollection container. Special considerations include the following:

- No tourniquet is needed. Instead, clasp the infant's wrist between your middle finger and forefinger, and allow the infant to encircle your thumb with its fingers. Flex the wrist gently downward while you examine the dorsal surface of the hand.
- Once blood begins to flow, you can release your hold on the needle and use your free hand to fill the microcollection containers.
- After withdrawing the needle, apply firm pressure with sterile gauze until the bleeding stops. Do not apply a bandage, as the child may remove it and place it in his or her mouth.

Scalp vein venipuncture can be used when other venipuncture sites are not accessible. The scalp vein is located by applying a large rubber-band tourniquet around the scalp at the level of the forehead and shaving the hair, if necessary. This procedure requires additional training and expertise.

GERIATRIC PATIENTS

With the aging of the population, many of your patients are likely to be geriatric patients. As with infants, collection from geriatric patients presents both physical and psychological challenges. Working with geriatric patients also can bring considerable rewards for a phlebotomist who takes the time to get to know his or her patients as people.

As do all patients, geriatric patients need and deserve respect from the health care professionals with whom they come in contact. Geriatric patients may feel less in control of their medical situations than other patients do, and some may feel apprehensive about having you perform a collection. As you would with any patient, treat your geriatric patients with consideration for their special concerns and needs. A little extra tender loving care (TLC) goes a long way in this population (Figure 12-4). You can help ease their anxiety by being friendly and cheerful. Taking the time to listen to your patients and to talk with them can make the experience not only easier for you both but also more rewarding.

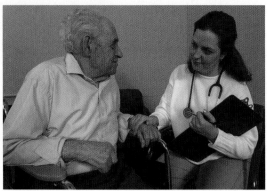

Figure 12-4
Phlebotomists should always be considerate and respectful of geriatric patients.

Physical Changes

As people age, their bodies undergo a number of changes that may have an impact on the safety and effectiveness of normal collection procedures. Skin changes are among the most important. The amount of collagen in the skin is reduced, so the skin becomes less elastic, and the layers of skin become thinner. Bruising is more likely, and it takes longer to replace cells, so that longer healing times are needed.

 Clinical Tip: Treat the skin of geriatric patients gently. Try massaging the site rather than slapping the arm for a vein or squeezing a finger.

Blood vessels, too, become less elastic and more fragile. Vessels may narrow due to atherosclerosis. Loss of supporting connective tissue leads to "loose skin," and loss of muscle tissue may allow veins to move from their usual locations. Veins are often closer to the skin; therefore, the penetration angle of the needle needs to be reduced.

Arteries are often closer to the surface in geriatric patients. Do not mistake an artery near the surface for a vein. Before sticking it, check your target "vein" to make sure it is not pulsing.

Common Disorders

Many conditions in geriatric patients may lead to the need for assistance in the draw, whether from other staff or from a family member.

Hearing loss is common among geriatric patients. Begin your encounter with a patient by speaking slowly and deliberately to be sure the patient under-

stands. (However, do not continue using this style once the patient clearly indicates that he or she understands your normal speaking voice.)

A number of conditions, including Parkinson's disease and stroke, can lead to unclear speech. Remember that difficulty speaking does not imply difficulty understanding.

Arthritis affects a large percentage of geriatric patients. Arthritis may prevent your patient from fully straightening his or her arm or fingers. Do not force a patient's arm flat; ask if the patient can do this or whether the action is uncomfortable. When the arm cannot be straightened, a butterfly may be useful in the antecubital area.

Many patients may be on anticoagulant therapy for previous heart attacks or strokes. Be aware of this possibility, especially because of the delay in clotting time it is likely to cause. These patients have an increased risk of hematoma.

Poor nutrition or chronic degenerative disease may lead to emaciation. Nutritional status can affect skin health, hemostasis, and ability to tolerate blood loss. Geriatric patients also may have increased susceptibility to infection due to disease or loss of immune function with age.

Tremor is common in advanced old age and may make it difficult for the patient to hold his or her arm steady during the blood collection process.

Mental Impairment

Forgetfulness, confusion, and dementia are more common among geriatric patients. Use the wristband, not the patient's response, to confirm patient identification. Some patients may be in restraints to prevent them from hurting themselves or others. Always check with a nurse before loosening restraints.

Special Considerations for Blood Collection

Identifying the Patient
Be especially careful with patient identification. Rely on the ID bracelet if there is any doubt that the patient understands you.

Limiting Blood Loss and Bruising
Be aware of the frequency of blood draws, as the risk for anemia is higher in geriatric patients. If possible, use a dermal puncture to reduce blood loss and bruising (however, poor circulation may make this inadvisable). Be especially gentle when milking the finger to limit bruising.

Applying the Tourniquet

If you are performing venipuncture, you can apply the tourniquet over clothing to limit bruising. Using a Velcro strip rather than latex may help as well. Do not apply the tourniquet as tightly, because veins in geriatric patients collapse more easily, and release the tourniquet immediately after inserting the needle.

Locating the Vein

To improve access and comfort, place the arm on a pillow, and have the patient grip a washcloth while the arm is supported on either side by rolled towels. Do not "slap" the arm to find a vein; rather, gently massage the area for several minutes to warm it and improve blood flow. The antecubital fossa may not be the best site. If not, look for veins in unusual locations.

Performing the Puncture

Anchor the vein firmly, as veins have a tendency to roll more easily in geriatric patients. Try immobilizing the vein on both sides rather than directly on it. Use a smaller needle or a butterfly and smaller tubes for more fragile veins. Do not probe to find the vein. After completing the venipuncture, apply pressure longer to ensure that bleeding has stopped.

PATIENTS REQUIRING BLOOD DRAWS FOR EXTENDED PERIODS OF TIME

Patients with certain conditions require regular blood testing over an extended, possibly indefinite, period of time. Box 12-1 lists some of the most common conditions. Frequent blood drawing in these patients often causes the most commonly used sites to become damaged from overuse. The veins may become hardened and difficult to penetrate with the needle, and the skin may develop scar tissue. In some diseases, the trauma to the skin from frequent needle puncture may cause it to become delicate and easily torn.

BOX 12-1 Conditions Requiring Blood Draws for Extended Periods of Time

Hepatitis C infection
HIV infection
Other chronic infections
Leukemia
Terminal cancers
Sickle cell disease
IV drug use

For these patients, try to minimize damage to the veins by frequently rotating the sites from which you draw, and using the smallest needle consistent with the tests required. Consider alternative sites such as on the forearm, on the underside of the arm, and on the wrist or fingers. If the antecubital vein has already been damaged from overuse, switch to these sites rather than attempting another draw from the damaged area.

SPECIAL EQUIPMENT USED IN THE INTENSIVE CARE UNIT AND EMERGENCY ROOM

Patients in the intensive care unit (ICU) or emergency room (ER) are likely to have some type of **vascular access device** (VAD) or indwelling line in place that may affect your collection. A VAD is a tube that is inserted into either a vein or an artery and is used to administer fluids or medications, monitor blood pressure, or draw blood.

Blood collection from a VAD is done only by trained personnel on the physician's order. The phlebotomist may be asked to assist with the collection or handle the sample after collection. Understanding the types of devices and the requirements they impose will improve your ability to work in these areas.

Types of Vascular Access Devices

The name of the VAD is based on the location of the tubing in the vascular system. A **central venous catheter** (CVC), also called a **central venous line,** is the most common type of VAD. "Central" refers to the large veins emptying into the heart, into which the CVC is inserted. CVCs are most commonly inserted into the subclavian vein and then pushed into the superior vena cava, proximal to the right atrium (Figure 12-5). Access is gained through the several inches of tubing that sit outside the entry site. Types of CVCs include **Broviac, Groshong, Hickman,** and **triple lumen**.

An **implanted port** is a chamber located under the skin and connected to an indwelling line. This reduces the risk of infection. To access this device, a noncoring needle is inserted through the skin into the chamber, through a self-sealing septum.

A **peripherally inserted central catheter** (PICC) is threaded into a central vein after insertion into a peripheral (noncentral) vein, usually the basilic or cephalic, accessed from the antecubital area. PICCs are most commonly used in angioplasty procedures, in which the lumen of an obstructed central vein is rewidened. They are not used for drawing blood,

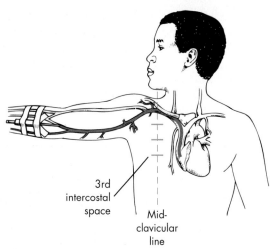

Figure 12-5
Central venous catheters are most commonly inserted into the subclavian vein and then pushed into the superior vena cava, proximal to the right atrium. (From Elkin MK, Perry AG, Potter PA: Nursing Interventions and Clinical Skills, ed 2. St. Louis, Mosby, 2000.)

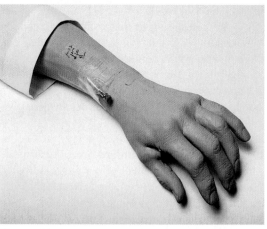

Figure 12-6
A heparin lock in place. (From Clayton BD, Stock YN: Basic Pharmacology for Nurses, ed 12. St. Louis, Mosby, 2001.)

however, because the tubing collapses easily when aspirated.

An **arterial line** is placed in an artery for continuous monitoring of blood pressure or frequent collection of samples for blood gas testing. The radial artery is the most common site; the brachial, axillary, and femoral arteries are alternative sites.

A **heparin** or **saline lock** is a tube temporarily placed in a peripheral vein to administer medicine or draw blood. A winged infusion or intravenous (IV) catheter set connected to the tubing provides the venous access; the other end has a port with a rubber septum through which a needle can pass. These devices are most commonly inserted in the lower arm just above the wrist and may be left in place up to 48 hours (Figure 12-6). To prevent a clot from blocking the line, it is flushed with either saline or heparin just before and after the procedure. Saline is becoming the more frequent choice over heparin.

An **arteriovenous** (AV) **shunt** is an artificial connection between an artery and a vein. AV shunts in the lower arm are used for dialysis patients to provide access for blood removal, purification, and return. Venipuncture should not be performed on an arm with an AV shunt. Nor should the arm be used for taking blood pressure or for any other procedure that would impair circulation.

An **external AV shunt** consists of a cannula with a rubber septum, through which a needle may be inserted for drawing blood. An **internal AV shunt** consists of a **fistula,** or permanent internal connection

between the artery and vein, using the patient's tissue, a piece of bovine tissue, or a synthetic tube. An arm containing a fistula is used for phlebotomy procedures only with the physician's permission.

Drawing from a Vascular Access Device

As stated earlier, only specially trained personnel can draw blood from a VAD, and usually only with the physician's order. Important considerations in the procedure include the following:

- Never use a syringe larger than 20 mL, because pulling on the plunger can create enough vacuum to collapse the line.
- VADs are often periodically flushed with heparin to keep the line open. For this reason, the first sample of blood collected through the line should not be used. The amount discarded is dependent on the dead-space volume in the line, the sample type, and the type of VAD. For non-coagulation specimens, discard twice the dead-space volume. For coagulation speciments, discard six times the dead-space volume, or 5 mL.
- The order of draw should be blood cultures, anticoagulated tubes, and then clotted tubes.

Working with Intravenous Lines

When a patient has an IV line in place in one arm, blood should be drawn from the other arm whenever possible. If this is impossible, or if there are lines in both arms, the following points should be kept in mind:

- Have the nurse turn off the IV drip before the draw. The drip should be turned off for at least 2 minutes.
- Apply a tourniquet distal to the IV insertion site.
- Select a vein distal to the IV insertion site, and in a different vein.
- Discard the first 5 mL of blood, because it will be contaminated with the IV fluid.
- Note on the requisition that the specimen was drawn from an arm with an IV, and identify the IV solution.

REVIEW FOR CERTIFICATION

Special considerations apply when drawing blood from pediatric patients, geriatric patients, and patients in the ER or ICU. Dermal puncture is the most common way to obtain samples from newborns and small children, as this minimizes blood loss. Dorsal hand or scalp venipuncture may be needed for larger blood volumes. Fears may be eased by a calm, soothing, and empathetic manner. Skin and vein changes are a prominent concern in geriatric patients, and careful technique is required to avoid bruising or collapsing the vein. The potential for hearing loss or mental impairment should be considered, but do not assume that a geriatric patient is impaired without evidence. In patients requiring chronic draws, such as those with HIV or cancer, rotate collection sites to avoid damaging veins and tissue. ER and ICU patients are likely to have some

type of VAD in place. Collection from a VAD is done only by specially trained personnel and on a physician's order. Venipuncture in such a patient takes place on the opposite arm whenever possible. If that is not possible, the puncture site should be distal to the IV site, and in a different vein.

BIBLIOGRAPHY

Clagg ME: Venous Sample Collection from Neonates Using Dorsal Hand Veins. Laboratory Medicine. April 1989.

Faber V: Communicating Trust, Empathy Helps in Collection. Advance for Medical Laboratory Professionals. January 27, 1997.

Faber V: Phlebotomy and the Aging Patient. Advance for Medical Laboratory Professionals. January 5, 1998.

Garza D: Tailoring Phlebotomy to the Patient. Advance for Medical Laboratory Professionals. February 22, 1999.

Haraden L: Pediatric Phlebotomy: Great Expectations. Advance for Medical Laboratory Professionals. November 1997.

Klosinski DD: Collecting Specimens from the Elderly Patient. Laboratory Medicine. August 1997.

National Committee for Clinical Laboratory Standards: H3-A3: Procedures for the Collection of Diagnostic Blood Specimens by Venipuncture. Villanova, PA, NCCLS, July 1991.

National Committee for Clinical Laboratory Standards: H21-A3: Collection, Transport, and Processing of Blood Specimens for Coagulation Testing and General Performance of Coagulation Assays, ed 3. Villanova, PA, NCCLS, December 1998.

Werner M (ed): Microtechniques for the Clinical Laboratory: Concepts and Applications. New York, John Wiley & Sons, 1976.

STUDY QUESTIONS

1. List and explain five strategies you can use to help reduce a child's anxiety before a draw.
2. What type of needle may be used for pediatric patients younger than 2 years old?
3. What is EMLA used for?
4. Name two safe ways that a child can be immobilized during a draw.
5. If an infant is under a Bili light, what must the phlebotomist do before collection?
6. How is a PKU sample collected?
7. Name four physical changes that geriatric patients undergo that the phlebotomist must consider when collecting blood.
8. Explain the procedure for drawing blood from a geriatric patient.
9. What is a VAD?
10. Explain the procedure for drawing blood from a patient who has an IV line.
11. List six types of VADs.
12. Name at least two psychological complications a child may experience during a phlebotomy procedure. List the actions you would take, as a phlebotomist, when drawing blood from a child.
13. List the special considerations to take when drawing blood from a newborn.
14. Name other diseases that neonates may be screened for, besides PKU.
15. List at least two common disorders associated with geriatric patients and special considerations to take when drawing blood from such patients.
16. Why is it important to rotate the collection site in a patient with HIV infection?

CERTIFICATION EXAM PREPARATION

1. Which of the following is *incorrect*?
   a. Newborns have a higher proportion of red blood cells compared with adults.
   b. More blood may be needed from newborns to provide enough serum or plasma for testing.
   c. Newborns have a higher proportion of plasma compared with adults.
   d. Newborns and infants are more susceptible to infection.

2. Crying causes an increase in:
   a. bilirubin
   b. platelet count
   c. white blood cell count
   d. creatinine

3. Which gauge needle is best to use for a draw on a child younger than 2 years?
   a. 18
   b. 21
   c. 23
   d. 25

4. Jaundice means:
   a. yellowing of the skin
   b. bruising of the skin
   c. swelling of the skin
   d. none of the above

5. Which lab test assays jaundice?
   a. glucose
   b. electrolytes
   c. bilirubin
   d. complete blood count (CBC)

6. Neonatal screening tests for which disorders are mandated by the United States?
   a. PKU and hyperthyroidism
   b. PKU and hypothyroidism
   c. PKU and sickle cell anemia
   d. PKU and biotinidase deficiency

7. Samples for PKU testing are typically collected:
   a. in a microcollection container
   b. in a collection tube
   c. on special filter paper
   d. in a micropipet

8. Which of the following occurs as we grow older?
   a. The layers of the skin become more elastic.
   b. Hematomas are more likely.

   c. Arteries move further away from the surface of the skin.
   d. Blood vessels widen due to atherosclerosis.

9. Which of the following is not a VAD?
   a. CVC
   b. IV
   c. PICC
   d. EMLA

10. Blood should *never* be collected from the arm of a patient containing:
    a. an AV shunt
    b. an IV
    c. an arterial line
    d. a CVC

11. Dermal punctures in pediatric patients are preferred for:
    a. crossmatch testing
    b. blood culture testing
    c. PKU testing
    d. serum testing

12. When warming an infant's heel for a dermal puncture, the heel should be warmed for:
    a. 30 seconds
    b. 1 to 2 minutes
    c. 3 to 5 minutes
    d. 6 to 8 minutes

13. Types of CVCs include all of the following *except:*
    a. Groshong
    b. triple lumen
    c. Broviac
    d. fistula

14. An arm containing _____ is never used for phlebotomy procedures.
    a. a heparin lock
    b. an arterial line
    c. a fistula
    d. an implanted port

15. Only specially trained personnel acting on a doctor's order are allowed to collect specimens from:
    a. geriatric patients
    b. VADs
    c. newborns
    d. mentally impaired patients

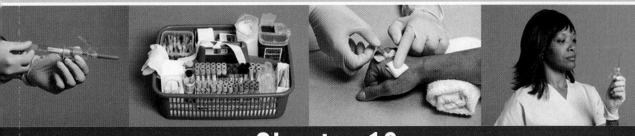

Chapter 13

Arterial Blood Collection

OUTLINE

OBJECTIVES

After completing this chapter, you should be able to:

1. Explain how arterial blood differs from venous blood.
2. Describe what is measured in arterial blood gas testing, and explain the significance of abnormal results.
3. List the equipment needed to collect arterial blood, and discuss the differences from routine venipuncture equipment.
4. List the arteries that can be used for blood gas collection, and describe the advantages and disadvantages of each.
5. Explain the principle and procedure for testing collateral circulation.

6. Define respiratory steady state, and list the steps that should be taken to ensure that it exists when blood is collected.
7. Describe the steps in arterial blood gas collection.
8. Discuss at least five complications that may occur with arterial puncture.
9. List at least seven sample collection errors that may affect arterial blood gas testing.
10. Describe capillary blood gas testing, including uses, limitations, and procedure.

KEY TERMS

arterial blood gases
arteriospasm
brachial artery
capillary blood gas testing
collateral circulation
dorsalis pedis artery

femoral artery
flea
hyperventilation
modified Allen test
partial pressure of carbon dioxide
partial pressure of oxygen

radial artery
respiratory steady state
scalp artery
thrombosis
umbilical artery

ABBREVIATIONS

ABG: arterial blood gas
COPD: chronic obstructive pulmonary disease
Pco$_2$: partial pressure of carbon dioxide

Po$_2$: partial pressure of oxygen
RT: respiratory therapist

Arterial blood is collected to determine the level of oxygen and carbon dioxide in the blood and measure the pH. Arterial collection is much more dangerous to the patient than venous collection is, and it requires in-depth training beyond routine phlebotomy skills. It is usually performed by physicians, nurses, or respiratory therapists (RTs). Phlebotomists occasionally are asked to perform or assist with this procedure, and because of the ongoing changes in health care delivery, it is likely that at some point you will have to collect an arterial sample. However, you will *not* be permitted to participate in actual arterial collection before you receive specialized training at a health care institution. Only a qualified registered nurse or RT may perform an arterial puncture. Arterial collection is most often performed in the radial artery, where collateral circulation from the ulnar artery can make up the loss to the supplied tissues. Arterial samples must be processed very quickly after collection to minimize changes in analyte values.

COMPOSITION OF ARTERIAL BLOOD

Arterial blood is rich in both oxygen and electrolytes; this is different from venous blood, in which the levels of these substances vary, depending on the metabolic activities of surrounding tissues. In addition, arterial blood is uniform in composition throughout the body. This makes arterial blood monitoring ideal for managing oxygen, electrolytes, and acid-base balance. Arterial collection is most often used for testing **arterial blood gases** (ABGs), ammonia, and lactic acid.

ARTERIAL BLOOD GAS TESTING

ABG testing determines the concentrations of oxygen and carbon dioxide dissolved in the blood and measures the pH. The absolute amount of oxygen is expressed as the **partial pressure of oxygen**, or Po_2. Similarly, the carbon dioxide level is expressed as the **partial pressure of carbon dioxide**, or Pco_2. Reference (normal) values for arterial blood gases are shown in Table 13-1.

ABGs measure the gas exchange ability of the lungs and the buffering capacity of the blood. A lower-than-normal Po_2 and a higher-than-normal Pco_2 indicate that gas exchange in the lungs is impaired. Abnormal values mean that the body's tissues are not getting adequate oxygen, a serious and potentially life-threatening situation. This may be due to many different conditions, including chronic

TABLE 13-1 Reference Values for Arterial Blood Gas Samples

Parameter	Normal Range	Description
pH	7.35–7.45	Measure of acidity or alkalinity of the blood
Po_2	80–100 mm Hg	Measure of amount of oxygen dissolved in the blood
Pco_2	34–45 mm Hg	Measure of carbon dioxide in the blood
HCO_3^-	22–26 mEq/L	Measure of bicarbonate in the blood
O_2 Saturation	97–100%	Percent of oxygen bound to hemoglobin

obstructive pulmonary disease (COPD), lung cancer, diabetic coma, shock, cardiac or respiratory failure, or neuromuscular disease, among others. Normal blood pH is 7.35 to 7.45. A lower pH indicates acidosis, and a higher pH indicates alkalosis. These too may be life threatening.

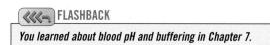 **FLASHBACK**

You learned about blood pH and buffering in Chapter 7.

Equipment for Arterial Puncture

Figure 13-1 displays some of the special equipment needed for arterial collection. Also needed are bandages and a thermometer to take the patient's temperature.

Heparinized Syringe and Needle

Arterial blood is collected in a syringe that has been pretreated with heparin to prevent coagulation. Syringes must be either glass or gas-impermeable plastic. The volume of blood required determines the syringe size; available syringe volumes range from 1 to 5 mL. Treated, prepackaged syringes are available. The choice of needle gauge and length is site dependent. The typical collection needle is usually 21 or 22 gauge, 1 to 1½ inches long. The 1-inch needle is used for either the brachial or radial arteries. The 1½-inch is used for the femoral artery. Either the needle or the syringe should have a safety device in order to comply with federal safety regulations.

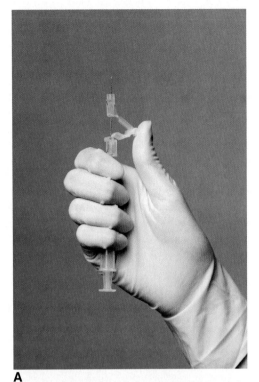

A

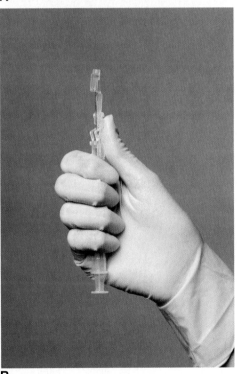

B

Figure 13-1

A, ABG syringe with safety engineered syringe–hinged safety shield. **B**, Sliding shield syringe. (From Bonewit-West K: Clinical Procedures for Medical Assistants, ed 6. Philadelphia, Saunders, 2004.)

You may be required to prepare a heparinized syringe when no commercial prepackaged product is available. To do this, follow these steps:

1. Use a solution of sodium heparin with a concentration of 1000 U/mL.
2. Calculate the volume of heparin to draw up. Use 0.05 mL heparin solution for each milliliter of blood to be drawn.
3. Attach a 20-gauge needle to the syringe, and draw up the heparin by slowly pulling back on the plunger.
4. Rotate the liquid in the syringe to coat the barrel.
5. Remove the 20-gauge needle, and replace it with the needle you will use for collection.
6. Expel the excess heparin and any air by depressing the plunger fully with the needle pointed down.

Antiseptic

The risk of serious infection is greater with arterial puncture than with venipuncture. For this reason, both alcohol and povidone-iodine or chlorhexidine are used to clean the site.

Lidocaine Anesthetic

Arterial collection can be painful. To lessen pain, 0.5 mL of lidocaine, a local anesthetic, is injected subcutaneously, using a 25- to 26-gauge needle on a 1-mL syringe.

Safety Equipment

Arterial blood is under pressure and may spray out of the puncture. You need a fluid-resistant gown, face protection, and gloves. You also need a puncture-resistant container for sharps.

Luer Tip

This plastic tip covers the syringe top after you have removed the needle. This keeps air from reaching the specimen and altering gas concentrations.

Other Equipment

Other equipment needed for arterial puncture includes the following:

- Transport container
- Crushed ice
- Ice and water
- Gauze pads
- Pressure bandages
- Thermometer (to take the patient's temperature)

No tourniquet is needed, because arterial blood is under pressure.

Site Selection

The artery used for collection must be located near the skin surface and be large enough to accept at least a 23-gauge needle. In addition, the region distal to the collection site should have **collateral circulation**, meaning that it receives blood from more than one artery. This allows the tissue to remain fully oxygenated during the collection procedure. Collateral circulation is tested using the modified Allen test (Procedure 13-1). Finally, the site should not be inflamed, irritated, edematous, or proximal to a wound.

Arteries Used for Arterial Puncture

The arteries used for arterial puncture are shown in Figure 13-2. Phlebotomists collect only from the radial or brachial arteries; other collections require a physician or other specially trained professional. Other arteries that can be used include the femoral and dorsalis pedis arteries.

The **radial artery**, supplying the hand, is the artery of choice. Although it is smaller than either the brachial or femoral artery, it has good collateral circulation and is easily accessible along the thumb side of the wrist. The ulnar artery provides collateral circulation to the hand. The radial artery can be compressed between the ligaments and bones, allowing easy application of pressure after puncture and reducing the chance of hematoma. Its small size is a disadvantage in patients with low cardiac output, because it is hard to locate.

The **brachial artery** is very large; therefore, it is easy to palpate and puncture. It is located in the antecubital fossa, below the basilic vein and near the insertion of the biceps muscle. It has adequate collateral circulation; however, not as much as the radial artery. Nevertheless, the brachial artery has important disadvantages. It is very deep and is close to the median nerve. Puncturing the median nerve is a significant risk in brachial artery collection. Also, unlike the radial artery, the brachial artery lies in soft tissue and therefore is more difficult to compress, increasing the risk of hematoma and bleeding into the puncture site.

The **femoral artery** is the largest artery used. It is located in the groin area above the thigh, lateral to the pubic bone. The femoral is used when the previously mentioned sites are not available for puncture. Its large size and high volume make it useful when cardiac output is low. However, it has poor collateral circulation. In addition, it is a difficult site to keep aseptic, increasing the risk of infection, and the puncture itself may dislodge accumulated plaque from the arterial walls. Only personnel with advanced training can perform femoral artery puncture.

Alternative sites in adults include the **dorsalis pedis artery** in the foot. In infants, the **umbilical artery** and **scalp artery** are used. When puncturing the dorsalis pedis the posterior tibial must be checked for an adequate pulse. These punctures, too, are performed only by qualified and trained personnel.

Testing Collateral Circulation

The **modified Allen test** is the most common method used to assess the adequacy of collateral circulation in the radial artery. Procedure 13-1 illustrates how to perform this test.

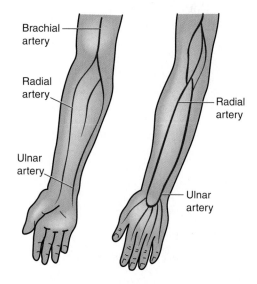

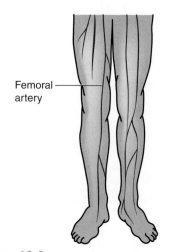

Figure 13-2

The arteries used for arterial collection include the radial artery, brachial artery, and femoral artery.

Procedure 13-1
Modified Allen Test

1. **Extend the patient's wrist over a towel, and have the patient make a fist.**

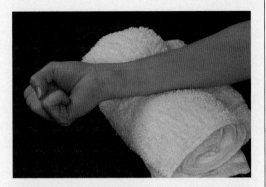

2. **Locate pulses of both the ulnar and the radial arteries, and compress both arteries.**

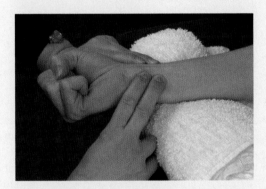

3. **Have the patient open and close the fist repeatedly.**
   This squeezes blood out of hand. The patient's palm should blanch (become lighter).

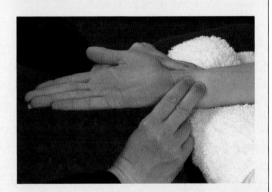

4. **Release the pressure from the ulnar artery.**
   Observe the color of the patient's palm within 5 to 10 seconds.
5. **Interpret the results.**
   Negative result: If no color appears during the 5 to 10 seconds, there is inadequate collateral circulation and the artery should not be used.
   Positive result: If color appears within 5 to 10 seconds, there is adequate collateral circulation and you may proceed with the radial puncture.

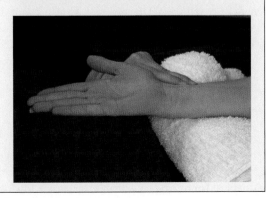

Radial Artery Puncture

Procedure 13-2 illustrates how to perform a radial artery puncture.

ARTERIAL PUNCTURE COMPLICATIONS

Complications from arterial puncture may include the following:

- **Arteriospasm**, the spontaneous constriction of an artery in response to pain. Arteriospasm may close the artery, preventing oxygen from reaching tissue.
- Nerve damage, caused by inadvertent contact with a nerve. This is more likely during arterial puncture, because the needle passes more deeply into tissue than in venipuncture.
- Hematoma, resulting from inadequate pressure on the site. This is more likely in elderly patients, whose artery walls are not as elastic and thus not as likely to close spontaneously.
- **Thrombosis**, or clot formation within the artery.
- Hemorrhage. This is more likely in patients who have coagulation disorders or are receiving anticoagulant therapy (heparin or Coumadin).
- Infection, from skin contaminants. Contaminants are easily carried to the rest of the body without encountering the immune system.

Sampling Errors

Arterial collections are particularly prone to technical errors that affect the values determined in the lab. The most significant source of error is failure to deliver the sample to the lab immediately or to properly store the sample on ice if delivery will be delayed. Blood cells continue to respire after collection, and this may cause considerable changes in the analyte values, including Po_2, Pco_2, and pH. A sample not on ice should be delivered to the lab within 5 to 10 minutes. Iced samples must be delivered within 1 hour. Ice should not be used if the sample is being tested for potassium because lower temperatures affect those levels.

Other sources of error include:

- Using too much heparin, which lowers the pH value.
- Using too little heparin, causing the specimen to clot.
- Insufficient mixing, causing the specimen to clot.

- Allowing air bubbles to enter the syringe, decreasing the carbon dioxide reading.
- Using an improper plastic syringe, which allows atmospheric gas to diffuse in and specimen gases to diffuse out through the plastic.
- Using an improper anticoagulant. pH is altered by EDTA, oxalates, and citrates.
- Puncturing a vein instead of an artery.
- Exposing the specimen to the atmosphere after collection. Prevent this by using a Luer tip to cover the syringe after you remove the needle.

Specimen Rejection

Specimens may be rejected by the lab for a variety of reasons, including:

- Inadequate volume of specimen for the test
- Clotting
- Improper or absent labeling
- Use of the wrong syringe
- Air bubbles in the specimen
- Failure to ice the specimen
- Too long a delay in delivering the specimen to the lab

CAPILLARY BLOOD GAS TESTING

Capillary blood gas testing is an alternative to ABG testing when arterial collection is not possible or is not recommended. Capillary blood is not as desirable a specimen for blood gas testing, because it is a mixture of blood from the capillaries, venules, and arterioles and is mixed with tissue fluid. In addition, this method of collection is open to the air, and the specimen may exchange gases with room air before it is sealed.

Capillary blood gas testing is most commonly performed on pediatric patients, as they generally should not be subjected to the deep punctures required for ABG testing.

The collection is done using a normal heel-stick procedure. Important points in the procedure are as follows:

1. Warm the site to 40 to 42° C for 5 to 10 minutes before the stick, to maximize the arterial character of the capillary blood.
2. Collect the sample in a heparinized glass pipet. Before collection, insert a metal filing, called a **flea**, into the tube. After collection, a magnet is used to draw the flea back and forth across the length of the tube to mix the contents with the heparin (Figure 13-3).

Procedure 13-2
Radial Artery Puncture

1. **Prepare the patient, and examine and complete the requisition form.**

   Take the patient's temperature and respiration rate and record on the requisition form. Also document the oxygen received by the patient and the device used to deliver the oxygen. (Example: "95% oxygen through nasal cannula" or "patient is on room air.")

   The patient should be in a **respiratory steady state**, meaning that he or she has received the specified amount of oxygen and has refrained from exercise for at least 30 minutes. It is important to maintain this steady state during collection. Keep the patient calm, and make sure that he or she is not experiencing **hyperventilation**, because this changes the arterial oxygen and carbon dioxide levels. Pediatric patients should not be crying or holding their breath. Reassurance and distraction help keep the patient from becoming agitated.

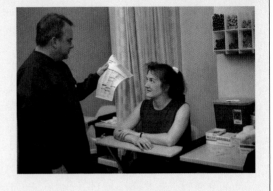

2. **Choose and prepare the site.**

   Perform the modified Allen test to assess collateral circulation in the hand. If the result is positive, proceed. Position the patient comfortably. Fully extend the arm with the anterior surface facing upward. Palpate for the artery with either the middle or index finger to locate the greatest maximum pulsation.

   Clean the site first with alcohol and then with povidone-iodine.

   Inject the local anesthetic. Wait 1 to 2 minutes for the anesthetic to begin working.

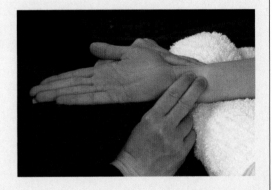

3. **Perform the puncture.**

   Cleanse the fingers of your nondominant hand, and place over the area where the needle should enter the artery, using the index finger and middle finger of your nondominant hand to stabilize the artery.

   Hold the syringe like a dart with your dominant hand, with the needle tip pointed bevel up toward the upper arm. Insert the needle 5 to 10 mm distal to the finger you placed on the artery. Insert it at an angle 45 to 60 degrees above the plane of the skin.

Procedure 13-2—cont'd

Radial Artery Puncture

As the needle is inserted into the artery, blood should appear in the hub. It should be bright red and move with the pulse. Do not withdraw the syringe plunger. Blood pressure should push the blood into the syringe without any assistance.

4. Withdraw the needle, apply pressure, and ice the syringe.

Withdraw the needle with your dominant hand.

With your nondominant hand, apply direct pressure to the site with a folded gauze square. Hold it for at least 5 minutes. You, not the patient, must continue to apply pressure until the bleeding stops. If the patient is on anticoagulant therapy, apply pressure for at least 15 minutes.

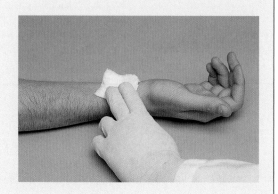

Meanwhile, with the hand holding the syringe, depress the plunger slightly, if necessary, to expel any air that may have entered the needle. Engage the safety device for the needle. Cap off the syringe with the Luer tip cap. To mix the blood with heparin, roll the syringe between your thumb and fingers for 5 seconds, followed by gentle inversion for 5 seconds. Place the syringe in the ice.

5. Examine the puncture site.

After 5 minutes (or 15 minutes for patients on anticoagulant therapy), check the site to ensure that the bleeding has stopped. A number of medications increase bleeding times, including anticoagulants (such as heparin and warfarin) and thrombolytics (such as tissue plasminogen activator, streptokinase, and urokinase). Once the bleeding has stopped, clean the site with alcohol to remove the iodine, and apply a bandage.

Check for a pulse distal to the site. If the pulse is absent or weak, contact the nurse immediately.

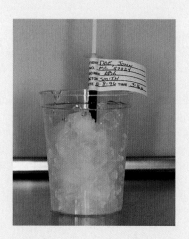

6. Label and ice the specimen.

Dispose of the needle in the sharps container.

Label the specimen with a waterproof pen, and return the syringe to the ice.

Deliver the specimen to the lab immediately.

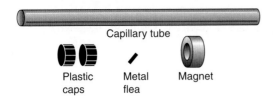

Capillary tube

Plastic caps · Metal flea · Magnet

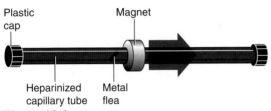

Plastic cap · Magnet

Heparinized capillary tube · Metal flea

Figure 13-3
A metal filing, called a flea, is inserted into the capillary tube before collection. A magnet is used to stir the sample after collection.

3. Fill the tube completely with blood, so that no air bubbles remain.
4. Seal both ends of the tube with clay or plastic caps, to prevent air contamination.
5. Mix well using the magnet and flea, and transport the specimen to the lab on ice.

REVIEW FOR CERTIFICATION

Because of the increased danger of arterial blood collection, special training is required beyond that needed for routine venipuncture. Arterial blood monitoring is ideal for managing oxygen, electrolytes, and acid-base balance. ABGs measure the gas exchange ability of the lungs and the buffering capacity of the blood. Arterial blood is collected in a syringe pretreated with heparin to prevent coagulation. The site is cleaned with both alcohol and povidone-iodine or chlorhexidine to minimize the serious risk of infection. Lidocaine is used as an anesthetic. The site is selected after testing the adequacy of collateral circulation using the modified Allen test. A rapid return of color indicates that the site has adequate collateral circulation and may be used for collection. In adults, the radial artery is the preferred site. The patient must be in a respiratory steady state and should be kept calm during the procedure. The specimen should be delivered immediately or kept on ice if a delay of more than 5 to 10 minutes is expected. Complications include arteriospasm, nerve damage, hematoma, hemorrhage, thrombosis, and infection. Sampling errors affecting test values may be introduced from improper cooling, delay in delivery, too much or too little heparin, insufficient mixing, exposure of the sample to air, and improper collection technique. Capillary blood gas testing is an alternative to ABG testing when arterial collection is not possible or recommended. A metal flea and magnet are used to mix the contents with the heparin.

BIBLIOGRAPHY

Bishop ML: Clinical Chemistry: Principles, Procedures, and Correlations. Philadelphia, JB Lippincott, 1992.
Burton GG, Hodgkin JE, Ward JJ: Respiratory Care: A Guide to Clinical Practice. Philadelphia, JB Lippincott, 1991.
National Committee for Clinical Laboratory Standards: H11-A4: Procedures for the Collection of Arterial Blood Specimens: Approved standard, ed 4. Wayne, PA, NCCLS, 2004.
Shapiro BA: Clinical Application of Blood Gases. ed 5. St Louis, Mosby, 1994.

STUDY QUESTIONS

1. Arterial collection is most often used for testing _____.
2. List four conditions that produce abnormal ABG values.
3. What is a normal blood pH?
4. What is the difference between acidosis and alkalosis?
5. Describe the difference between a syringe used for venipuncture and a syringe used for ABG collection.
6. Besides alcohol, which other antiseptic must be used for arterial puncture?
7. What local anesthetic may be used to numb the site?
8. What safety precautions must be taken by the phlebotomist when collecting blood from an artery?
9. What gauge needle is most often used for blood gas collection?
10. Define collateral circulation, and state which test is used to determine whether this is present.
11. For an arterial collection, at what angle is the needle inserted into the artery?
12. How long must pressure be applied to the puncture site after an arterial collection?
13. Define arteriospasm.
14. List five ABG sampling errors.
15. Name five reasons that ABG specimens may be rejected.
16. In which population is capillary blood gas testing most commonly performed, and on what part of the body is this procedure usually done?
17. Why is capillary blood not as desirable as arterial blood for testing blood gases?

CERTIFICATION EXAM PREPARATION

1. Arterial blood collection monitors all of the following *except:*
   a. ammonia
   b. glucose
   c. lactic acid
   d. blood gases

2. A normal blood pH is:
   a. 7.35
   b. 7.00
   c. 7.60
   d. 7.75

3. The ABG syringe is coated with:
   a. sodium citrate
   b. sodium fluoride
   c. EDTA
   d. heparin

4. A typical needle gauge for ABG collection is:
   a. 16
   b. 20
   c. 22
   d. 18

5. Which artery is most frequently used for ABG collection?
   a. brachial
   b. femoral
   c. dorsalis pedis
   d. radial

6. All of the following are ABG sampling errors *except:*
   a. delivery of an un-iced sample to the lab 15 minutes after collection
   b. use of the anticoagulant EDTA
   c. air bubbles in the syringe
   d. use of a gas-impermeable plastic syringe

7. The modified Allen test determines:
   a. partial pressure of oxygen
   b. partial pressure of carbon dioxide
   c. collateral circulation
   d. pH

8. In an arterial collection, the needle should be inserted at:
   a. 90 degrees
   b. 45 degrees
   c. 30 degrees
   d. 70 degrees

9. If lidocaine is injected before an arterial blood collection, wait _____ minutes for the anesthetic to begin working.
   a. 1 to 2
   b. 2 to 3
   c. 3 to 4
   d. 4 to 5

10. The modified Allen test is performed on the:
    a. ulnar and brachial arteries
    b. brachial and radial arteries
    c. ulnar and radial arteries
    d. radial and femoral arteries

11. All of the following are complications of ABG collection *except*:
    a. petechiae
    b. arteriospasm
    c. thrombosis
    d. hematoma

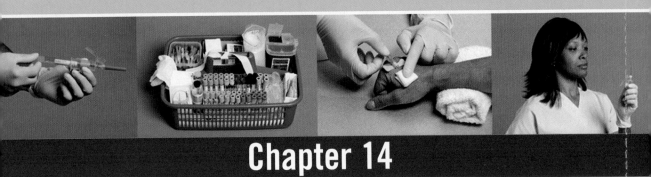

Chapter 14

Special Collections and Procedures

OUTLINE

OBJECTIVES

After completing this chapter, you should be able to:

1. Define basal state.
2. Define and explain the uses of:
   a. fasting specimens
   b. timed specimens
   c. 2-hour postprandial specimens
3. Describe the procedure for performing the various tolerance tests.
4. Define diurnal variation, and list the blood constituents that may be affected by it.
5. Define therapeutic drug monitoring, describe the differences among a random level and peak and trough levels, and explain how TDM samples are collected.
6. Describe the reasons and procedures for collecting blood for culture.
7. Explain the steps in collecting blood from donors for transfusion.

8. Define and explain the uses of autologous donation and therapeutic phlebotomy.
9. Explain how samples to be tested for or suspected of containing cold agglutinins, cryofibrinogen, or cryoglobulin should be handled.
10. List samples that should be chilled until tested.
11. List samples that are light sensitive, and explain how they should be handled.
12. Describe the precautions to be taken when collecting legal or forensic specimens.
13. List samples that are time sensitive, and explain how they should be handled.
14. Explain how to prepare blood smears, describe features of unacceptable smears, and list the possible causes.
15. Explain how to prepare smears to be examined for malaria.

KEY TERMS

aerobic bacteria	differential count	lactose tolerance test
agglutination	diurnal variation	oral glucose tolerance test
anaerobic bacteria	epinephrine tolerance test	peak level
autologous donation	fasting specimen	polycythemia
bacteremia	feathered edge	septicemia
basal state	fever of unknown origin	SPS
blood culture	glucagon tolerance test	therapeutic drug monitoring
chain of custody	half-life	therapeutic phlebotomy
cold agglutinins	hemochromatosis	trough level
cryofibrinogen	hyperglycemia	2-hour postprandial test
cryoglobulin	hypoglycemia	

ABBREVIATIONS

BC: blood culture
COC: chain of custody
FUO: fever of unknown origin
HIV: human immunodeficiency virus

NIDA: National Institute on Drug Abuse
OGTT: oral glucose tolerance test
TDM: therapeutic drug monitoring

Although routine venipuncture is the most common procedure you will perform as a phlebotomist, special collecting or handling procedures are needed in many situations for samples that involve one or more special circumstances. Fasting specimens, timed specimens, blood cultures, and blood donor specimens all require collection procedures specific to the sample being collected. A variety of samples require special handling, which may involve keeping the sample warm, cool, or away from light, or providing immediate delivery or legal documentation. In this chapter, you will learn when and why these special procedures are needed and the details of how to perform them.

> **BOX 14-1** Factors That Influence Blood Composition
>
> Age
> Altitude
> Dehydration
> Environment
> Gender
> Pregnancy
> Stress
> Diet
> Diurnal variation
> Drugs
> Exercise
> Body position
> Smoking

FASTING SPECIMENS AND THE BASAL STATE

As detailed in Box 14-1, many factors influence the composition of blood. **Diurnal variation** refers to the normal daily fluctuations in body chemistry related to hormonal cycles, sleep-wake cycles, and other regular patterns of change.

To minimize the variations introduced by normal fluctuations in blood composition, reference ranges for blood tests are based on healthy patients in what is known as the basal state. The basal state is defined as the body's state after 12 hours of fasting and abstention from strenuous exercise. Routine phlebotomy rounds are scheduled for the early morning, because most patients are in the basal state at that time.

Some test results are more affected than others when a patient has not been scrupulously fasting for 12 hours. Glucose and triglycerides are especially affected. For this reason, a fasting specimen may be requested that is drawn after a 12-hour complete fast. Caffeine and nicotine are also prohibited during the fasting period, as these are metabolic stimulants. If a fasting specimen is requested, the phlebotomist must ask the patient if he or she has had *anything* to eat or drink other than water, or has had any caffeine or nicotine, within the past 12 hours. It is better to ask the question in this form than to ask, "Have you been fasting for 12 hours?" because some patients may not consider an evening snack or morning juice to be a violation of their fast. If the patient has violated the fast, you can still draw the sample, but make a note on the requisition.

Timed Specimens

Timed specimens are taken to determine changes in the level of some substance of interest over time. Timed specimens are most often used to monitor:

- Medication levels (e.g., digoxin for heart disease, levodopa for Parkinson's disease).
- Changes in the patient's condition (e.g., a decrease in hemoglobin level).
- Normal diurnal variation in blood levels at different times of the day (e.g., cortisol or other hormones).

2-Hour Postprandial Test

The **2-hour postprandial test** is used to test for diabetes mellitus. It compares the fasting glucose level with the level 2 hours after consuming glucose, either by eating a meal or ingesting a measured amount of glucose. In patients with diabetes mellitus, the glucose level will be higher than normal, whereas the level in normal patients will have returned to the fasting level. After obtaining a fasting specimen, patients are instructed to eat a full meal and return to the lab 2 hours after eating, for the second specimen.

Oral Glucose Tolerance Test

The **oral glucose tolerance test** (OGTT) tests for both diabetes mellitus and other disorders of carbohydrate metabolism. **Hyperglycemia**, or abnormally elevated blood sugar, is most commonly caused by diabetes; **hypoglycemia**, or abnormally lowered blood sugar, may be due to one of several endocrine disorders or other metabolic disruptions. Hyperglycemia is detected with a 3-hour OGTT, and hypoglycemia is detected with a 5-hour OGTT (Figure 14-1). Longer testing periods are sometimes used as well to identify a variety of metabolic disorders.

The OGTT has fallen out of general use for the diagnosis of diabetes mellitus, and has been replaced by either a fasting glucose sample (at least 18 hours without caloric intake) or a random glucose sample. A 1-hour OGTT is still used to screen for gestational diabetes in pregnant women at risk.

Patients will be instructed by their physicians regarding pretest preparation, which includes eating high-carbohydrate meals for several days and then fasting for 12 hours immediately before the test.

Testing begins between 0700 (pronounced "oh-seven-hundred") and 0900 (7 A.M. to 9 A.M.), with the collection of a fasting blood specimen and sometimes a urine specimen. These specimens should be tested before the OGTT proceeds. In the event that the glucose level is severely elevated, the physician may decide not to proceed with the test.

 Clinical Tip: Times are given in military time. To get clock time, subtract 1200 for times of 1300 or later. Example: 1430 = 2:30 P.M.

The patient then drinks a standardized amount of glucose solution within 5 minutes. Timing for the rest of the procedure begins after the drink is finished. The phlebotomist gives the patient the collection schedule and instructs the patient to return to the collection station at the appropriate times (Table 14-1). Patients also should be instructed to continue to fast and drink plenty of water, so they will remain adequately hydrated throughout the test.

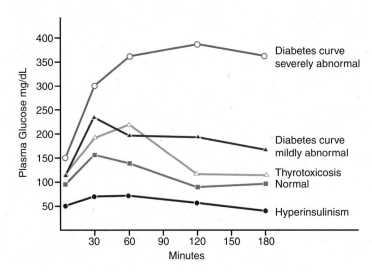

Figure 14-1

Results from oral glucose tolerance tests are graphed to determine the level of serum glucose over time. In a person with normal glucose metabolism, serum glucose returns to baseline (starting value) by 2 hours. Prolonged elevation may indicate diabetes.

TABLE 14-1 Collection Schedule for Oral Glucose Tolerance Tests

Test	Schedule
2-Hour OGTT	Fasting, 30 minutes, 1 hour, 2 hours
3-Hour OGTT	Fasting, 30 minutes, 1 hour, 2 hours, 3 hours
5-Hour OGTT	Fasting, 30 minutes, 1 hour, 2 hours, 3 hours, 4 hours, 5 hours

BOX 14-2 Representative Blood Constituents That Show Marked Diurnal Variation

Hormones
   Cortisol
   Testosterone
   Estradiol
   Progesterone
   Serum iron
   Glucose
White blood cells (eosinophils show especially pronounced variation)

Some patients do not tolerate the test well. Any vomiting should be reported to the physician ordering the test. If the patient vomits shortly after the test begins, the procedure will have to be started again.

All collections should be made on time and using the same collection method (i.e., venipuncture or dermal puncture) and anticoagulant for each sample. A urine specimen may be collected at the same time. Samples should be labeled with the time from test commencement (30 minutes, 1 hour, and so forth).

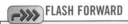**FLASH FORWARD**

Urine specimen collection is covered in Chapter 15.

Other Tolerance Tests

Similar procedures are used for other tolerance tests. The **epinephrine tolerance test** determines the patient's ability to mobilize glycogen from the liver. In response to a dose of the hormone epinephrine, glycogen is converted to glucose and released into the bloodstream. The test begins with a fasting specimen, followed by the epinephrine injection administered by the physician. Specimen collection begins 30 minutes later. The **glucagon tolerance test** is identical in purpose and procedure, except that the hormone glucagon is injected instead of epinephrine.

The **lactose tolerance test** determines whether the lactose-digesting enzyme lactase is present in the gut. A 3-hour OGTT is performed first, to produce a baseline glucose uptake graph. The following day, a lactose tolerance test is performed. The procedure is identical to the OGTT, except that lactose is consumed. Because lactose is broken down into glucose and galactose, the timed samples should produce an identical glucose uptake graph. Lower glucose levels indicate a problem with lactose metabolism.

Diurnal Variation

Many substances in the blood (especially hormones) show diurnal variation, or regular changes throughout the day (Box 14-2). Cortisol, for instance, is usually twice as high in the morning as in the late afternoon. The time for the draw is usually scheduled for the diurnal peak or trough. Cortisol is usually drawn at 1000 or 1600, for instance.

Therapeutic Drug Monitoring

Patients differ greatly in the rate at which they metabolize or excrete medications. In addition, the margin of safety, or the difference between the level at which a drug is therapeutic and the level at which it becomes toxic, may be very narrow. In order to maintain constant therapeutic plasma drug levels and ensure that the drug does not reach toxic levels, a patient may require timed specimens to measure the levels of the medication. This is known as **therapeutic drug monitoring** (TDM). Results of TDM are used by the pharmacy to adjust drug dosing. Table 14-2 lists some commonly monitored drugs. The rate of metabolism is often given in terms of the drug's **half-life**, the time for half the drug to be metabolized. Drugs with long half-lives, including digoxin, often require only one timed specimen. Drugs with short half-lives, such as

TABLE 14-2 Commonly Monitored Therapeutic Drugs

Drug Name	Therapeutic Purpose
Procainamide and digoxin	Heart medication
Gentamicin	Antibiotic
Tobramycin	Antibiotic
Vancomycin	Antibiotic
Theophylline	Antiasthmatic
Dilantin and valproic acid	Anticonvulsant

the aminoglycoside antibiotics (including gentamicin, tobramycin, and vancomycin) require the most careful monitoring. Monitoring for these rapidly metabolized antibiotics is done with a pair of specimens, known as a peak and a trough.

Collection is usually timed to coincide with either the trough or the peak serum level. The trough level is the lowest serum level and occurs immediately before the next dose of medicine is given. The requisition will specify the actual collection time, which is usually 30 minutes before the dose. The peak level, or highest serum level, occurs sometime after the dose is given; exactly when depends on the characteristics of the drug, the patient's own metabolism, and the method of administration. The tube should be labeled with the draw time in all cases. TDM results are needed promptly, because the pharmacy is usually waiting for the results to determine both the time and concentration of the next dose of drug.

BLOOD CULTURES

A **blood culture** (BC) is ordered to test for the presence of microorganisms in the blood. **Septicemia** refers to a blood infection by any pathogenic microorganism, and **bacteremia** refers specifically to a bacterial infection. Patients with symptoms of chills and fever, or **fever of unknown origin** (FUO), may require a BC. BCs are ordered as stat or timed specimens.

Isolating pathogenic organisms from blood is difficult, because the number of organisms may be low (leading to false-negative results), and the potential for sample contamination is high (leading to false-positive results). To increase the likelihood of finding pathogens and decrease the number of false-positives, collection is performed at timed intervals and from multiple sites. *Aseptic collection technique is critical for meaningful results.* Drawing the correct volume is also critical, because the ratio of blood to culture media depends on the system used. Always check your institution's guidelines. Volumes for pediatric patients differ from those for adults.

Types of Collection Containers

There are three basic types of containers for collecting blood cultures:

1. A long-necked bottle, which accepts a BD Vacutainer® needle and tube holder.
2. A shorter bottle, which accepts a winged infusion device using a special adapter.

3. A standard evacuated tube with sodium polyanethole sulfonate (**SPS**) anticoagulant.

Figure 14-2 shows these three types of collection containers.

Timing

The number of organisms in the bloodstream is often highest just before a spike in the patient's temperature. By frequently recording the temperature, these spikes can often be predicted, and collection scheduled accordingly. In other situations, collection may be timed at regular intervals, often hourly or just before antibiotic administration.

Multiple Sites

Contamination by skin bacteria is a frequent complication of BC collection. However, distinguishing contaminants from true pathogens can be difficult because some contaminants can grow on indwelling devices, therefore causing infection in the patient. To reduce errors caused by this contamination, a known skin contaminant must be cultured from at

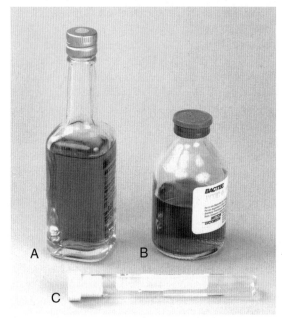

Figure 14-2

Examples of culture systems used in the collection of blood cultures. **A**, Specially designed BD Vacutainer® tube for collecting a blood culture (direct method). **B**, BD Bactec™ blood culture bottle (indirect method). **C**, Vacuum tube (yellow top) for collecting blood cultures. (From Flynn JC Jr: Procedures in Phlebotomy, ed 3. Philadelphia, Saunders, 2005.)

least two different sites to be considered a blood pathogen. It is even better to collect two pairs of samples, with the second pair following the first by 30 minutes or more.

Sample Collection

Procedure 14-1 outlines the steps in blood culture collection. As noted earlier, samples are collected either directly into a bottle containing culture media or into a sterile anticoagulated tube for later transfer at the lab. The ratio of blood to culture media is crucial to the culture, so be sure to collect the sample size indicated on the bottle. In addition to culture media, some tubes contain activated charcoal, which absorbs antibiotics from the patient's blood so they won't inhibit growth of the bacteria in the culture tube.

For direct collection, two samples are collected from each site. The first sample is tested for **anaerobic bacteria**, and the second (which is more likely to have been exposed to air) is tested for **aerobic bacteria**. Be sure to label the samples to reflect their order of collection.

For anticoagulated tube collections, one tube is collected per site. At the lab, the specimen is cultured onto the appropriate media. When a syringe collection must be performed, one syringe of blood is collected, and the transfer is made to the anaerobic bottle first. It was once standard procedure to change syringe needles before this transfer, but this is no longer recommended.

> **Clinical Tip:** Aerobic bacteria use oxygen to grow; anaerobic bacteria are killed by exposure to oxygen.

BLOOD DONOR COLLECTION

Blood donation is a vital link in the health care system, and the phlebotomist plays a central role in the collection of donated blood. Blood banks collect and store donated blood for use in both emergency and scheduled transfusions. Guidelines for uniform collection procedures and safeguards have been established by the American Association of Blood Banks (AABB) and the U.S. Food and Drug Administration (FDA).

Potential donors must be screened to ensure that the donation is not harmful to the donor or the recipient. Donors must be at least 17 years old (16 in some states), weigh a minimum of 110 pounds, and

not have donated blood in the past 8 weeks. Donor screening is usually done by the phlebotomist. All information provided during the screening is confidential. The screening process is performed every time a person donates blood. Screening involves the following:

- Registration: The donor must provide his or her name, date of birth, address, other identifying information, and written consent. All information must be kept on file for 5 years.
- Interview and medical history: This is done in private by a trained interviewer. All responses are kept completely confidential. Potential donors may be rejected for a variety of reasons, including exposure to human immunodeficiency virus (HIV) or hepatitis, current drug use, or cardiovascular conditions.
- Physical exam: The donor's weight, temperature, blood pressure, pulse, and hemoglobin level are determined. Hemoglobin is usually measured with a drop of whole blood from a dermal puncture. The blood is placed into a copper sulfate solution of known density. Blood that sinks (because it is weighted with enough hemoglobin) is acceptable for donation (Figure 14-3). A hematocrit may be substituted for the hemoglobin determination.

Collection Procedure

Blood is collected by the "unit," whose volume is 405 to 495 mL, or approximately one-half liter (Figure 14-4). It is collected directly into a sterile plastic bag, which hangs below the collection site and fills by gravity. The weight of the filled bag triggers a clamp that stops the collection. A 16- to 18-gauge needle is used for collection. This large needle speeds the collection and prevents hemolysis.

A large vein in the antecubital area is used for donor collection. The site is cleaned first with soap and water and then with iodine. After the puncture, the needle is secured to the arm with tape, to prevent motion during the collection. The donor is instructed to pump his or her fist, to increase flow. (Hemoconcentration may result from this action, but this is not a concern with blood collected for transfusion.) The phlebotomist stays with the donor during the collection and observes for any signs of distress, anxiety, or pale skin. After needle removal, the phlebotomist instructs the patient to apply firm pressure to the site and bandages the site when the bleeding has stopped.

Procedure 14-1
Blood Culture Collection

1. Prepare the site.

Proper site preparation is critical to obtain a valid blood culture specimen. After identifying the site, scrub it vigorously with alcohol to clean at least 1½ to 2 inches beyond the intended puncture site.

Scrub vigorously with 2% iodine or povidone-iodine swab stick. Using a new swab stick, clean the site, moving outward in a concentric circle. An alternative is to use a one-step Medi-flex ChloraPrep® applicator instead of the two steps outlined here.

Allow the site to dry for 1 minute. This ensures enough time for the iodine to kill surface bacteria.

Avoid touching the site once it has been cleaned. If you must touch it, reclean the site afterward.

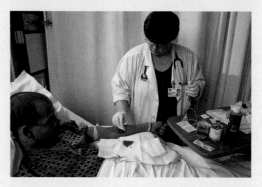

2. Prepare your collection equipment.

Clean the tops of collection bottles with iodine (if they have plastic tops, you may use alcohol). Place a clean alcohol pad on top of each bottle until they are inoculated. Immediately before inoculation, wipe the top with the pad to prevent iodine contamination of the sample. Be sure not to touch the bottle tops directly.

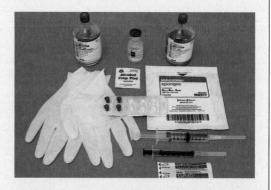

3. Collect the sample.

Reapply the tourniquet, and perform the venipuncture. Collect two samples. Label the first "anaerobic" and the second "aerobic," and indicate the site of the puncture.

4. Attend to the patient.

After collection, remove the iodine from the patient's arm with alcohol.

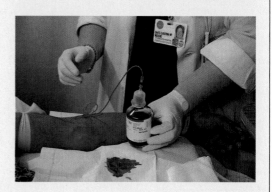

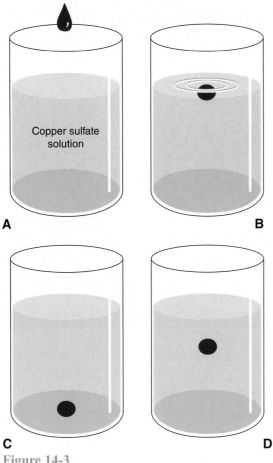

Figure 14-3

Hemoglobin determination for blood donation. **A** and **B**, A drop of the donor's blood is placed into a copper sulfate solution. **C** and **D**, Blood that sinks to the bottom of the solution is acceptable for donation. Blood that remains on top or sinks very slowly to the bottom is not acceptable.

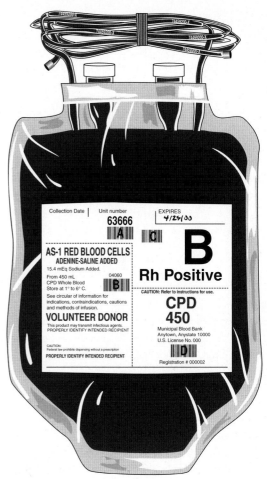

Figure 14-4

A unit of blood has a volume of approximately 400 to 500 mL.

Autologous Donation

An **autologous donation** is blood donated by a patient for his or her own use later. Patients planning surgery often make autologous donations before the procedure. This may reduce the likelihood of complications and may be especially useful for patients with rare blood types. Because multiple units might be needed during surgery, patients may need to donate several times. A patient can donate as often as every 72 hours, assuming that his or her health is good. Hemoglobin is checked during the donation series and should not fall below 11 g/dL.

Therapeutic Phlebotomy

Therapeutic phlebotomy is the removal of blood from a patient's system as part of the treatment for a disorder. The principal disorders treated by therapeutic phlebotomy are **polycythemia**, a malignancy characterized by excessive production of red blood cells, and **hemochromatosis**, an excess of iron in the blood. In both cases, periodic removal of a unit of blood may be part of the treatment program. Because such a large volume must be removed, therapeutic phlebotomy is performed in the donor center, although a special area may be set aside for this purpose. This blood cannot be used for transfusion.

SPECIAL SPECIMEN HANDLING

Cold Agglutinins

Cold agglutinins are antibodies often formed in response to infection with *Mycoplasma pneumoniae*, a cause of atypical pneumonia. The antibodies created by the immune system during the infection may also react with red blood cells at temperatures below body temperature, causing them to stick together, hence "cold agglutinins" (**agglutination** is the process of sticking together). Because the agglutinins attach to red blood cells at cold temperatures, the specimen must be kept warm until the serum is separated from the cells, to avoid falsely lowering the agglutinin levels.

To collect a cold agglutinin sample, prewarm a plain red-topped tube (containing no gel) in a 37° C incubator for 30 minutes. To keep the specimen warm, it can be wrapped in an activated heel-warmer pack or placed in the incubator. Deliver the specimen as quickly as possible to the laboratory.

Cryofibrinogen and Cryoglobulin

Warm collection and storage are also required for two other types of samples: **cryofibrinogen** (an abnormal type of fibrinogen) and **cryoglobulin** (an abnormal serum protein). Both precipitate when cold and redissolve when warmed. These samples should be collected and handled in the same manner as a cold agglutinin sample.

Chilled Specimens

A number of tests require that the specimen be chilled immediately after collection (Box 14-3). Chilling is used to prevent chemical changes that would alter test results. The sample should be placed in crushed ice or in an ice and water mixture and immediately delivered to the lab. The temperature should be 1° to 5° C, and the sample should be transported to the lab for testing within 5 minutes of collection (Figure 14-5).

Light-Sensitive Specimens

Exposure to light can break down or alter certain blood constituents (Box 14-4). Specimens to be tested for these constituents must be protected from light after collection. This is done by wrap-

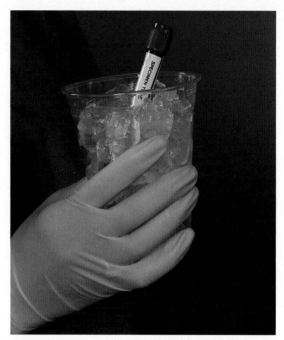

Figure 14-5

Samples that must be kept cold should be placed in crushed ice or in an ice and water mixture with a temperature of 1 to 5° C.

ping the tube in aluminum foil immediately after collection (Figure 14-6). An amber-colored microtube can be used for dermal collection (e.g., of bilirubin samples).

Time-Sensitive Specimens

Some analytes are very unstable or volatile. Because of this, the tests must be performed rapidly after the sample is taken. Box 14-5 lists analytes that are time-sensitive.

Legal and Forensic Specimens

Blood specimens may be collected for use as evidence in legal proceedings, including alcohol and drug testing, DNA analysis, or paternity or parentage

---

BOX 14-3 Tests Requiring Chilled Specimens

Arterial blood gases
Ammonia
Lactic acid
Pyruvate
Glucagon
Gastrin
Adrenocorticotropic hormone
Parathyroid hormone

BOX 14-4 Blood Constituents That Are Light Sensitive

Bilirubin
Beta-carotene
Vitamin A
Vitamin B_6
Porphyrins

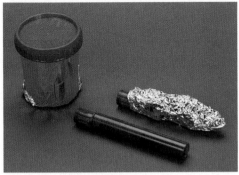

Figure 14-6

Samples that must be protected from light should be wrapped in aluminum foil immediately after collection. Amber-colored tubes also can be used.

testing. Such samples must be handled with special procedures designed to prevent tampering, misidentification, or interference with the test results.

The most important concept in handling forensic specimens is the **chain of custody** (COC), a protocol that ensures that the sample is always in the custody of a person legally entrusted to be in control of it. The chain begins with patient identification and continues through every step of the collection and testing process. COC documentation includes special containers, seals, and forms, as well as the date, time, and identification of the handler (Figure 14-7).

The National Institute on Drug Abuse (NIDA) has established requirements for patient preparation and specimen handling in COC samples. These requirements include the following:

- The purpose and procedure of the test must be explained to the patient.
- The patient must sign a consent form.
- The patient must present picture identification.
- The specimen must be labeled appropriately to establish a COC.
- The specimen must be sealed in such a way that any tampering can be identified.
- The specimen must be placed in a locked container before transport to the testing site.

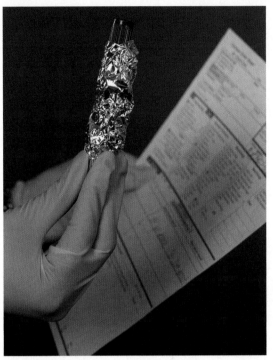

Figure 14-7

Chain of custody documentation includes special containers, seals, and forms, as well as the date, time, and identification of the handler.

Legal Alcohol Collection

Collection for alcohol testing requires special handling to prevent alteration of the test results. Important features of alcohol testing include the following:

- The site must not be cleaned with alcohol, as this would falsely elevate the result. Instead, use sterile soap, water, and gauze or another nonalcoholic antiseptic solution.
- Tubes must be filled as full as the vacuum allows to minimize the escape of alcohol from the specimen into the space above.
- The specimen should not be uncapped, because that also allows alcohol to escape and compromises the integrity of the sample before testing.

BLOOD SMEARS

Blood smears are made to allow microscopic examination of the blood cells. The blood smear is used for determining the proportion of the various blood cell types, called a **differential count**; counting reticulocytes; and special staining procedures.

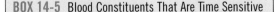

BOX 14-5 Blood Constituents That Are Time Sensitive

Ammonia
Lactate
Platelet aggregation
Brain natriuretic peptide
Prostatic acid phosphatase
ACTH: Adrenocorticotropic hormone
Aldolase

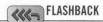

Blood Smear Preparation

Blood smears are usually prepared following dermal puncture. Slides are made in pairs. Figure 14-8 illustrates a good smear as well as several examples of unacceptable smears. Procedure 14-2 outlines how to prepare blood smears.

Malaria Smears

Malaria is caused by blood-borne protozoa of the genus *Plasmodium*. A patient with malaria has cycles of fever and chills that coincide with the life

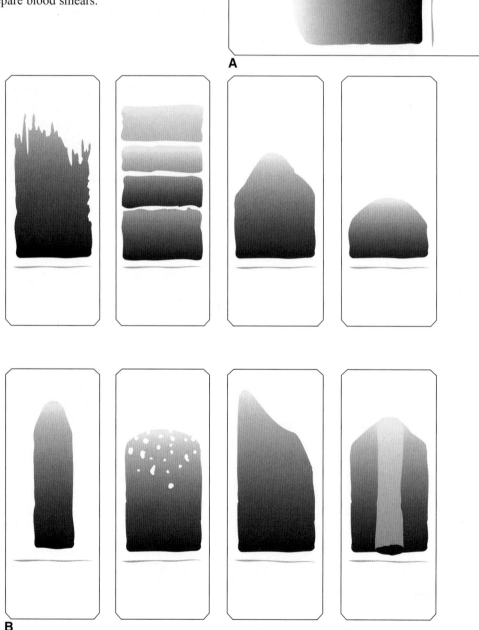

Figure 14-8
Blood smear slides. **A**, A good smear. **B**, Several examples of unacceptable smears. (From Rodak BF: Hematology: Clinical Principles and Applications, ed 3. Philadelphia, Saunders, 2007.)

Procedure 14-2

Blood Smear Preparation

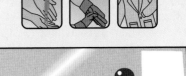
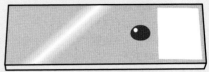

1. Prepare the smears.

Place one drop of blood on a clean slide, ½ to 1 inch from the end, centered between the two sides.

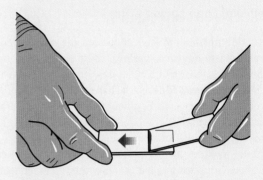

Place the edge of a second slide, the "spreader," onto the first slide, in front of the blood at a 25- to 30-degree angle, and draw it back to just contact the drop.

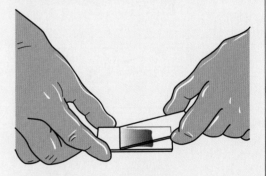

Move the spreader slide forward, away from the drop, in one continuous movement to the end of the slide. The blood will be drawn along over the slide.

To make the second slide, place a drop of blood onto the spreader slide. Using the first slide as the spreader, repeat the procedure.

Dry and label the slides. Use pencil on the frosted end; do not use pen, as ink may run when the slide is stained.

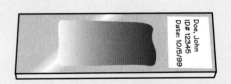

2. Examine the smears.

An acceptable smear must have a **feathered edge**, meaning that the cells appear to thin out farther from the original drop. At the far end, you should see a *very thin* transparent layer. This is the area from which the differential count is made. See Figure 14-8 for examples of blood smears. Table 14-3 describes common problems with smears and their likely causes.

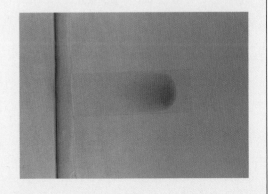

cycle of the parasite in the bloodstream. Malaria is diagnosed with a blood smear, drawn as a stat or timed collection just before the onset of fever or chills. The test requires two to three regular smears, plus a thick smear. To make the thick smear, use a larger drop of blood, and spread it out to only about the size of a dime (Figure 14-9). The sample must be allowed to dry for at least 2 hours; it is then stained to reveal the parasites.

REVIEW FOR CERTIFICATION

Routine phlebotomy specimens are often collected in the early morning, because most patients are in the basal state at that time. A 12-hour complete fast may be required for some tests, especially glucose and triglycerides. The phlebotomist must ensure that the patient has complied with the fast and note any irregularities on the requisition. Timed specimens include the 2-hour postprandial test for diabetes mellitus and the oral glucose tolerance test for diabetes mellitus, hyperglycemia, and hypogly-

TABLE 14-3 Unacceptable Smears and Their Causes

Result	Cause
Uneven distribution of blood	Uneven pressure on spreader slide
	Uneven movement of spreader slide
Holes in smear	Dirty slide
No feathered edge	Drop too large
	Drop not placed close enough to far edge of slide
	Spreader slide lifted before it reached end of sample slide
Streaks in feathered edge	Chipped or dirty spreader slide
	Spreader slide not placed flush against smear slide
	Drop of blood in front of spreader slide
Smear too thick and long	Drop of blood too big
	Angle of spreader slide >30 degrees
Smear too thin and short	Drop of blood too small
	Angle of spreader slide <25 degrees

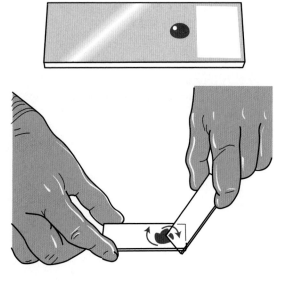

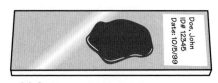

Figure 14-9

The thick smear for a malaria sample uses a larger drop of blood and is spread out only to about the size of a dime.

cemia. Therapeutic drug monitoring tests are timed to coincide with the peak or trough of serum drug levels. Testing for the presence of microorganisms in the blood requires a blood culture, with collection at timed intervals from multiple sites, using aseptic collection of the proper volume. Units of blood may be collected for donation to the blood bank or for use by the patient during later surgery. Therapeutic phlebotomy removes blood from the patient, most often to treat polycythemia or hemochromatosis. Samples to test for cold agglutinins, antibodies formed against *Mycoplasma pneumoniae*, must be kept warm after collection, as must those for cryofibrinogen and cryoglobulin. Other specimens may require chilling or protection from light.

Legal or forensic samples require documentation of the chain of custody, a protocol that ensures that the sample is always in the custody of a person legally entrusted to be in control of it. Alcohol specimens must be handled carefully to avoid contamination of the sample with alcohol and prevent escape of alcohol from the blood.

Blood smears are used for differential counts, counting reticulocytes, and special staining procedures. An acceptable smear must have a feathered edge, prepared by careful drawing of the blood drop across the slide using another slide.

BIBLIOGRAPHY

American Diabetes Association: Report of the Expert Committee on the Diagnosis and Classification of Diabetes Mellitus. Diabetes Care. 2002.

Blaney KD, Howard PR: Basic and Applied Concepts of Immunohematology. St. Louis, Mosby, 2000.

Burtis CA, Ashwood ER: Tietz Fundamentals of Clinical Chemistry, ed 5. Philadelphia, WB Saunders, 2000.

Clinical and Laboratory Standards Institute (CLSI). Procedures for the Collection of Diagnostic Blood Specimens by Venipuncture; Approved Standard—Sixth Edition. CLSI Document H3-A6. November, 2007.

Ernst DJ: Controlling Blood Culture Contamination Rates. Medical Laboratory Observer. May 2000.

Forbes BA, Sahm DF, Weissfeld AS: Bailey & Scott's Diagnostic Microbiology, ed 10. St. Louis, Mosby, 1998.

Koneman EW, et al: Color Atlas and Textbook of Diagnostic Microbiology, ed 5. Philadelphia, JB Lippincott, 1997.

Mahon CR, Manuselis G: Textbook of Diagnostic Microbiology, ed 2. Philadelphia, WB Saunders, 2000.

Murray PR, et al: Manual of Clinical Microbiology, ed 7. Washington, DC, ASM Press, 1999.

Rodak BF: Diagnostic Hematology. Philadelphia, WB Saunders, 1995.

Stiene-Martin EA, Lotspeich-Steininger CA, Koepke JA: Clinical Hematology: Principles, Procedures, Correlations, ed 2. Philadelphia, JB Lippincott, 1998.

STUDY QUESTIONS

1. Define basal state.
2. List 10 factors that influence blood composition.
3. What three things are timed specimens most often used to monitor?
4. What is an OGTT?
5. What is TDM, and why would this be ordered?
6. Why are blood cultures ordered?
7. What collection technique is critical for meaningful blood culture results?
8. Describe the screening process a potential blood donor goes through.
9. What special handling procedure is necessary for cold agglutinin samples?
10. List five tests that require transport on ice.
11. Explain chain of custody.
12. Describe the important features of blood alcohol testing.
13. Explain the procedure for preparing a blood smear.
14. Describe the procedure for preparing a thick smear to test for malaria.
15. List the disorders for which therapeutic phlebotomy is used. Define the diseases based on the word roots, prefixes, and/or suffixes.

CERTIFICATION EXAM PREPARATION

1. Timed specimens are most frequently collected to monitor:
   a. bilirubin
   b. medication levels
   c. cold agglutinins
   d. cryoglobulins

2. A 2-hour postprandial test is used to test for:
   a. blood alcohol
   b. medication levels
   c. malaria
   d. diabetes mellitus

3. Hyperglycemia means:
   a. decreased glucose
   b. decreased hemoglobin
   c. increased glucose
   d. increased hemoglobin

4. For a 3-hour OGTT, how many samples will be collected?
   a. 3
   b. 4
   c. 5
   d. none of the above

5. Within what time period should a patient drink the glucose solution required for an OGTT?
   a. 5 minutes
   b. 10 minutes
   c. 15 minutes
   d. 20 minutes

6. The epinephrine tolerance test determines the patient's ability to:
   a. mobilize glycogen from the liver
   b. digest lactose
   c. metabolize carbohydrates
   d. metabolize medications

7. Blood culture collection involves:
   a. a peak and trough sample
   b. an aerobic and anaerobic sample
   c. a chilled sample
   d. an accompanying urine sample

8. Therapeutic phlebotomies are commonly performed on patients with:
   a. hemochromatosis
   b. leukemia
   c. polycythemia
   d. a and c

9. To collect a cold agglutinin sample:
   a. Warm the sample tube for 30 minutes before collection.
   b. Pack the sample tube in ice before collection.
   c. Wrap the sample in aluminum foil after collection.
   d. Pack the sample tube in ice after collection.

10. Which specimen requires chilling during transfer to the lab?
    a. cryofibrinogen
    b. cryoglobulin
    c. ammonia
    d. cold agglutinins

11. When making smears for malaria:
    a. Prepare two regular smears only.
    b. Prepare two to three regular smears and one thick smear.
    c. Prepare one thick smear only.
    d. Prepare one regular smear and one thick smear.

12. It is necessary for a patient to fast for 12 hours before:
    a. blood donation
    b. blood culture
    c. glucose tolerance test
    d. therapeutic phlebotomy

13. Factors influencing blood composition include all of the following *except*:
    a. altitude
    b. gender
    b. age
    d. weight

14. Specimens that are sensitive to light include all of the following *except*:
    a. vitamin A
    b. lactic acid
    c. beta-carotene
    d. bilirubin

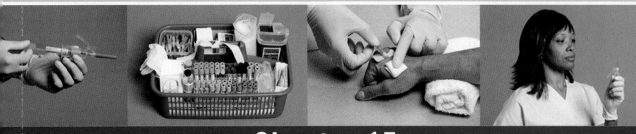

Chapter 15

Special Nonblood Collection Procedures

OUTLINE

OBJECTIVES

After completing this chapter, you should be able to:

1. Describe six kinds of urine samples, explain how each is collected, and state one use for each.
2. Instruct a patient how to collect a midstream clean-catch urine specimen.
3. Explain how a urine sample can be collected from an infant, and state at least one limitation.
4. Discuss why a fecal sample may be requested, list three types of samples, and describe collection methods.

5. Discuss how and why semen samples may be collected.
6. Explain the proper procedure for collecting a throat sample and a nasopharyngeal sample.
7. Explain the reason and the procedure for collecting a sweat chloride sample.
8. Describe how cerebrospinal fluid is collected, and explain how the tubes collected should be distributed.

Continued

OBJECTIVES—cont'd

9. Define each of the following terms and list at least one reason for collecting each fluid:
   a. synovial fluid
   b. peritoneal (ascitic) fluid
   c. pleural fluid
   d. pericardial fluid

10. Explain how amniotic fluid is formed, and describe three reasons for testing it.

KEY TERMS

amniocentesis
catheterized urine sample
8-hour specimen
first morning specimen
iontophoresis

iontophoretic pilocarpine test
midstream clean catch
nasopharyngeal culture
occult blood specimens
random specimen

72-hour stool specimen
suprapubic aspiration
sweat electrolytes
timed specimens

ABBREVIATIONS

C&S: culture and sensitivity
CSF: cerebrospinal fluid
NP: nasopharyngeal

O&P: ova and parasites
SE: sweat electrolytes

A phlebotomist is rarely just a phlebotomist today. In addition to collecting blood, you may be called on to collect nonblood specimens, assist the nurse or physician in doing so, or instruct patients regarding the procedures for collecting or handling such specimens. Nonblood specimens can provide valuable information about a patient's health or disease state. Each of the specimen types discussed in this chapter is collected to provide specific information about the physiologic processes occurring in the body or about the presence of infection or foreign substances. Strict adherence to collection protocols is as important for these procedures as it is for blood collection. Nonblood specimens include urine, feces, semen, and other bodily fluids. Special handling procedures are needed for some specimens to maintain sterility, preserve specimen integrity, or ensure chain of custody.

URINE SPECIMENS

Why Collect a Urine Specimen?

Urine is created by the kidneys as they filter the blood. Urine contains excess salts, waste products, and small amounts of the many types of molecules that naturally circulate in the bloodstream. For this reason, urine provides a valuable snapshot of the inner workings of the body. As with blood, normal values and ranges have been established for the various substances expected to be found in urine. These values are different from those for blood, and the normal ranges are often wider, because concentrations are significantly affected by fluid intake. Urine samples should be delivered to the lab within 1 hour of collection, to prevent the breakdown of unstable compounds. **Timed specimens**, which are specimens collected at specific times, are the exception, as discussed later.

> **◀◀◀ FLASHBACK**
>
> *You learned about the kidney's role in urine formation in Chapter 6.*

Types of Urine Specimens

Random Specimen

A **random specimen** can be collected at any time. It is used to screen for obvious abnormalities in the concentration of proteins, glucose, and other significant constituents of urine.

First Morning Specimen

A **first morning specimen**, also called an **8-hour specimen**, is collected immediately after the patient awakens. It is a very concentrated specimen that ensures the detection of chemicals that may not be found in a more dilute, random sample. Among other tests, this specimen is used for pregnancy testing. This sample should be delivered to the lab within 1 hour of collection, to prevent breakdown of unstable compounds.

Timed Specimen

This is a series of samples often collected over 24 hours and combined to provide a single large specimen (Figure 15-1). It is used to detect low levels of certain proteins and hormones, including creatine, a protein released from muscle. In addition, some compounds are excreted in varying amounts over the course of a day, so a timed specimen is used to determine an average value. The typical procedure is to have the patient void and discard the first morning sample, then collect and combine all urine for the next 24 hours, ending with the first morning sample of the next day. Exact timing and collection of samples are critical. If delivery of the urine sample will not be made within 1 hour, refrigeration of the sample will preserve it. Some samples need to be preserved, either with an added preservative or by refrigeration. Specific instructions for each test should be given in the laboratory manual at your health care facility.

Collection Procedures for Urine Specimens

The most common procedure for collecting many types of urine specimen is known as the **midstream clean catch**. It is collected after the patient has passed several milliliters of urine. This allows

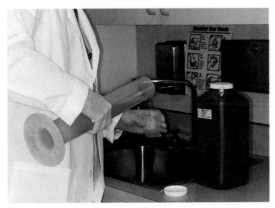

Figure 15-1
The timed urine specimen is often collected over 24 hours and combined to provide a single large specimen. (From Stepp CA, Woods MA: Laboratory Procedures for Medical Office Personnel. Philadelphia, WB Saunders, 1998.)

microorganisms from the urethra to be flushed out and not collected in the sample. When properly collected, the specimen is sterile or nearly so, unless the patient has a urinary tract infection. This sample can be used for urine culture as well as for chemical analysis. Procedure 15-1 outlines the steps for collecting a "midstream" urine specimen. In many cases, the patient can perform the collection himself or herself. The procedure instructions can be adapted to the situation you encounter. Other types of procedures may be more appropriate for special populations.

Pediatric Collection

Pediatric specimens for routine urinalysis can be collected using a soft, clear plastic bag with an adhesive that fits over the genital area of the child (Figure 15-2). This is not a sterile collection.

Catheter Collection

A **catheterized urine sample** is collected by a physician, nurse, or medical assistant. A catheter is inserted through the urethra into the bladder. This technique may be used for a culture and sensitivity (C&S) test when a urinary tract infection is suspected and obtaining a normal clean-catch specimen is not possible. It may also be used if the patient is unable to collect a sample independently. The phlebotomist may assist in processing the sample after collection.

Suprapubic Aspiration

A **suprapubic aspiration** sample is collected by a physician. A needle is inserted through the abdominal wall into the bladder for collection of a sample. The specimen is used for bacterial culture of anaerobes (bacteria that do not grow in the presence of oxygen) and for cytologic (cell) examination in cases of suspected bladder cancer.

Urine Samples for Drug Testing

Urinalysis can reveal the presence of many different types of drugs and metabolites in the bloodstream. Drug testing is becoming increasingly common in outpatient settings, driven by the concern for a drug-free workplace. In addition, drug testing may be performed on athletes to monitor the use of performance-enhancing drugs such as anabolic steroids or on patients to determine whether prescription drugs have been misused.

Samples for drug testing are collected in a chemically clean container, usually as a random

Procedure 15-1

Midstream Clean Catch

1. Clean the genitalia.

For women, use sterile soap to cleanse the area surrounding the urethra. The labia should be separated to improve access.

For men, use towelettes with benzalkonium and alcohol. For uncircumcised men, retract the foreskin for cleaning. For both men and women, begin at the urethra and work outward. Avoid using strong bactericidal agents such as povidone-iodine (Betadine) or hexachlorophene.

2. Collect the sample.

Have the patient begin voiding into the toilet.

Without stopping the urine flow, bring the container into the urine stream until sufficient urine has been collected (the container should be about three quarters full). Be sure not to touch the inside of the container. Have the patient void the rest of the urine into the toilet.

3. Finish the collection.

Cap the container. Refrigerate or add preservatives if necessary. Label the specimen with the patient's name and the date and time of collection.

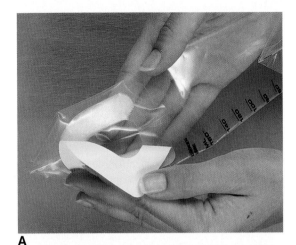

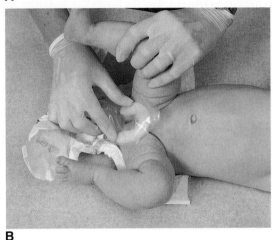

Figure 15-2
Pediatric specimens for routine urinalysis can be collected using a soft, clear plastic bag with an adhesive that fits over the genital area of the child. (From Bonewit-West K: Clinical Procedures for Medical Assistants, ed 5. Philadelphia, WB Saunders, 2000.)

sample via a clean catch. The collection of the sample is usually performed by the patient alone, but in a room without running water to prevent alteration of the specimen. The collection container also has a temperature-sensitive strip on the outside. A freshly collected sample will have a temperature similar to body temperature. The collection and handling procedures must follow chain of custody guidelines, because the sample may be used in a legal proceeding or in decision making regarding employment or athletic participation. The chain of custody is documented with special forms, seals, and containers.

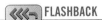 **FLASHBACK**

You learned about chain of custody in Chapter 14.

FECAL SPECIMENS

Why Collect a Fecal Specimen?

The two most common reasons for ordering a fecal sample are to look for intestinal infection and to screen for colorectal cancer. Microscopic examination of feces reveals the presence of intestinal ova and parasites (O&P) from organisms such as *Giardia* and tapeworm. Feces can be cultured to look for diarrhea-causing bacterial diseases such as cholera or salmonella. Cancer of the colon or rectum causes bleeding, and this blood, called *occult blood,* can be detected chemically. Feces also can be chemically analyzed to reveal digestive abnormalities such as excess fat, which may indicate a gallbladder disorder or other fat digestion abnormality.

Types of Fecal Specimens

Random Specimen

A random specimen is used for most determinations, including bacterial cultures, O&P, and fats and fibers.

Occult Blood Specimen

Occult blood specimens are collected after 3 days of a meat-free diet. Patients are instructed to avoid aspirin and vitamin C as well, as these can interfere with test results. Several types of special test cards are available, which may be prepared by the patient at home and sent in (Figure 15-3).

Seventy-two-Hour Stool Specimen

A **72-hour stool specimen** is used for quantitative fecal fat determination. A special large container is provided for collection.

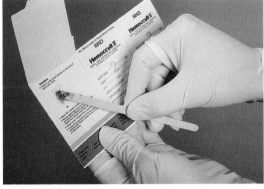

Figure 15-3
Fecal specimens are collected on special test cards, which may be prepared by the patient at home and sent in. (From Bonewit-West K: Clinical Procedures for Medical Assistants, ed 5. Philadelphia, WB Saunders, 2000.)

Collection Procedure for Fecal Specimens

Patients should be given the appropriate collection container and instructed to defecate into it, not the toilet, which would contaminate the sample with cleaning compounds. Patients should also be instructed to avoid contamination of the specimen with urine. Containers resemble a gallon-sized paint can, and are typically plastic or wax-coated cardboard. The container should be tightly sealed and then wrapped in a plastic bag for transport. Specimens should be kept at room temperature or refrigerated until delivery to the lab. If the sample cannot be analyzed immediately, it may be necessary to transfer a portion of the stool to vials containing a preservative. This is especially important when it is to be examined for O&P. Kits with such vials are available commercially, or they may be prepared locally. They can be given directly to the patient, who is responsible for adding the appropriate amount of stool. O&P containers use formalin as a preservative, which is a carcinogen, and should not be sent home with the patient. Instead, the patient delivers the sample to the lab soon after collection, where it is transferred to the vials according to the laboratory's instructions.

SEMEN SPECIMENS

Why Collect a Semen Specimen?

Semen specimens are used to determine whether viable sperm are present in the semen, either for fertility testing or to assess the success of a vasectomy. Semen may also be collected as a forensic specimen from a rape victim.

Collection Procedure for Semen Specimens

The patient should be instructed to avoid ejaculation for 3 days before the collection. The sample should be ejaculated into a sterile plastic container. A condom containing spermicide is an unacceptable collection container. The time of the collection should be recorded, because sperm die quickly, and viability analysis is based on the time elapsed since collection. For fertility testing, the volume of semen is also important, so the patient should report whether the sample collected is complete or partial. The sample should be kept close to body temperature and delivered to the lab within 30 minutes of collection. It is best if the sample is collected in a private room in the health care facility and delivered to the lab immediately.

THROAT SPECIMENS

Why Collect a Throat Specimen?

A throat culture sample (throat swab) is used to diagnose a throat infection. In particular, the sample is used to determine whether the infection is due to *streptococcus A* bacteria, for which antibiotics are an effective treatment. Diagnosis is performed with either a standard bacterial culture or a rapid strep test.

Collection Procedure for Throat Specimens

Procedure 15-2 outlines the procedure for collecting a throat culture.

NASOPHARYNGEAL SPECIMENS

Why Collect a Nasopharyngeal Specimen?

The nasal passages and pharynx are host to many types of infectious organisms, particularly in children. A **nasopharyngeal** (NP) **culture** is used to diagnose whooping cough, croup, pneumonia, and other upper respiratory tract infections.

Collection Procedure for Nasopharyngeal Specimens

The sample is collected using a cotton- or Dacron-tipped sterile wire (Figure 15-4). This swab is passed carefully through the nostril to reach the back of the nasopharynx. It is rotated gently to collect a mucus sample and then removed. The swab is placed in either transport media or growth media, depending on the test to be performed.

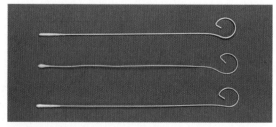

Figure 15-4
A nasopharyngeal culture specimen is collected using a cotton- or Dacron-tipped sterile wire passed carefully through the nostril to reach the back of the nasopharynx.

Procedure 15-2

Throat Swab

1. Assemble your equipment.
You will need a tongue depressor, a flashlight, a sterile collection swab, and a transport tube with transport media (as shown in the photo).

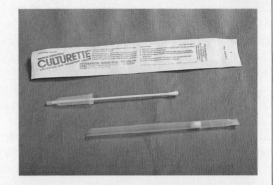

2. Collect the sample.
The patient is usually sitting upright. Ask the patient to tilt his or her head back with the mouth opened wide.

Gently depress the tongue with the tongue depressor. Inspect the back of the throat with the flashlight to locate the areas of inflammation.

Touch the tip of the swab quickly to the tonsils and any other inflamed area. Speed is essential, because the patient may gag involuntarily and touch the swab with the tongue. Be careful not to touch the inside of the cheek, the tongue, or the lips, as this will contaminate the sample and necessitate another collection with a new swab.

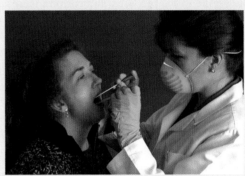

3. Process the sample.
Return the swab to the holder.

Crush the ampule (containing a preservative) at the bottom of the holder containing the transport media, allowing the media to soak into the pledget, or barrier pad that separates the media and swab. Label the sample, and deliver it to the lab.

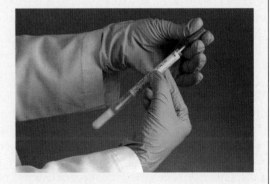

SWEAT ELECTROLYTE SPECIMENS

Why Collect a Sweat Electrolyte Specimen?

Sweat electrolytes (SE) are the salts present in normal sweat. The SE test is performed as part of the diagnosis for cystic fibrosis. A person with cystic fibrosis has elevated levels of chloride in the sweat.

Collection Procedure for Sweat Electrolyte Specimens

SE specimens are subjected to the **iontophoretic pilocarpine test,** which requires special training. Sweating is induced by applying a weak electrical current (known as **iontophoresis**) and the drug pilocarpine to the test area. Pilocarpine increases sweating. Sweat is collected on a piece of sterile filter paper, which is then weighed and analyzed coulometrically (using an electric charge to measure conductivity) to determine the chloride level. The filter paper must be covered with paraffin during collection to prevent evaporation and handled with forceps or gloves to prevent contamination.

CEREBROSPINAL FLUID SPECIMENS

Why Collect a Cerebrospinal Fluid Specimen?

Cerebrospinal fluid (CSF) circulates in the brain and spinal cord, where it provides nourishment and removes wastes from the central nervous system. It is most commonly collected by lumbar puncture (spinal tap), in which a needle is inserted between the vertebrae at the base of the spine. CSF is used most commonly to diagnose meningitis or other central nervous system infections.

Collection Procedure for Cerebrospinal Fluid Specimens

CSF collection is done only by a physician. The phlebotomist may be asked to process and deliver samples after collection. Three tubes are collected and numbered in the order of collection. Tube 1 is delivered to the microbiology lab. Tubes 2 and 3 are delivered to the chemistry and hematology labs; which lab gets which tube is determined by your institution's policy. The hematology sample should be refrigerated until analysis, while the other samples should remain at room temperature. CSF specimens are always handled as stat collections.

TABLE 15-1 Common Body Fluid Collections

Site	Fluid	Typical Reason for Collection
Joint space	Synovial fluid	Diagnosis of arthritis; pain reduction
Peritoneal (abdominal) cavity	Peritoneal fluid	Diagnosis of ascites (abnormal increase of peritoneal fluid)
Pleural cavity (surrounding the lungs)	Pleural fluid	Diagnosis of pleural pneumonia
Pericardium (surrounding the heart)	Pericardial fluid	Diagnosis of pericarditis

BODY FLUID SPECIMENS

Fluid from various body cavities may be withdrawn for analysis or therapy. Table 15-1 lists the most common collection sites and the fluid removed. These collections are always performed by physicians. Fluid is collected in a sterile container, labeled, and transported to the lab for analysis as a stat specimen.

AMNIOTIC FLUID SPECIMENS

Why Collect an Amniotic Fluid Specimen?

Amniotic fluid is the fluid within the amniotic sac, developed within the uterus, that bathes and cushions the developing fetus. It is formed by the metabolism of fetal cells, the transfer of water across the placental membrane, and, in the third trimester, by fetal urine. Amniotic fluid contains fetal cells, which may be analyzed for the presence of certain genetic disorders, such as Down syndrome. In the third trimester of pregnancy, the amniotic fluid can be analyzed for lipids that indicate the degree of development of the fetus' lungs. Bilirubin can also be determined at this stage, to test for hemolytic disease of the newborn. Fluid may be tested for proteins associated with other abnormalities such as spina bifida.

Collection Procedure for Amniotic Fluid Specimens

Amniotic fluid is collected by a physician, in a procedure known as **amniocentesis**. The amniotic fluid is removed by a needle inserted through the mother's abdominal wall into the amniotic sac. The fluid is transferred into a sterile container protected from the light and is immediately transported to the lab for analysis.

REVIEW FOR CERTIFICATION

Nonblood specimens can provide valuable information about a patient's health or disease state. The most common procedure for urine specimen collection is the midstream clean catch, which can be done by the patient or assisted by the phlebotomist. Urine samples should be delivered to the lab within 1 hour of collection, except for timed specimens, which typically involve 24-hour collection, or stat specimens. Fecal specimens are most commonly analyzed for the presence of ova and parasites or occult blood. These specimens may be collected by the patient, who may also deliver the sample card to the lab for processing. Semen specimens are typically collected for fertility testing or rape determination. For fertility testing, prompt delivery is necessary for the determination of sperm viability. Throat culture swabs are carefully introduced through the mouth to the back of the throat; the specimens are used to culture infectious organisms. A nasopharyngeal sample is taken through the nostril to assess upper respiratory tract infections. Cystic fibrosis is diagnosed with the aid of a sweat electrolytes test, which a phlebotomist with special training may assist in performing. Internal bodily fluids, including cerebrospinal fluid, joint fluids, peritoneal fluid, and amniotic fluid, are collected only by doctors. Phlebotomists may be involved in handling and transporting these samples.

BIBLIOGRAPHY

Brunzel NA: Fundamentals of Urine and Body Fluid Analysis. Philadelphia, WB Saunders, 1994.

Haraden LA: Iontophoresis: No sweat. Advance for Medical Laboratory Professionals. December 7, 1998.

National Committee for Clinical Laboratory Standards: GP8-P: Collection and Transportation of Single Collection Urine Specimens. Villanova, PA, NCCLS, 1985.

National Committee for Clinical Laboratory Standards: GP13-P: Collection and Preservation of Timed Urine Specimens. Villanova, PA, NCCLS, 1987.

National Committee for Clinical Laboratory Standards: GP16-A: Routine Urinalysis. Villanova, PA, NCCLS, 1995.

Williams RH, Leiken JB: Medicolegal Issues and Specimen Collection for Ethanol Testing. Laboratory Medicine. August 1999.

STUDY QUESTIONS

1. Define a random urine specimen and what it is used to screen for.
2. Explain the differences between a first morning specimen and a timed specimen.
3. Describe the procedure for collecting a midstream clean-catch specimen.
4. Explain why fecal specimens may be collected.
5. Explain why semen specimens may be collected.
6. Explain why nasopharyngeal specimens may be collected.
7. Explain the purpose of the SE test.
8. In CSF collections, how many tubes are collected, and which departments receive which tubes?
9. Explain why amniotic fluid may be collected.
10. Explain the difference between a throat culture and a nasopharyngeal culture.
11. Define the body areas where the following body fluids are found, and whether the phlebotomist, the nurse, or the physician would be responsible for obtaining the specimen:
    Pleural fluid
    Synovial fluid
    Cerebrospinal fluid
12. Give some of the findings that a 24-hour urine specimen will yield and at least one method of yielding the results.
13. Explain two methods used to induce sweating in the Sweat Electrolytes test, and the equipment used to collect, preserve, and process the specimen in the lab.

CERTIFICATION EXAM PREPARATION

1. An 8-hour specimen is typically collected:
   a. in the morning
   b. before going to bed
   c. after a meal
   d. any time during the day

2. Which urine test is most commonly used to determine pregnancy?
   a. random
   b. fasting
   c. first morning
   d. timed

3. The sweat electrolytes test is typically used to screen for:
   a. multiple sclerosis
   b. myasthenia gravis
   c. cystic fibrosis
   d. spina bifida

4. A urine specimen is labeled:
   a. before collection
   b. after collection
   c. by the patient
   d. on the lid of the specimen

5. Which of the following samples may not be used for a C&S?
   a. catheterized
   b. clean catch
   c. suprapubic
   d. random

6. A 72-hour stool specimen is collected to determine:
   a. fat quantities
   b. occult blood
   c. protein concentrations
   d. creatine levels

7. A semen analysis must be:
   a. delivered to the lab within 30 minutes of collection
   b. kept refrigerated
   c. collected in a condom
   d. obtained after a 5-day period of abstinence

8. The following are always treated as stat specimens, *except:*
   a. urine
   b. peritoneal fluid
   c. cerebrospinal fluid
   d. synovial fluid

9. The test used to diagnose whooping cough, croup, and pneumonia is:
   a. SE test
   b. NP culture
   c. throat swab
   d. urinalysis

10. The following specimens are always collected by a physician, *except:*
    a. amniotic fluid
    b. NP culture
    c. synovial fluid
    d. CSF

UNIT 4

Specimen Handling

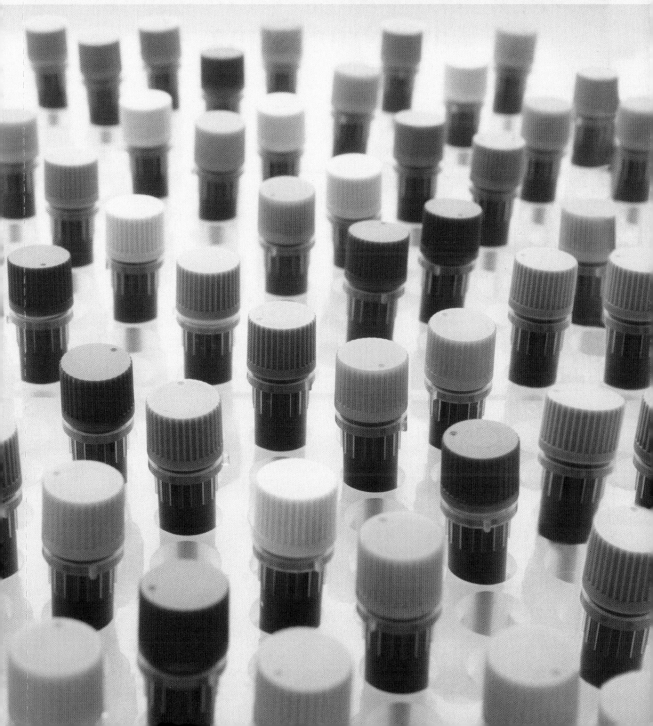

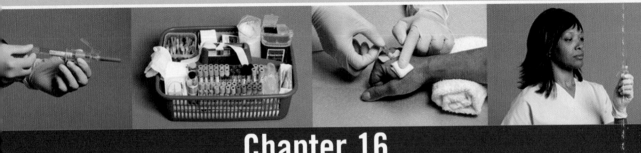

Chapter 16

Specimen Transport, Handling, and Processing

OUTLINE

OBJECTIVES

After completing this chapter, you should be able to:

1. Discuss what might happen to a sample that is not properly handled and processed.
2. Describe four ways in which samples can be safely transported to the lab.
3. Explain why tubes should be transported in an upright position.
4. State the acceptable time between specimen collection and separation of cells from plasma or serum, and explain why this is necessary.
5. List two exceptions to this rule, and state the maximum time that each may be held.
6. List two tests for which the samples must be kept warm, and explain how to do this.
7. Describe how to handle samples that must be chilled.
8. List at least three analytes that are light sensitive, and explain how to protect them.
9. Describe four ways that a sample may be transported to the laboratory.
10. Describe the safety equipment that must be used when processing samples.
11. Explain why samples must be allowed to clot fully before processing, and state the average time for complete clotting to occur in a red-topped tube and when clot activators are used.
12. Explain the principle and proper operation of a centrifuge.
13. Describe the proper procedure for removing a stopper.
14. List at least five reasons for specimen rejection.

KEY TERMS

accession number
aerosol

aliquot
analyte

centrifuge
glycolysis

pneumatic tube system

Proper handling of specimens after collection is critical to ensure the accuracy of the test results obtained from them. Analytes may change in composition and concentration over time and with temperature changes or exposure to light. The best drawing technique in the world is meaningless if the sample is not processed according to established guidelines. Transport systems may be as simple as direct delivery to the lab or as complex as motorized carrier systems routed through a central distribution site. In the lab, the central processing station catalogs the sample, centrifuges it, and prepares aliquots for distribution to other departments. Rejection of specimens can be avoided with proper attention to collection technique, handling, and transport.

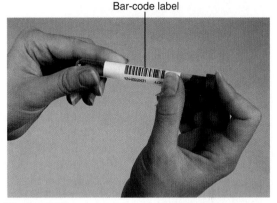

Bar-code label

Figure 16-1

Bar code labels are becoming the standard for specimen labeling in most hospitals. (From Bonewit-West K: Clinical Procedures for Medical Assistants, ed 5. Philadelphia, WB Saunders, 2000.)

GENERAL GUIDELINES FOR SPECIMEN TRANSPORT

Tubes with additives should be inverted gently and completely 5 to 10 times immediately after being drawn. Thorough mixing allows the additives to be evenly distributed throughout the sample. Gentle inversion minimizes hemolysis.

Specimens must be correctly labeled. Bar code labels are becoming the standard in most hospitals (Figure 16-1). An efficient and safe way to transport samples is the use of a leak-resistant bag (Figure 16-2). Some bags have a separate front pouch for requisitions to prevent contamination of the requisition should the specimen leak. Specimens transported from outside a hospital lab are carried in crush-resistant containers with absorbent material inside and biohazard labels outside the container.

Tubes should remain upright during transport. This accomplishes several purposes: It promotes complete clot formation when there is no additive present; it prevents sample contamination due to prolonged contact with the stopper; and it reduces the likelihood of aerosol formation during uncapping, as there is no residual blood clinging to the stopper (see page 237 for discussion of aerosols).

Time Constraints

The quality of test results depends heavily on the time between drawing the sample and analyzing it. Ongoing **glycolysis** (metabolic sugar breakdown within cells) within the specimen is a primary cause of inaccurate test results. Many different tests can be affected by glycolysis, including those for glucose, calcitonin, phosphorus, aldosterone, and a number of enzymes.

As a general rule, a sample should be delivered to the lab within 45 minutes of being drawn. Stat requisitions should be delivered to the lab immediately after being drawn.

According to the Clinical and Laboratory Standards Institute (CLSI), no more than 2 hours should pass between collection and separation of cells from plasma or serum. Once separated, the specimen can be held for longer periods. The appropriate storage temperature depends on the sample type and tests ordered.

A few sample types can wait longer before processing without loss of viability. Because fluoride inhibits glycolysis, glucose samples collected in gray-topped tubes can be held for 24 hours at

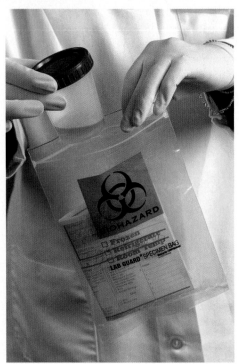

Figure 16-2
A leakproof bag is an efficient and safe way to transport samples.

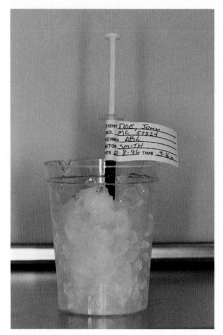

Figure 16-3
Samples needing to be chilled can be transported in shaved ice. (From Stepp CA, Woods MA: Laboratory Procedures for Medical Office Personnel. Philadelphia, WB Saunders, 1988.)

room temperature and for 48 hours at 2 to 8° C. Whole blood specimens collected in ethylenediaminetetraacetic acid (EDTA) are stable for 24 hours. However, blood smears made from such samples must be done within 1 hour of collection, because EDTA will eventually distort cell morphology.

Temperature Considerations

Temperature extremes can cause hemolysis. Samples that do not require cooling or warming should be kept at room temperature during transport.

Keeping Specimens Warm

Specimens that must be maintained at 37° C during transport and handling include cold agglutinins and cryofibrinogen. The tubes for these specimens should be warmed in a heel warmer before collection, and the sample should be transported in a heel warmer as well. Some tests require warming of the sample in a 37° C incubator before testing. The phlebotomist should alert the lab staff of the arrival of a warm sample to make sure that it is held at the correct temperature until testing. Patients with certain types of blood disorders may have acquired

cold agglutinins, which can cause problems with automated instruments. To prevent this, the EDTA tube for a complete blood count (CBC) must be prewarmed and kept warm.

Keeping Specimens Cool

Chilling a specimen slows down metabolic processes and keeps **analytes** (the substances being tested) stable during transport and handling. Samples that need to be chilled include blood gases and lactic acid. To chill a sample, place it in a slurry of chipped or shaved ice and water (Figure 16-3). This promotes complete contact between the sample and the ice bath. Avoid large ice cubes, as these may cause part of the sample to freeze.

Protecting Specimens from Light

Exposure to light can break down light-sensitive analytes. Bilirubin is the most common light-sensitive analyte; others include vitamin B_{12}, carotene, folate, and urine porphyrin. To prevent light exposure, samples are collected in amber-colored microtubes, wrapped in aluminum foil (Figure 16-4), or placed inside a brown envelope or heavy paper bag.

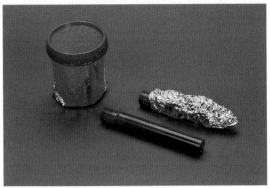

Figure 16-4

Samples needing to be protected from light exposure are collected in amber-colored microtubes or wrapped in aluminum foil.

TRANSPORTING SAMPLES TO THE LAB

How a sample is transported to the lab depends on the size of the institution and the degree of specialization within it. In many institutions, samples are hand carried by the phlebotomist or another member of the lab team. Samples may be dropped off at designated areas within the hospital for transportation and delivery by the lab staff. This system works best when there are clear standards for documentation. A typical system uses a logbook at the drop-off and pickup area in which information about the specimen is documented. Minimum information should include the patient's name, hospital number and room number, specimen type, date and time of delivery to the drop-off area, and name of the person depositing it.

Larger hospitals may have a transportation department that is responsible for patient escort as well as sample delivery. In addition to the standard information concerning patient identification and sample type, specimens should be labeled with the lab as the destination.

Some institutions use a **pneumatic tube system,** in which samples are carried in sealed containers within a network of tubes. Shock-absorbing foam inserts can be placed in carriers to reduce the impact a sample experiences during transport. Samples are first routed to a central station and then sent on to the lab. Pneumatic systems are often used for the delivery of paperwork and other items but are not always appropriate for blood samples, and the lab must assess how well this system meets its needs. Factors may include the reliability of the system, the speed of delivery, the likelihood of specimen damage during transport, and the cost

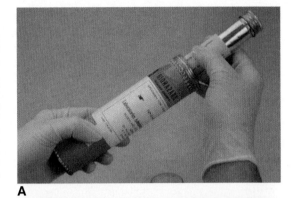

A

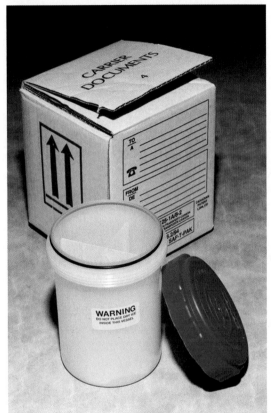

B

Figure 16-5

Courier and overnight mail services use a variety of specialized containers to protect samples and to prevent the contamination of other materials during transport. (*A* from Zakus SM: Clinical Procedures for Medical Assistants, ed 4. St. Louis, Mosby, 2001; *B* from Kinn ME, Woods MA: The Medical Assistant: Administrative and Clinical, ed 8. Philadelphia, WB Saunders, 1999.)

of the alternative. Some institutions use small, self-contained motorized vehicles running on tracks in place of pneumatic systems.

Samples may arrive at the lab from sites outside of the hospital, such as a community clinic or private doctor's office. These samples usually arrive by courier. Because of the short time allowed between collection and serum or plasma separation, the sample should be centrifuged at the collection site before transport. Samples also may arrive by overnight mail. Special containers are used to protect the sample and prevent contamination of other material during transport (Figure 16-5).

PROCESSING

Safety

The Occupational Safety and Health Administration (OSHA) requires personal protective equipment to be worn during sample processing. Required equipment consists of gloves; a full-length lab coat, buttoned or snapped, with closed cuffs; and protective face gear, including either goggles and mask or a chin-length face shield.

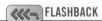

FLASHBACK

You learned about OSHA's role in regulating workplace safety in Chapter 3.

Central Processing

Specimens entering the lab are usually first handled by central processing, an area devoted to cataloging and sorting samples as they arrive. The date and time of arrival are logged, often with a time and date stamping machine. Each sample is marked with an **accession number**, a unique identifying number used for cataloging the sample in the lab. Samples are also labeled with bar codes that are read by an electronic reader, which also records the time the sample is received and stores it in the computer system. Samples are then sorted by sample type and destination within the lab. Central processing is also usually responsible for centrifuging samples, to separate plasma or serum from cellular elements, and for preparing **aliquots,** which are small portions of the specimen transferred into separate containers for distribution to a variety of lab departments.

Before centrifuging, the stopper should remain on the sample to prevent its contamination or alteration. Cap removal releases carbon dioxide, which raises the pH and allows sample evaporation, causing increased concentration of analytes. An open tube is likely to pick up dust, sweat, powder from gloves, or other contaminants. It also creates the possibility of infectious aerosols during centrifugation.

Clotting

Serum specimens must be completely clotted before centrifugation. Incompletely clotted samples continue to clot after serum separation, interfering with testing. Plasma specimens, in contrast, can be centrifuged immediately, because they have anticoagulants to prevent clotting.

Complete clotting may take 30 to 45 minutes at room temperature. Samples from patients on anticoagulants such as heparin or dicumarol have longer clotting times, as do chilled specimens and those from patients with high white blood cell counts. Samples with clot activators (including serum separator tubes) clot more rapidly, usually within 15 minutes. If thrombin is used, complete clotting may occur within 5 minutes. Activators are also available that can be added to the tube after collection.

Centrifuging

A **centrifuge** spins the sample at a very high speed, separating components based on density. Cellular elements, which are denser, move to the bottom; the less dense plasma or serum is pushed to the top. Centrifuges come in a variety of sizes, from small tabletop models designed to hold 6 to 8 specimens to large floor models that can hold 20 or more (Figure 16-6).

The most important principle of centrifuge operation is that every sample must be balanced by another of equal weight (Figure 16-7). Failure to balance the load causes the rotor of the centrifuge to spin out of center. This can damage the centrifuge and may allow it to move during operation, possibly causing it to fall off the table or move across the floor. In addition to the direct danger this poses to lab personnel, the resulting breakage of samples presents a biohazard. When necessary, an extra tube containing water should be added to balance an odd number of tubes.

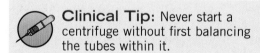

Clinical Tip: Never start a centrifuge without first balancing the tubes within it.

The lid of the centrifuge must be closed and secured during operation; and it must stay closed until the rotor comes to a stop. Never try to bring the centrifuge to a premature halt by touching the rotor; this is dangerous and can also disrupt the sample. Specimens should be centrifuged only once, as repeated centrifugation can cause hemolysis and deterioration of analytes.

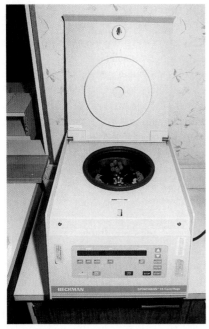

Figure 16-6
A tabletop centrifuge. (From Stepp CA, Woods MA: Laboratory Procedures for Medical Office Personnel. Philadelphia, WB Saunders, 1998.)

Removing a Stopper

The major risk of stopper removal is formation of an **aerosol,** a microscopic mist of blood that forms from droplets inside the tube. Aerosols are especially likely if the tube or rim has been contaminated by blood during collection or transport. Many automated instruments allow for testing without stopper removal. In these cases the instrument removes the sample by piercing the stopper of the tube.

Careful stopper removal reduces the risk of aerosol formation. To remove a stopper, place a 4- by 4-inch piece of gauze over the top, and pull the stopper straight up, twisting it if necessary. Do not rock it from side to side or "pop" it off. The Hemogard top is a plastic top that fits over the stopper to reduce aerosol formation and spattering. Commercial stopper removers are available as well.

Preparing Aliquots

All tubes into which aliquots are placed should be labeled before filling and then capped before delivery to the appropriate department. Aliquots are not poured off, because this may allow splashing and aerosol formation. Instead, an aliquot is removed with any one of several types of disposable pipetting systems (Figure 16-8).

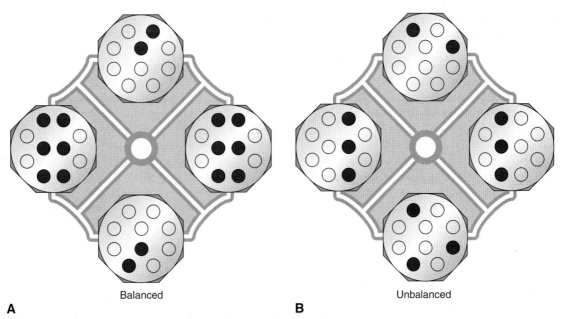

Balanced

A

Unbalanced

B

Figure 16-7
Tubes must be balanced in the centrifuge to avoid creating a hazard and damaging the machine.
A, A balanced centrifuge arrangement. **B,** An unbalanced arrangement.

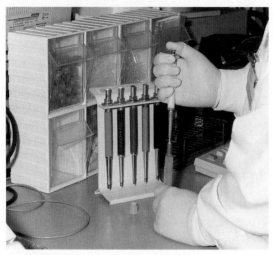

Figure 16-8
The specimen is divided into aliquots for distribution to lab departments. Several types of disposable pipetting systems are available for the removal of aliquots. (From Stepp CA, Woods MA: Laboratory Procedures for Medical Office Personnel. Philadelphia, WB Saunders, 1998.)

TRANSPORT AND PROCESSING OF NONBLOOD SPECIMENS

Microbiology samples must be transported to the lab immediately to increase the likelihood of recovering pathogenic organisms. Most specimens are collected in transport media and do not require additional processing after collection. Most samples go in the refrigerator, but the phlebotomist should always check the lab manual, because some do not.

Twenty-four-hour urine samples must have their volume measured and recorded before aliquoting. Stool samples are kept at room temperature or refrigerated during transport and after delivery.

SPECIMEN REJECTION

All specimens received by the lab must be evaluated for acceptability before further processing. Criteria for rejection include:

1. Improper or inadequate identification
2. Hemolysis
3. Incorrect tube for the test ordered (e.g., EDTA for a chemistry test)
4. Tubes used past their expiration date
5. Inadequate ratio of blood to additive (e.g., a short draw for sodium citrate)

6. Insufficient volume for testing (known quantity not sufficient, or **QNS**)
7. Specimen drawn at the wrong time (e.g., a therapeutic drug level sample)
8. Contaminated specimen (e.g., urine for culture and sensitivity testing collected in a nonsterile container)
9. Improper handling (e.g., cold agglutinins not kept warm)

REVIEW FOR CERTIFICATION

Proper specimen handling is essential for obtaining accurate test results. Tubes with additives should be inverted gently and completely 5 to 10 times immediately after being drawn. All specimens must be properly labeled, and tubes should remain upright during transport. As a general rule, a sample should be delivered to the lab within 45 minutes of being drawn, with no more than 2 hours between collection and centrifuging. Stat requisitions should be delivered to the lab immediately after being drawn. The phlebotomist should alert the lab staff regarding samples that must be kept warm, to make sure that they are held at the elevated temperature until testing. Samples that require chilling should be placed in a slurry of chipped or shaved ice and water. To prevent light exposure, samples are collected in amber-colored microtubes or wrapped in aluminum foil. Transport systems vary in complexity, but all rely on scrupulous documentation at every stage. Samples may arrive at the lab via direct transport by the phlebotomist, pneumatic tube, collection department staff, courier, or overnight mail. Processing begins with assigning an access number, centrifuging, and preparing aliquots. Safety precautions include the use of personal protective equipment and careful stopper removal to minimize the formation of and exposure to aerosols. Rejection of specimens can be avoided through careful attention to labeling, proper collection and handling techniques, and prompt delivery to the lab.

BIBLIOGRAPHY

Beckala HR: Regulations for Packaging and Shipping Laboratory Specimens. Laboratory Medicine. October 1999.

King D: Is Your Lab's Specimen Delivery System up to Speed? Advance for Medical Laboratory Professionals. February 14, 2000.

National Committee for Clinical Laboratory Standards: H 18-A: Procedures for the Handling and Processing of Blood Specimens. Villanova, PA, NCCLS, June 1994.

STUDY QUESTIONS

1. Describe how tubes with anticoagulant should be inverted.
2. What tests can be affected by glycolysis?
3. How soon after collection should cells be separated from plasma or serum?
4. How can specimens be maintained at 37°C during transport and handling?
5. What is the purpose of chilling a specimen?
6. What minimal documentation should be included with each specimen delivered to the lab?
7. What are some disadvantages to the pneumatic tube system?
8. What is the purpose of an accession number?
9. Explain why it is important that a centrifuge carry a balanced load.
10. Describe what aliquots are and how they are prepared.
11. Describe the procedure for removing a stopper.
12. How should stat specimens be transported to the lab as opposed to routine specimens?
13. Explain the purpose of maintaining tubes in an upright position during transportation.
14. List the reasons why specimens should be delivered under time constraint to the lab.
15. Name the light-sensitive analytes and describe how to handle these specimens.

CERTIFICATION EXAM PREPARATION

1. Hemolysis can be minimized by:
   a. specimen tubes remaining upright
   b. vigorous mixing
   c. immediate separation of cells from plasma or serum
   d. prewarming of the sample

2. Cold agglutinins and cryofibrinogen samples should be:
   a. chilled before collection
   b. transported on ice to the lab
   c. warmed before collection and transported warmed
   d. transported at room temperature

3. Infant bilirubins are transported:
   a. on ice
   b. in amber-colored microtubes
   c. in a heel warmer
   d. No special transport measures are necessary.

4. Once a cap is removed from a blood tube, the pH:
   a. may decrease
   b. may increase
   c. will not change
   d. becomes alkaline

5. Which of the following can be centrifuged immediately after collection?
   a. serum separator tubes
   b. clot tubes
   c. thrombin tubes
   d. sodium citrate tubes

6. All of the following are reasons for specimen rejection, *except:*
   a. a CBC collected in a lithium heparin tube
   b. an EDTA tube used for a chemistry test
   c. a sodium level collected in a sodium heparin tube
   d. a cold agglutinin sample transported in a heel warmer

7. Complete blood clotting may take _____ at room temperature.
   a. 10 to 15 minutes
   b. 20 to 30 minutes
   c. 30 to 45 minutes
   d. 1 hour

8. The major risk of stopper removal is:
   a. glycolysis
   b. hemolysis
   c. aerosol
   d. clotting

9. All of the following are assigned to a specimen, *except:*
   a. name of collector of the specimen
   b. accession number
   c. specimen type
   d. name of person depositing specimen in the lab

Professional Issues

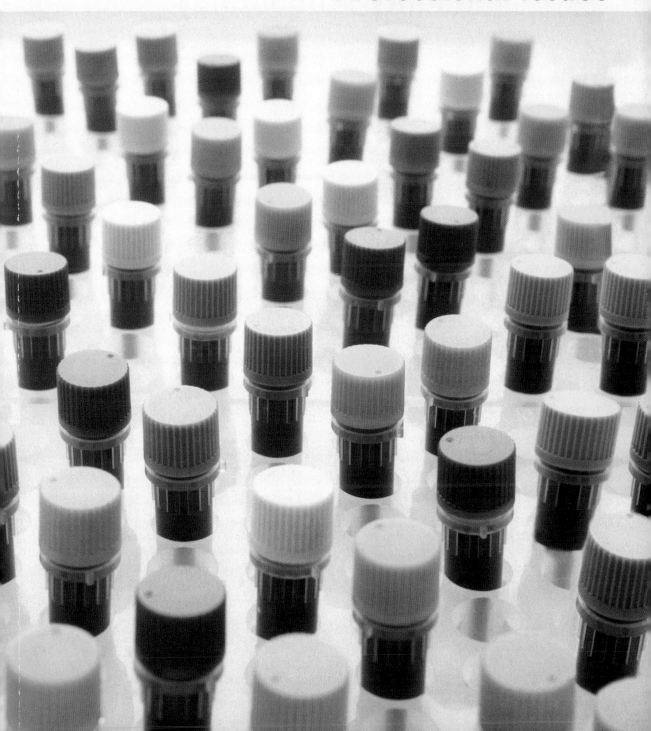

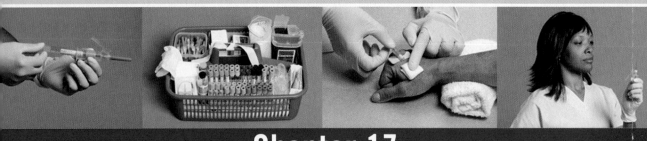

Chapter 17

Quality Phlebotomy

OUTLINE

OBJECTIVES

After completing this chapter, you should be able to:

1. Define quality assurance, quality control, total quality management, and continuous quality improvement, and discuss their differences and roles in quality phlebotomy.
2. Describe the contents of the procedure manual and explain how the phlebotomist can use it.
3. Explain the role of the floor book, and describe the information it contains.
4. List three types of analytical variables.
5. Describe at least five errors that may occur as a result of improper requisition handling, and explain quality assurance procedures to monitor for them.
6. Describe procedures that should be followed for the quality control of phlebotomy equipment.
7. Explain why expired tubes should not be used.
8. Define delta check and explain its use in quality assurance.
9. List nine patient activities that may affect laboratory test results, and give at least one example of a test affected by each.

10. List at least four blood collection sites that may lead to sample contamination, and list six sites that may result in pain or injury to the patient.
11. Discuss at least two errors that may result from improper tourniquet application.
12. Explain the risks of failing to cleanse the puncture site carefully, and discuss one method to monitor for such errors.
13. Describe precautions that must be taken when iodine is used as a cleansing agent, and list at least two laboratory tests that can be affected.
14. Discuss at least eight precautions that must be taken in collecting and labeling specimens.
15. Explain the phlebotomist's role in ensuring a positive patient perception of the level of care received.
16. Explain the steps to be followed in the case of an accidental needle stick, and describe quality assurance procedures that may be used.
17. Discuss the monitoring of variables during sample transport.

Continued

OBJECTIVES—cont'd

18. Explain the effects of sample-processing variables on sample quality (e.g., separation times, centrifugation).
19. Describe how refrigerators and freezers are monitored.
20. Explain how multiple aliquots prepared from a single sample should be handled.

KEY TERMS

continuous quality
  improvement
delta check
floor book

Joint Commission on
  Accreditation of
  Healthcare
  Organizations

preanalytical variables
procedure manual
quality assurance
quality control

quality phlebotomy
total quality management

> ## ABBREVIATIONS
> **CQI:** continuous quality improvement
> **JCAHO:** Joint Commission on Accreditation of Healthcare Organizations
> **QA:** quality assurance
> **QC:** quality control
> **TQM:** total quality management

Quality phlebotomy is a set of policies and procedures designed to ensure the highest quality patient care and consistent specimen analysis. Continual, gradual improvement in the standard of care delivered is the goal of quality phlebotomy. The phlebotomist is best able to control preanalytical variables, which are those that influence patient care and sample integrity before analysis in the lab. Patient preparation, specimen collection, and transport and processing are critical areas for quality phlebotomy. Throughout this book, you have learned important precautions and techniques designed to maintain both patient comfort and safety and the quality of the sample collected. We review those items here and discuss the lab procedures that have an impact on the quality of test results.

of methods used to guarantee quality patient care, including the methods used for patient preparation and collection and transportation protocols. Both QC and QA are included in **total quality management** (TQM), the entire set of approaches used by the institution to provide patient satisfaction. **Continuous quality improvement** (CQI) is the major goal of TQM programs.

Quality assurance programs are mandated by the **Joint Commission on Accreditation of Healthcare Organizations** (JCAHO). JCAHO standards require that a systematic process be in place to monitor and evaluate the quality of patient care. The direct involvement of workers is a requirement of TQM programs. The team approach improves production by reducing errors and waste, thereby resulting in a reduction in healthcare cost.

FEATURES OF QUALITY PHLEBOTOMY

Quality phlebotomy refers to a set of policies and procedures designed to ensure the delivery of the highest quality patient care and consistent specimen analysis. Quality phlebotomy ensures better patient care by reducing errors and increasing efficiency, making the delivery of care more cost efficient.

There are several aspects to quality phlebotomy. **Quality control** (QC) refers to the quantitative methods used to monitor the quality of procedures, such as regular inspection and calibration of equipment, to ensure accurate test results. Quality control is part of **quality assurance** (QA), the larger set

Total Quality Management

TQM focuses on gradual, continual improvements in the quality of services provided by the lab. Rather than merely setting a minimum standard to be met, the TQM philosophy sees the potential for improvement in every area, no matter how high the current performance level, in order to improve the services provided to "customers." For the clinical laboratory, the customers are the patients, the physicians and other health care providers who order tests, and the personnel who use test results to provide treatment. The phlebotomist is the member of the lab team with the most direct patient contact and is therefore most responsible for customer satisfaction in this area.

Quality Assurance

QA guarantees quality patient care through a specific program, including both technical and nontechnical procedures. QA programs use written documentation to set standards for the performance of procedures, monitor compliance with the written procedures, and track patient outcomes with scheduled evaluations of all lab activities. Documentation provides written policies and procedures covering all services and provides evidence that standards have been met and that work is being performed efficiently. In the event of a problem, documentation provides a means of monitoring the actions taken to resolve the problem. Documentation includes a procedure manual for laboratory procedures, a floor book distributed to nursing stations and other departments detailing schedules and other information, the identification of variables that may affect patient care and test results, and continuing education for all members of the lab staff.

Procedure Manual

The **procedure manual** is present in the department at all times. It contains protocols and other information about all the tests performed in the lab, including the principle behind the test, the purpose of performing it, the specimen type the test requires, the collection method, and the equipment and supplies required. QA procedures relevant to the procedure manual include updating the standards and protocols to comply with advances in the field, training for lab members in the proper performance of procedures, scheduled testing of standard samples, and monitoring of results.

Floor Book

The **floor book** contains a variety of information pertinent to the smooth coordination of nursing staff and lab personnel. It includes laboratory schedules, sweep times, and written notification of any changes, plus information on patient preparation, specimen types and handling, and normal values. The floor book is also called the directory of services. QA procedures relevant to the information in the floor book include monitoring the numbers of incomplete or duplicate requisitions received, collecting statistics on the number of missed or delayed collections, and recording the time between a test request and reporting of the results.

Monitoring of Variables

A variable is any factor that can be measured or counted that affects the outcome of test results and therefore patient care. Once identified, a variable is controlled through the institution of a set of written procedures. Monitoring of the variable is performed and documented to ensure that its impact on test results is minimized.

There are three types of variables: preanalytical, analytical, and postanalytical. The phlebotomist is most responsible for controlling **preanalytical variables**, those that occur before analysis of the specimen (Figure 17-1). Analytical variables, those that occur during specimen analysis, can be affected by preanalytical variables, such as collection time or transport conditions. Postanalytical variables, such as delays in reporting results or improper entry of results in the data bank, also may be part of the phlebotomist's responsibilities.

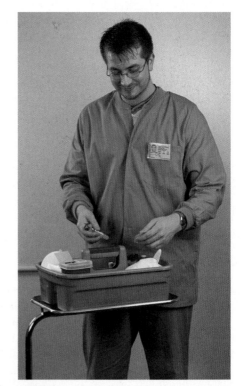

Figure 17-1
Phlebotomists are most responsible for controlling preanalytical variables, such as ensuring that the equipment they use is free of defects.

PREANALYTICAL VARIABLES

Requisition Handling

Preanalytical variables occur in each area of the phlebotomist's duties, beginning with test ordering and requisition handling. Requisitions must be accurately and completely filled out with the patient number, tests ordered, and priority (Figure 17-2). Variables to be controlled include duplicate or missing requisitions, tests left off the requisition, missing patient number, missing doctor name, or priority not indicated. When demographic, diagnostic, and insurance information is omitted or is inaccurate, there is a delay in the reporting results, introducing a postanalytical variable. QA procedures for these variables include recording and counting the numbers of each type of requisition error.

Equipment

Phlebotomy equipment is designed and manufactured to be free of defects and minimize variability. Nonetheless, errors do occur, and it is up to the phlebotomist to identify and eliminate them before they interfere with patient care. QA procedures include the following:

- Tubes should be checked for lot number and expiration date. Never use an expired tube.
- Stoppers should be checked for cracks or improper seating. Reject any tube with a defective stopper.
- Tubes may lose vacuum without any visible sign of defect. When filling a tube, be aware of incomplete filling because of loss of vacuum.
- Needles should always be inspected for defects, including blunted points or burrs (Figure 17-3). Never use a defective needle or one from a package with a broken seal.
- Syringe plungers must move freely in the barrel. Reject a syringe with a sticky plunger.

Patient Identification

It cannot be emphasized too strongly that proper patient identification is the most important procedure in phlebotomy. Improper identification can lead to injury or death. Proper identification is made when the patient number on the requisition matches the number on the patient's identification band *and* that band is attached to the patient.

A **delta check** is a QA procedure that helps spot identification errors. This check compares previous patient results with current results. If the difference ("delta") between the two sets of results is outside the limit of expected variation, it alerts lab personnel to the possibility of an error.

PATIENT PREPARATION AND SPECIMEN COLLECTION

Many preanalytical variables arise during patient preparation and specimen collection. Although not all of them can be completely controlled in every procedure, developing skill as a phlebotomist in large part means minimizing the effect of these variables to the greatest extent possible.

Patient Preparation

The patient's physical condition at the time of the collection has a significant effect on the sample quality. The phlebotomist has little or no control over most of these variables, but may note their presence to aid in the interpretation of test results. Factors include:

- Posture: A sample collected from an erect patient has higher concentrations of large molecules such as enzymes and albumin, as well as white and red blood cells, compared with a sample collected from a supine patient (Figure 17-4). This is due to a gravity-induced shift in fluids upon standing.
- Short-term exercise: Exercise increases levels of muscle enzymes such as creatine kinase, as well as white blood cells, creatinine, and fatty acids.
- Long-term exercise: A prolonged exercise regimen increases sex hormones and aldolase, as well as many of the values increased by short-term exercise.
- Medications and medical treatments: Certain medications affect test results directly. Aspirin is the most common one, prolonging bleeding times. Other treatments to be aware of include the administration of radiographic dyes, blood transfusions, or intravenous fluids. Anticoagulants (warfarin and heparin) cause prolonged bleeding after the puncture. It is important to know this since it requires extra time after the puncture to apply pressure at the site, to avoid compartment syndrome.

 FLASHBACK

You learned about the risk of compartment syndrome in Chapter 11.

- Alcohol consumption: Although moderate amounts of alcohol do not affect test results (except, of course, for the alcohol test), glucose is slightly

Biomedical Laboratories, Inc.
100 Main Street
Athens, Georgia 45760

☐ Fax — Send additional copy of report to:
_____ ( )_____

☐ Call — Client Number/Physician's Name — Phone/Fax Number

☐ Mail — Physician's Address — City, State, Zip

Patient's Name (Last)	(First)	(M)	Sex	Date of Birth MO	DAY	YR	Collection Time AM / PM	Fasting ☐ YES ☐ NO	Collection Date MO	DAY	YR

NPI/UPIN	Physician's ID #	Patient's SS #	Patient's ID #	Urine hrs/vol hrs____ vol____

Physician's Name (Last, First) — X _____ Physician's Signature

Patient's Address — Phone

Medicare # (Include prefix/suffix) — ☐ Primary ☐ Secondary

City — State — ZIP

Medicaid # — State — Physician's Provider #

Name of Responsible Party (if different from patient)

Diagnosis/Signs/Symptoms in ICD-9 Format(Highest Specificity)

R E Q U I R E D

Address of Responsible Party — APT #

City — State — ZIP

RESP. PARTY / **PATIENT**

Patient's Relationship to Responsible Party ■ 1 - Self ■ 2 - Spouse ■ 3 - Child ■ 4 - Other

INSURANCE			
Insurance Company Name	Plan	Carrier Code	
Subsciber/Member #	Location	Group #	
Insurance Address		Physician's Provider #	
City	State	ZIP	
Employer's Name or Number	Insured SS# (If Not Patient)	Worker's Comp ☐ Yes ☐ No	

Perform-ance Lab — Carrier — Group # — Employee # — Mem

I hereby authorize the release of medical information related to the service described herein and authorize payment directed to LabCorp.
X _____ Patient's Signature — Date

MEDICARE ADVANCE BENEFICIARY NOTICE (ABN)
I have read the ABN on the reverse. If Medicare denies payment, I agree to pay for the identified test(s).
X _____ Patient's Signature — Date

INDIVIDUAL COMPONENTS OF TEST COMBINATIONS/PROFILES LISTED IN THE SECTION ABOVE CAN BE ORDERED BELOW.

@ : Carrier-specific limited coverage test
# : Investigational test per Medicare

NOTE: WHEN ORDERING TESTS FOR WHICH MEDICARE OR MEDICAID REIMBURSEMENT WILL BE SOUGHT, PHYSICIANS SHOULD ONLY ORDER TESTS THAT ARE MEDICALLY NECESSARY FOR THE DIAGNOSIS OR TREATMENT OF THE PATIENT. COMPONENTS OF THE ORGAN OR DISEASE PANELS/COMBINATIONS PRINTED BELOW ARE SHOWN ON THE REVERSE SIDE AND MAY ALSO BE ORDERED INDIVIDUALLY BELOW. COMPONENTS MAY BE BILLED SEPARATELY PER CARRIER POLICY.

ORGAN OR DISEASE PANELS (See reverse for components)

Code	Test	#	Tube
303758	Basic Metabolic Panel	80049	SST
302085	Comp Metabolic Panel	80054	SST
303754	Electrolyte Panel	80051	SST
303755	Hepatic Function Panel	80058	SST
303744	Hepatitis Panel	80059	SST
303756	Lipid Panel	80061	SST
235010	Lipid Panel w/LDL/HDL Ratio	80061	SST
000455	Thyroid Panel	80091	SST
000620	Thyroid Panel w/ TSH	80092	SST

HEMATOLOGY

Code	Test	#	Tube
005009	CBC w Diff w Plt	85025	LAV
115907	CBC w Diff w/o Plt	85022	LAV
028142	CBC w/o Diff w Plt	85027	LAV
005017	CBC w/o Diff w/o Plt	85021	LAV
005058	Hematocrit	85014	LAV
005041	Hemoglobin	85018	LAV
005249	Platelet Count	85595	LAV
005033	RBC Count	85041	LAV
005025	WBC Count	85048	LAV
005090	WBC Differential	85007	LAV

ALPHABETICAL/COMBINATION TES

Code	Test	#	Tube
006049	ABO and Rh (see reverse)	86900 / 86901	LAV
001081	Albumin	82040	SST
001107	Alkaline Phosphatase	84075	SST
001545	ALT (SGPT)	84460	SST
001396	Amylase	82150	SST
006254	Antinuclear Antibodies	86038	SST
001123	AST (SGOT)	84450	SST
000810	B12 and Folate (see reverse)	82607 / 82746	SST
001099	Bilirubin, Total	82250	SST

ALPHABETICAL TESTS CON'T

Code	Test	#	Tube
001040	BUN	84520	SST
001016	Calcium	82310	SST
007419	Carbamazepine (Tegretol®)	80156	SER
002139	CEA	82378	SST
001065	Cholesterol, Total	82465	SST
001370	Creatinine	82565	SST
007385	Digoxin (Lanoxin)	80162	SER
004515	Estradiol	82670	SST
004598	Ferritin	82728	SST
100800	Fructosamine	82985	SST
004309	FSH	83001	SST
028480	FSH and LH (see reverse)	83001 / 83002	SST
001958	GGT	82977	SST
001818	Glucose, Plasma	82947	GRY
001032	Glucose, Serum	82947	SST
002022	Glucose, 2-hr. PP	82950	SST
001693	Glycohemoglobin, Total	83036	LAV
004556	hCG, Beta Subunit, Qual	84703	SST
004416	hCG, Beta Subunit, Quant	84702	SST
001925	HDL Cholesterol	83718	SST
162289	Helicobacter pylori, IgG	86677	SST
006395	Hep B Surface Antibody	86706	SST
006510	Hep B Surface Antigen	87340	SST
140608	Hep C Antibody	86803	SST
001453	Hemoglobin A1c	83036	LAV
083824	HIV Antibodies *	86701	SST
001339	Iron	83540	SST
001321	Iron and IBC (see reverse)	83540 / 83550	SST
001115	LDH	83615	SST

ALPHABETICAL TESTS CON'T

Code	Test	#	Tube
004283	LH	83002	SST
001404	Lipase	83690	SER
007708	Lithium (Eskalith®)	80178	SER
001537	Magnesium	83735	SST
007823	Phenobarbital (Luminal®)	80184	SER
0007401	Phenytoin (Dilantin®)	80185	SST
001180	Potassium	84132	SST
004465	Prolactin, Serum	84146	SST
010322	Prostate-Specific Antigen	84153	SST
004747	Prostatic Acid Phos	84066	SST
001073	Protein, Total	84155	SST
005199	Prothrombin Time (PT)	85610	BLU
020321	PT and PTT Activated	85610 / 85730	BLU
005207	PTT Activated	85730	BLU
006502	Rheumatoid Arthritis Factor	86431	SST
006072	RPR	86592	SST
006197	Rubella Antibodies, IgG	86762	SST
005215	Sed Rate, Westergren	85651	LAV
001198	Sodium	84295	SST
004226	Testosterone	84403	SST
007336	Theophylline	80198	SER
001149	Thyroxine (T4)	84436	SST
001172	Triglycerides	84478	SST
002188	Triiodothyronine (T3)	84480	SST
004259	TSH, High Sensitivity	84443	SST
001057	Uric Acid	84550	SST
003038	Urinalysis Microscopic on Positives	81003	URN
003772	Urinalysis with Microscopic	81001	URN
007260	Valproic Acid (Depakene®)	80164	SER

MICROBIOLOGY - See Reverse Side

■ ENDOCERVICAL ■ THROAT ■ URINE
■ STOOL ■ URETHRAL INDICATE SOURCE
OTHER

Code	Test	#	
008649	Aerobic Bacterial Culture †	87070	Bact Tmspt
164160	Chlamydia/GC DNA Probe w/ Confirmation on Positives *	87490 / 87590	Probe Tmspt
096479	Chlamydia/GC DNA Probe without Confirmation	87490 / 87590	Probe Tmspt
164202	Chlamydia DNA Probe *	87490	Probe Tmspt
180745	Genital, Beta-Hemolytic Strep Cult, Group B	87081	Bact Tmspt
008334	Genital Culture, Routine †	87070	Bact Tmspt
180810	Lower Respiratory Culture †	87070	Steril Tmspt
164210	N. gonorrhoeae DNA Probe *	87590	Probe Tmspt
008623	Ova and Parasites	87015 / 87211	O & P Kit
008144	Stool Culture †	87081 X2 / 87045	Fecal Tmspt
008169	Throat, Beta-Hemolytic Strep Cult, Group A	87081	Bact Tmspt
008342	Upper Respiratory Culture, Routine	87060	Bact Tmspt
008847	Urine Culture, Routine †	87086	Urn Cul Tmspt

† = ID/Susceptibility at Additional Charge
* = Confirmation at Additional Charge

Clinical Information/Comments

OTHER TESTS/INDIVIDUAL PROFILE COMPONENTS
TEST# — TEST NAMES

LABCORP USE ONLY	STAT ☐ 998074	VENIPUNCTURE ☐ 998085	TRAVEL ☐ 998096	NON LABCORP ☐ 998239	VERBAL ORDER ☐ 998250	CHART ORDER ☐ 998261	HANDWRITTEN ☐ 998272	24 HR TUV ☐ 998283	PST/PSC #

CONTAINERS RECEIVED → SST SPUN | USST UNSPUN | SER SERUM TRNSPT | FRZ FRZ TRNS | RED RED | LAV LAVENDER | SLD SLIDE | BLU LT. BLUE | GRY GREY | GRN GREEN | RYL BLU RYL BLU | YEL ACD | PLS PLASMA | URN URINE | 24U 24 HR URINE | TA-U TART. ACID | FL FLUID | OT OTHER | BACT TRNSP | O & P KIT | PROBE TRNSP | URN CUL TRNSP | STERIL TRNSP | FECAL TRNSP | VIRAL TRNSP

300-0384

Figure 17-2
Laboratory requisition form. (From Bonewit-West K: Clinical Procedures for Medical Assistants, ed 5. Philadelphia, Saunders, 2000.)

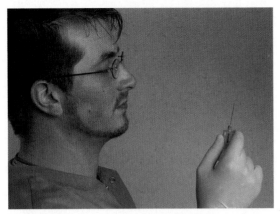

Figure 17-3
Always ensure that phlebotomy equipment is not defective.

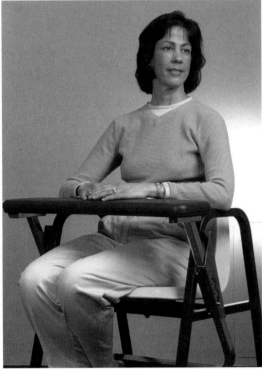

Figure 17-4
Collecting a specimen from an erect patient, as opposed to a supine patient, produces different test results.

elevated, and chronic consumption can lead to increased values on liver function tests, as well as interfering with platelet aggregation studies.

- Smoking: Smoking increases catecholamines, cortisol, white blood cells, mean corpuscular volume, and hemoglobin, and decreases eosinophils. Smoking also affects arterial blood gases.
- Stress: Anxiety, crying, or hyperventilating may affect test results, including the stress hormones

produced by the adrenal cortex. Prolonged crying or hyperventilating alters arterial blood gases, and crying can increase white blood cells.

- Diurnal variation: Certain specimens must be collected at specific times of day, because of significant changes throughout the day. Such specimens include cortisol and iron.
- Fasting: Prolonged fasting increases bilirubin and fatty acids. Overnight fasting concentrates most analytes. A fasting specimen should be taken 8 to 12 hours after the last intake of food. It is the phlebotomist's responsibility to ascertain that the patient has had no food during that time. Caffeinated beverages, such as coffee, tea, and soda, must be avoided as well. Caffeine causes a transient rise in blood sugar levels. A patient not in the fasting state may produce a *lipemic sample*, in which the serum or plasma appears turbid. This turbidity, which is caused by an increase in blood triglycerides, interferes with many tests that rely on photometry, or the passage of light through the sample. High-speed centrifugation may be used to pretreat lipemic specimens to overcome interference, but in cases of gross lipemia, the sample may have to be recollected.

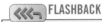

‹‹‹↰ FLASHBACK

You learned about fasting specimens in Chapter 14.

- Age: There are many lab values that vary with age. For instance, because organ function declines with advancing age, values affected by kidney or liver function are different for the elderly than for younger patients. Cholesterol and triglyceride values increase with age, whereas the sex hormones may rise and then fall. Both red and white blood cell values are higher in infants than adults. For all these reasons, it is important that the patient's date of birth be documented on the requisition form (Figure 17-5).
- Altitude: Patients living at higher altitudes have less oxygen available to breathe, so the body compensates by producing a higher red cell mass. Therefore, patients living in mountainous regions have higher red cell counts, hemoglobins, and hematocrits.
- Dehydration: Prolonged diarrhea or vomiting causes loss of fluid from the intravascular circulation. This results in hemoconcentration because of loss of plasma. Hemoconcentration produces a false increase in red blood cells, enzymes, calcium, and sodium.

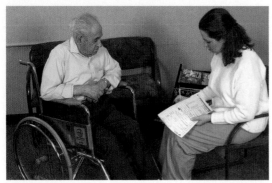

Figure 17-5
The patient's birth date should be documented by the phlebotomist on the requisition, as age can affect lab values.

- Sex: The normal ranges of some analytes differ for males and females. Males, for example, have higher hemoglobin, hematocrit, and red cell counts than do females.
- Pregnancy: The changes that occur in pregnancy affect lab values. The presence of the fetus and increased water retention cause a dilution effect that is reflected in falsely lower hemoglobin and red cell counts, as well as other analytes.

Specimen Collection

The phlebotomist has almost complete control over the variables that arise during specimen collection. These include the following:

- Site selection: Sites that can cause specimen contamination include hematomas or areas with edema and the side of the body that has undergone mastectomy or is currently receiving intravenous fluids. Sites that can cause pain or injury to the patient include burns or scars, previous puncture sites, the arm near a mastectomy, sites near fistulas or shunts, and the back of the heel or other regions close to the bone. In addition, accidental puncture of an artery during a venous procedure, or use of an artery for routine collection, carries a significant risk of infection.
- Tourniquet application: Tourniquets should be left on no longer than 1 minute, to reduce hemoconcentration of large molecules such as proteins and cholesterol (Figure 17-6). Tourniquets applied too tightly can cause petechiae.
- Site cleansing: Proper cleansing reduces the risk of infection. Blood culture collections require special care to prevent contamination of the sample with skin flora. As part of its QA program,

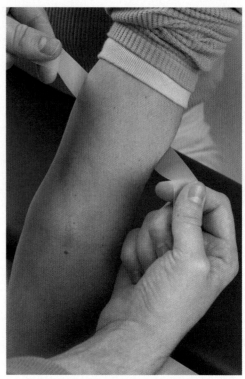

Figure 17-6
Application of the tourniquet is one preanalytical variable over which the phlebotomist has complete control.

the microbiology department keeps records of contaminated samples. Iodine must be removed from the site after collection, because it can irritate the skin. Iodine should not be used for dermal puncture, because it is virtually impossible to keep it out of the sample. Iodine interferes with bilirubin, uric acid, and phosphorus tests.
- Specimen collection: Specimens must be collected in the right tube for the test ordered and in the right order (Figure 17-7). The sample volume must be matched to the quantity of additives in the tube, and the tube size should be chosen to provide adequate volume for the test required. The specimen must be mixed gently and thoroughly by inversion immediately after being drawn.

 FLASHBACK

You learned the order of draw in Chapter 8.

- Labeling: Incorrect or incomplete labeling makes a specimen useless and requires redrawing the specimen at a later date. Label tubes immediately after they are drawn, before leaving the patient's room (Figure 17-8). Be sure that the labeling is

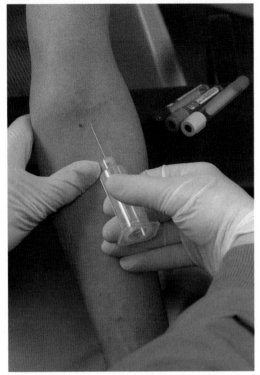

Figure 17-7
The phlebotomist should always ensure the correct order of draw.

complete, and note any special patient conditions on the requisition.

Patient's Perception

The patient's perception of the level of care he or she receives is directly affected by the skill, professionalism, and care you show as a phlebotomist. This perception reflects not only on you but on the entire lab as well. You should strive to avoid painful probing, unsuccessful punctures, and repeated draws and be scrupulously careful regarding site selection, accidental arterial puncture, and nerve injury. In addition, infection control procedures must always be followed. Break the chain of infection by perform-

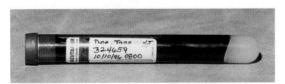

Figure 17-8
Make sure that specimens are properly labeled. (From Kinn ME, Woods MA: The Medical Assistant: Clinical and Administrative, ed 8. Philadelphia, Saunders, 1999.)

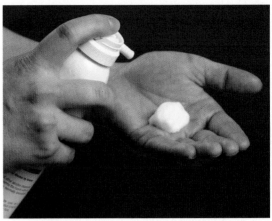

Figure 17-9
Infection control procedures are a vital part of quality phlebotomy. Hand hygiene and gloving should be performed for every procedure. (From Bonewit-West K: Clinical Procedures for Medical Assistants, ed 6. Philadelphia, Saunders, 2004.)

ing hand hygiene upon entering the room and after finishing the procedure and by wearing gloves during the procedure (Figure 17-9).

Accidental Puncture

Accidental puncture with a used needle must be reported immediately to a supervisor. Immediate and follow-up testing for blood-borne pathogens, plus counseling, is standard protocol for accidental needle sticks. QA procedures include monitoring the number of accidental punctures and instituting additional training or equipment modifications in the event of frequent accidents.

TRANSPORTATION

Specimen transportation variables include the method of delivery, the treatment of the sample during transportation, and the timing of delivery. Samples requiring either cold or warm temperatures during transport must be placed in the appropriate container and must be handled so that the appropriate temperature is maintained throughout the transport process (Figure 17-10). A heel warmer gradually loses its heat, for instance, and if the sample is not delivered before then, the sample will be compromised. Stat specimens require prompt delivery and analysis, and the on-time record of the phlebotomist and the lab is analyzed in QA programs to determine whether changes must be made in transportation procedures.

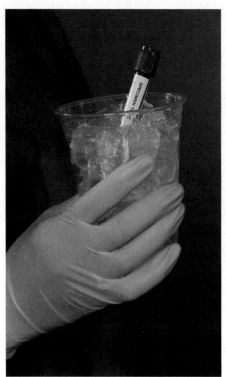

Figure 17-10
It is the phlebotomist's responsibility to ensure the proper handling of specimens.

Pneumatic tube systems require special monitoring to ensure that the sample is not overly agitated during transport, causing hemolysis. Some samples cannot travel by pneumatic tube, and it is the phlebotomist's responsibility to ensure their proper handling. The procedure manual contains precisely this type of information.

PROCESSING

Specimen processing is another area in which the phlebotomist and other lab staff have almost complete control over the variables that arise. These include the time between collection and processing, the centrifugation process, the possibility of contamination and evaporation, proper storage conditions, and processing of aliquots.

Separation Times

No more than 2 hours should elapse between the time a specimen is collected and the time serum or plasma is separated from formed elements. After this time, the sample will begin to show falsely lowered glucose and falsely elevated potassium and

lactate dehydrogenase. Even less time should be allowed for determinations of potassium, ammonia, adrenocorticotropic hormone, or cortisol. The exception is serum separator tubes, which are stable once they are spun and a good gel seal is in place.

Centrifuge Maintenance

Centrifuges must be calibrated every 3 months with a tachometer to ensure that they are running at the reported speed. Variation may indicate the need to replace worn parts. Spinning samples below the required speed may result in incomplete separation of liquid from formed elements, affecting test results (Figure 17-11).

Evaporation and Contamination

Specimens should not be left uncovered any longer than absolutely necessary during processing. Evaporation of liquid, especially from small samples, can affect arterial blood gases, alcohol, and ammonia, among other tests. Contamination may occur while the sample is uncovered, from airborne dust or talc from gloves. Contamination may also occur from

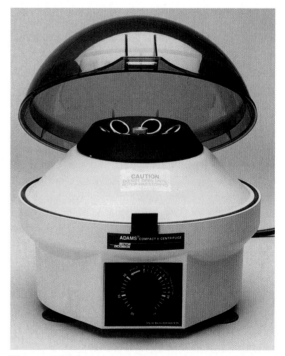

Figure 17-11
Correct use and maintenance of the centrifuge are important in quality specimen processing. (From Kinn ME, Woods MA: The Medical Assistant: Clinical and Administrative, ed 8. Philadelphia, Saunders, 1999.)

incomplete separation, such as when red blood cells are left in the sample after incomplete centrifugation.

Refrigerators and Freezers

Fluctuations in cold storage units can degrade sample quality. Temperatures of refrigerators and freezers must be monitored daily, with temperatures recorded either automatically or manually at specified times of day. Temperatures that are too high or low indicate that the unit needs maintenance or replacement.

Aliquot Handling and Labeling

Multiple aliquots prepared from a single specimen allow different departments to share a single sample for multiple tests. Each aliquot must be properly labeled as to the source and additives present. Specimens with different additives should never be combined in a single aliquot.

REVIEW FOR CERTIFICATION

Quality phlebotomy refers to a set of policies and procedures designed to ensure the delivery of consistently high-quality patient care and specimen analysis. Quality phlebotomy includes quality control, the quantitative methods used to monitor the quality of procedures. Quality control is part of quality assurance, the larger set of methods used to guarantee quality patient care. Total quality management is the entire set of approaches used by the institution to provide customer satisfaction. Continuous quality improvement is the major goal of TQM programs. QA programs use written documentation to set standards for the performance of procedures and monitor compliance. Two important documents are the procedure manual, which contains protocols and other information about all the tests performed in the lab, and the floor book, which contains a variety of information pertinent to the smooth coordination of nursing staff and lab personnel. Within the scope of TQM, the phlebotomist is most responsible for controlling preanalytical variables, those that occur before the specimen is analyzed. These variables include test ordering and requisition handling, equipment integrity, patient identification and preparation, specimen collection, and transportation. The patient's physical condition at the time of the collection has a significant effect on the sample quality and may be influenced by fasting, dehydration, and other states. Specimen collection variables include site selection, tourniquet application, and site cleansing. Postcollection variables include labeling, method of delivery, treatment of the sample during transportation, and timing of delivery. Specimen processing variables include the time between collection and processing, centrifugation process, possibility of contamination and evaporation, proper storage conditions, and processing of aliquots.

BIBLIOGRAPHY

Becan-McBride K: Pre-analytical Phase: An Important Requisite of Laboratory Testing. Advance for Medical Laboratory Professionals. September 28, 1998.

Clark C: Phlebotomy: Beyond the Basics. Advance for Medical Laboratory Professionals. September 22, 1997.

Dale JC: Pre-analytic Variables in Laboratory Testing. Laboratory Medicine. September 1998.

Drew N: Monitoring Specimen Collection Errors. Advance for Medical Laboratory Professionals. July 31, 2000.

Triana M, Coughlin WJ: Don't Overlook Phlebotomy QC. Medical Laboratory Observer. June 1983.

STUDY QUESTIONS

1. Explain the purpose of quality assurance (QA).
2. Describe how quality assurance differs from quality control (QC).
3. What is the role of the Joint Commission on Accreditation of Healthcare Organizations (JCAHO)?
4. List the four criteria that make up documentation processes.
5. What information does a procedure manual contain?
6. What is the purpose of a delta check?
7. If a patient presents with the smell of cigarettes on his or her breath, why should this be noted on the requisition?
8. What information should be labeled on aliquoted specimens?
9. Explain quality phlebotomy and its purpose.
10. Describe the philosophy, role, and purpose of TQM.
11. The procedure manual is present in the department at all times. Describe the information contained in the manual.
12. Explain the difference between the procedure manual and the floor log book.
13. Explain analytical variables and give examples of how to control or monitor such variables.
14. Describe a negative outcome of improper patient identification. Give two examples of how you would ensure that proper patient identification is achieved.
15. Give four variables of which a phlebotomist must be aware during a phlebotomy procedure, and examples of how to control or prevent such variables.

CERTIFICATION EXAM PREPARATION

1. What organization mandates quality assurance programs?
   a. OSHA
   b. NPA
   c. ASCP
   d. JCAHO

2. If there is a question concerning the principle behind a particular specimen collection, consult the:
   a. quality control logbook
   b. floor book
   c. policy manual
   d. procedure manual

3. If a phlebotomist wants to know the turn-around time for a specific procedure, it can be found in the:
   a. policy manual
   b. patient's chart
   c. floor book
   d. *Physician's Desk Reference*

4. Which of the following compares previous patient data with current data?
   a. postanalytical variables
   b. delta check
   c. accession numbers
   d. collection logbook

5. Fasting specimens should be collected:
   a. 24 hours after the fast
   b. 2 hours after waking up
   c. 8 to 12 hours after eating
   d. any time after midnight

6. The phlebotomist usually has complete control over all of the following variables, *except:*
   a. collection equipment
   b. patient preparation
   c. specimen collection
   d. specimen labeling

7. No more than _____ should elapse between the time a specimen is collected and the time serum or plasma is separated from formed elements.
   a. 30 minutes
   b. 1 hour
   c. 2 hours
   d. 3 hours

8. _____ refers to a set of policies and procedures designed to ensure the delivery of consistently high-quality patient care and specimen analysis.
   a. Quality phlebotomy
   b. Quality assurance
   c. Quality control
   d. Total quality management

9. The phlebotomist is most responsible for controlling _____.
   a. analytical variables
   b. postanalytical variables
   c. total quality management
   d. preanalytical variables

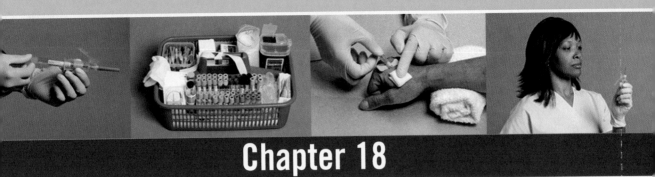

Chapter 18

Legal Issues in Phlebotomy

OUTLINE

Why Study Legal Issues?
The Legal System
   Laws
   Settlement and Judgment
Professional Liability
   Medical Malpractice

Other Examples of Potential
   Malpractice
   in Phlebotomy
Defense against Malpractice
Liability Insurance

Confidentiality
   HIPAA
Review for Certification

OBJECTIVES

After completing this chapter, you should be able to:

1. Discuss why legal issues are important to the phlebotomist.
2. Differentiate the following types of laws: statutory, case, administrative, public, and private.
3. Define plaintiff, defendant, felony, misdemeanor, and tort.
4. Define liability, and give examples of situations in which a phlebotomist may be held accountable for the consequences of an action.
5. Explain how the accepted standard of care is determined, and give examples of these standards as they relate to phlebotomy.
6. Define malpractice, and explain what is necessary to prove it.
7. Differentiate between punitive and compensatory damages.
8. Describe steps the phlebotomist can take to avoid being accused of malpractice.
9. Explain the importance of confidentiality.
10. Define protected health information under HIPAA regulations.
11. Describe how the phlebotomist can safeguard a patient's privacy.

KEY TERMS

accepted standard of care
administrative law
assault
battery
case law
civil action
criminal action
damages

dereliction
incident report
liability insurance
liable
malpractice
negligence
out-of-court settlement
plaintiff

protected health information
private law
public law
statutory law
tort
unintentional torts

ABBREVIATIONS

HIPAA: Health Insurance Portability and Accountability Act

IRS: Internal Revenue Service

OSHA: Occupational Safety and Health Administration

PHI: protected health information

Legal and ethical considerations form an important underpinning to the practice of medicine, and phlebotomy is no exception. An increasingly complex and litigious health care environment has made familiarity with legal issues an important part of the phlebotomist's training. Medical malpractice is the most common legal claim in the health care field. Injuries that arise from failure to follow the standard of care may be grounds for a finding of malpractice. Careful observance of the standard of care, and documentation of that practice, is the best defense against malpractice. New and comprehensive federal regulations governing the privacy of medical information have affected every sector of health care delivery. In addition to the legal requirement to protect patient confidentiality, there is an ethical duty to do so. Although full consideration of all the relevant legal issues is beyond the scope of this chapter, we introduce some important legal and ethical concepts that have an impact on the profession.

WHY STUDY LEGAL ISSUES?

The health care system has become increasingly complex in the last two decades. This complexity stems from the interplay of technologic advances, associated increased costs of delivering care, and fear of litigation.

Several factors have led to the dramatic rise in health care costs in recent decades. First, of course, is the gradual inflation in the price of all goods and services. More important has been the growing sophistication of medical technology, with consequent higher costs for equipment purchase and maintenance, plus the need for highly trained operators at all levels of health care delivery. For instance, the cost of drawing a blood sample has risen significantly since the development of safety needles and other systems designed to protect the phlebotomist. The simple compound microscope that was used to do a differential blood count in the 1940s cost perhaps a few hundred dollars and required only occasional adjustment and cleaning.

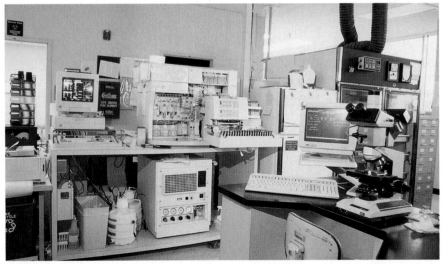

Figure 18-1

The invention of automated hematology equipment, though improving the quality of care, has also contributed to the rising costs of health care. (From Chester GA: Modern Medical Assisting. Philadelphia, Saunders, 1998.)

In contrast, today's automated cell counters cost many thousands of dollars and require frequent calibration and regular maintenance, as well as a higher level of training to operate (Figure 18-1). Similarly, the fast pace of drug discovery and development has increased the cost of medical treatment for the typical patient. All these advances have enhanced the quality of patient care, but at a significant price. In addition to these sources of cost increase, more stringent regulations designed to safeguard health care providers have led to higher costs for service delivery.

Even more significantly, the availability of sophisticated technology has meant that more doctors order more tests on more patients, and more patients expect them to order the tests. As the standard of care has risen, multiple sophisticated and expensive tests have been prescribed to supplement (and sometimes substitute for) a physician's clinical judgment. Increased fear of litigation has also fueled the rise in the use of multiple tests, often as much to protect against future lawsuits as to provide crucial medical information. Such "defensive medicine" is understandable, given the very high cost of malpractice insurance and the potential for a ruinous liability judgment in the event of an oversight or mistake.

The rising cost of health care has led to efforts to keep costs under control, including reimbursement restrictions on diagnostic tests and limitations on prescription drugs. Meanwhile, the rights of patients have been increasingly recognized and expanded, and the level of care expected by patients has grown.

Because of the conflicts arising from the interplay of these factors, along with the general rise in litigation in our society, the health care professions have been subjected to more and more lawsuits. Understanding your legal obligations and rights in this complex system is an important part of your professional training.

THE LEGAL SYSTEM

To understand your rights and obligations under the law, it is helpful to know a little bit about how the legal system operates.

Laws

Laws are created in a variety of ways. **Statutory law** is created by a legislative body. At the federal level, this is Congress, made up of the Senate and House of Representatives. State legislative bodies vary from state to state but usually follow the federal model.

Case law is law determined by court decisions, usually as an interpretation of existing statutory law. State courts rule on state laws, and federal courts rule on federal laws. The U.S. Supreme Court has ultimate jurisdiction over all laws, both federal and state.

Administrative law is created by administrative agencies, such as the Internal Revenue Service (IRS) or the Occupational Safety and Health Administration (OSHA). The regulations promulgated by these agencies are given the force of law by the statutory laws that created the agencies.

Laws are also classified as either public or private. When a **public law** is violated, the offense leads to a **criminal action**, and the violator is prosecuted by the public, in the person of the government's attorney (the district attorney). The offense may be either a felony or a misdemeanor, depending on the seriousness of the crime.

Phlebotomists can be charged with violations of public law. Therefore, blood must never be drawn without first obtaining the patient's consent. If a patient refuses to have his or her blood drawn, the phlebotomist must not attempt to force the patient to comply. To persist can lead to criminal charges of assault and battery. **Assault** is an unjustifiable attempt to touch another person, or the threat to do so. **Battery** is the intentional touching of another person without consent. Phlebotomists may also be liable for assault and battery for the use of dirty needles or damage to nerves from improper drawing techniques. Cases have been prosecuted in which the phlebotomist did not correctly identify the patient and, as a result, the patient received incorrect test results and improper care. If the patient dies as a consequence, the phlebotomist could be charged with murder or manslaughter.

In contrast to public law, when a **private law** is violated, the offense may lead to a **civil action**, in which the defendant is sued in civil court by the **plaintiff**, the person claiming to have been harmed by the defendant. Civil wrongs include torts. A **tort** is an injury to one person for which another person who caused the injury is legally responsible. Torts can be either intentional or unintentional. **Unintentional torts** are the basis for most medical malpractice suits.

A patient may choose to bring a civil action in a case for which a criminal action was also brought, whether or not the defendant was found guilty in the criminal action. For instance, a patient with a damaged nerve may sue for malpractice even if the case was not strong enough to sustain a criminal action. Other causes of action could include reusing needles, careless probing for a vein, accidental artery stick, drawing samples not requested by the physician, or releasing test results to someone not authorized to receive them.

Settlement and Judgment

Almost all civil and criminal actions are settled out of court. In an **out-of-court settlement**, the two parties reach an agreement without the intervention of a judge or jury. When a civil case is settled out of court, the settlement often includes a condition stating that neither party may discuss the amount of the settlement.

When the parties cannot reach agreement, the case goes to court for trial and judgment. A judgment against the defendant in a civil case usually results in a fine, which may be only compensatory (to pay for costs incurred because of the injury, such as further medical care) or punitive. Headline-making damage awards are most often for punitive damages. Judgments in either civil or criminal actions can be appealed if the losing party feels that some part of the court proceeding was in error. Judgments may be upheld, reversed, or modified on appeal.

PROFESSIONAL LIABILITY

To be **liable** for an action means that you are legally responsible for it and can be held accountable for its consequences. As a medical professional, you are liable for both your actions and, in some cases, your failure to act. For instance, if you damage a nerve while performing routine venipuncture, you may be held liable. If a physician orders a test that you fail to perform and, as a result, the patient suffers harm, you may be held liable.

You are legally responsible for *any* action you perform as a medical professional, whether or not it is a duty assigned to you or you have received training for it (Figure 18-2). For instance, if you perform an arterial puncture, you are liable for any injuries that may result from it, whether or not you have been properly trained to perform it. Therefore, *a professional should not attempt to perform duties for which he or she is not trained*. By performing a duty normally assigned to someone with a higher level of training and expertise, you are legally liable for that higher level of care. Your institution has policies and procedures regarding the duties you are expected to perform.

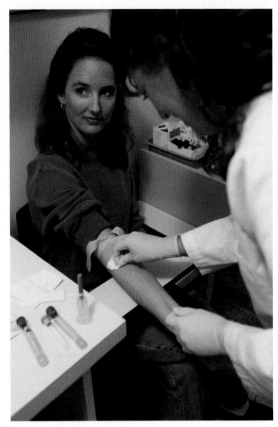

Figure 18-2

The phlebotomist is legally responsible for any injuries that result from venipuncture.

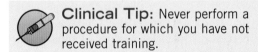
Clinical Tip: Never perform a procedure for which you have not received training.

Judgments regarding medical liability revolve around the concept of the accepted standard of care, which represents the consensus of medical opinion on patient care in a particular situation. The failure to perform an action consistent with the accepted standard of care is negligence.

When the standard of care is not followed, those professionals who were responsible for decision making in that situation are liable for injuries incurred by the patient. For instance, most institutions allow a phlebotomist to make only two unsuccessful attempts at routine venipuncture before seeking the assistance of a more senior phlebotomist. If this is the accepted standard of care in your institution and you violate that policy, a patient who experiences harm or suffering as a result may have grounds to sue you and your hospital. In a trial, the jury decides exactly what constitutes the accepted standard of care, whether that standard was followed, and whether the medical professionals were negligent. These decisions are usually made after listening to a variety of expert witnesses.

Medical Malpractice

Malpractice is the delivery of substandard care that results in harm to a patient. It is the most common liability in medicine and is sometimes called medical professional liability. A malpractice suit is brought by the plaintiff and usually names one or more professionals, as well as the institution, as the defendants. The suit alleges professional negligence as the cause of specific harms, which may include both physical and emotional distress, as well as lost income or potential income, as the result of specific actions.

In a civil suit, the plaintiff asks for **damages**, or monetary compensation. Damages may be awarded to cover only the actual costs of the injury, such as lost wages or further medical care. Damages can also be awarded to compensate for legal costs or pain and suffering. Punitive damages may be awarded to punish the defendant, usually for gross violations of accepted standards of care.

In a malpractice case, the burden of proof is on the plaintiff to show the four elements of negligence.

Duty

The plaintiff must prove that the defendant owed the plaintiff a duty of care. For example, if a phlebotomist had a requisition for a patient and was expected by his or her supervisors to draw blood, the phlebotomist owed the patient a duty of care.

Dereliction

The plaintiff must prove that the defendant breached the duty of care to the plaintiff. This determination revolves around the accepted standard of care and the specific action or inaction of the plaintiff. For example, if a phlebotomist mislabeled the sample specified on the requisition, this may constitute **dereliction.**

Injury

The plaintiff must prove that a legally recognizable injury to the patient actually occurred. For instance, if mislabeling led to improper care that harmed the patient, injury occurred. If the time of draw for a therapeutic drug monitoring sample was written incorrectly, and the patient received too much medication as a result, the patient may be able to prove injury.

Direct Cause

The plaintiff must prove that the injury was sustained as a direct result of the defendant's actions or inactions. For example, if overmedication can be shown to be a direct result of mislabeling, direct cause is demonstrated.

Other Examples of Potential Malpractice in Phlebotomy

The standard of care when drawing blood from a patient is to perform no more than two unsuccessful punctures before calling for assistance. A phlebotomist who continues to attempt venipuncture without calling for assistance at this point is derelict in his or her duty. A patient who subsequently experiences pain and swelling in the arm may have a cause of action, if it can be shown that the injury resulted from the excess number of attempts.

The standard of care when drawing at a patient's bedside is not to place the phlebotomy tray on the bed. A phlebotomist who does so is derelict in his or her duty. If a patient's movements subsequently cause the tray to spill and filled tubes to break, the patient may be exposed to blood-borne pathogens (assuming the samples were from a different patient who was infected). In order to establish injury, the patient would then have to become infected. In order to establish direct cause, the patient would need to show that the infection was the result of the exposure (and not the result of exposure from some other source, for example).

The standard of care when leaving a patient's bedside is to raise the bed rail if it was lowered for the draw. Therefore the phlebotomist has a duty to perform this action. If he or she fails to do so, this is a dereliction of duty. If the patient subsequently falls from bed and is injured, the question becomes whether the phlebotomist's failure to raise the bed rail was the direct cause of the injury. Mitigating factors might include whether the patient had been visited by a nurse in the meantime and whether the fall was the actual cause of the injury.

Defense against Malpractice

As the preceding examples illustrate, deviation from the standard of care leaves the phlebotomist exposed to charges of malpractice. Conversely, the principal defense against a malpractice suit is to show that the standard of care was followed. This requires not only the actual practice of good care but the documentation of it as well. Clear, complete medical records are the cornerstone of the defense, because they show exactly what was done, when, and by whom. If good care is delivered and good medical records document this, a malpractice suit has little chance of succeeding.

Similarly, if a situation arises in which observation of the standard of care is called into question, all parties should carefully document exactly what happened—who did what when. For instance, if a patient complains of a shooting pain during a draw, the phlebotomist has a responsibility to follow institutional protocol to deal with the injury or the complaint; he or she should not try to avoid reporting it. Each institution has a set of protocols for reporting such incidents, which usually involve prompt and complete documentation of the circumstances of the incident in an **incident report**.

 Clinical Tip: Always maintain clear, complete medical records. Whenever an unusual incident occurs during a phlebotomy procedure, report it to your supervisor immediately and fill out an incident report.

Patient communication is also an important aspect of preventing malpractice claims. For instance, clear communication with the patient is essential for obtaining informed consent for medical procedures (Figure 18-3). Procedures must be explained in a way that the patient can understand, and the patient must give a positive consent ("Yes," or "I understand"), not merely a nod of the head or a look of agreement. For a patient who does not speak English, an interpreter must be present to explain the procedure. As another example, the phlebotomist must remember to ask

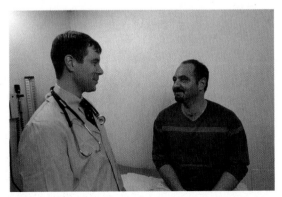

Figure 18-3
Clear communication with patients can help avoid malpractice claims.

specifically whether the patient is taking blood-thinning medications such as heparin. Without this information, the phlebotomist may not apply pressure long enough after the draw, possibly leading to compartment syndrome, a potentially very serious complication.

 Clinical Tip: Always obtain positive informed consent before performing a procedure.

 FLASHBACK
You learned about asking about medications in Chapter 9.

Liability Insurance

Liability insurance covers monetary damages that must be paid if the defendant loses a liability suit. Most hospitals require a doctor to show proof of insurance in order to have admitting privileges. Phlebotomists are usually covered by their institution's liability insurance, although some phlebotomists also obtain their own.

CONFIDENTIALITY

In addition to his or her legal obligations, a phlebotomist is bound by both legal and ethical responsibilities, especially in the area of confidentiality. With the passage of the Health Insurance Portability and Accountability Act (HIPAA), the privacy of medical information has taken on legal ramifications as well.

HIPAA

HIPAA defines a set of standards and procedures for protection of privacy of health information. **Protected health information** (PHI) is any part of a patient's health information that is linked to information that identifies the patient, such as date of birth, name, or address. PHI includes information in the patient's medical record, the results of tests, and other related information, in any form. Under HIPAA, patients have the right to control their protected health information, and disclosing PHI without the patient's consent is illegal. Upon intake, patients are informed of their rights under HIPAA. Your institution should have defined procedures for protecting private health information while allowing that information to be disclosed to those who need to know it and have a right to know it.

Safeguarding a patient's privacy requires several precautions:

- Never discuss a patient's condition, tests, or financial information in a public place, such as a hallway, elevator, or eating area. Be careful to keep phone conversations private. Avoid using the patient's name if possible.
- Never discuss information concerning a patient with someone not directly involved in that patient's care.
- Never release medical information concerning a patient to anyone not specifically authorized to acquire it. Disclosure of information to a third party (such as an employer, the news media, or a relative other than the parent of a minor) requires written authorization from the patient.
- Never leave patient records out where patients or visitors can glance at them.

In addition to protecting the patient's right to privacy, the phlebotomist has an obligation to maintain the integrity of the doctor–patient relationship. This means that the phlebotomist should not reveal test results to the patient, but should leave this to the physician.

A patient is also entitled to privacy out of ethical considerations alone. The Patient Care Partnership (Box 18-1) was developed by the American Hospital Association to encompass not only the right to confidentiality but other important aspects of ethical patient care. While it does not carry the force of law, it represents an ideal that health care institutions may use to evaluate their own practices.

BOX 18-1 The Patient Care Partnership

THE PATIENT CARE PARTNERSHIP
Understanding Expectations, Rights and Responsibilities

What to expect during your hospital stay:
- High quality hospital care.
- A clean and safe environment.
- Involvement in your care.
- Protection of your privacy.
- Help when leaving the hospital.
- Help with your billing claims.

When you need hospital care, your doctor and the nurses and other professionals at our hospital are committed to working with you and your family to meet your health care needs. Our dedicated doctors and staff serve the community in all its ethnic, religious and economic diversity. Our goal is for you and your family to have the same care and attention we would want for our families and ourselves.

BOX 18-1 The Patient Care Partnership—cont'd

The sections explain some of the basics about how you can expect to be treated during your hospital stay. They also cover what we will need from you to care for you better. If you have questions at any time, please ask them. Unasked or unanswered questions can add to the stress of being in the hospital. Your comfort and confidence in your care are important to us.

What to Expect During Your Hospital Stay
High Quality Hospital Care
Our first priority is to provide you the care you need, when you need it, with skill, compassion and respect. Tell your caregivers if you have concerns about your care or if you have pain. You have the right to know the identity of doctors, nurses and others involved in your care, and you have the right to know when they are students, residents or other trainees.

A Clean and Safe Environment
Our hospital works hard to keep you safe. We use special policies and procedures to avoid mistakes in your care and keep you free from abuse or neglect. If anything unexpected and significant happens during your hospital stay, you will be told what happened, and any resulting changes in your care will be discussed with you.

Involvement in Your Care
You and your doctor often make decisions about your care before you go to the hospital. Other times, especially in emergencies, those decisions are made during your hospital stay. When decision-making takes place, it should include:

Discussing your medical condition and information about medically appropriate treatment choices.
To make informed decisions with your doctor, you need to understand:
- The benefits and risks of each treatment.
- Whether your treatment is experimental or part of a research study.
- What you can reasonably expect from your treatment and any long-term effects it might have on your quality of life.
- What you and your family will need to do after you leave the hospital.
- The financial consequences of using uncovered services or out-of-network providers.

Please tell your caregivers if you need more information about treatment choices.

Discussing your treatment plan.
When you enter the hospital, you sign a general consent to treatment. In some cases, such as surgery or experimental treatment, you may be asked to confirm in writing that you understand what is planned and agree to it. This process

---

BOX 18-1 The Patient Care Partnership—cont'd

protects your right to consent to or refuse a treatment. Your doctor will explain the medical consequences of refusing recommended treatment. It also protects your right to decide if you want to participate in a research study.

Getting information from you.
Your caregivers need complete and correct information about your health and coverage so that they can make good decisions about your care. That includes:

- Past illnesses, surgeries or hospital stays.
- Past allergic reactions.
- Any medicines or dietary supplements (such as vitamins and herbs) that you are taking.
- Any network or admission requirements under your health plan.

Understanding your health care goals and values.
You may have health care goals and values or spiritual beliefs that are important to your well-being. They will be taken into account as much as possible throughout your hospital stay. Make sure your doctor, your family and your care team know your wishes.

Understanding who should make decisions when you cannot.
If you have signed a health care power of attorney stating who should speak for you if you become unable to make health care decisions for yourself, or a "living will" or "advance directive" that states your wishes about end-of-life care, give copies to your doctor, your family and your care team. If you or your family need help making difficult decisions, counselors, chaplains and others are available to help.

Protection of Your Privacy
We respect the confidentiality of your relationship with your doctor and other caregivers and the sensitive information about your health and health care that are part of that relationship. State and federal laws and hospital operating policies protect the privacy of your medical information.

©2003 American Hospital Association. All rights reserved.

BOX 18-1 The Patient Care Partnership—cont'd

You will receive a Notice of Privacy Practices that describes the ways that we use, disclose and safeguard patient information and that explains how you can obtain a copy of information from our records about your care.

Preparing You and Your Family for When You Leave the Hospital
Your doctor works with hospital staff and professionals in your community. You and your family also play an important role in your care. The success of your treatment often depends on your efforts to follow medication, diet and therapy plans. Your family may need to help care for you at home.

You can expect us to help you identify sources of follow-up care and to let you know if our hospital has a financial interest in any referrals. As long as you agree that we can share information about your care with them, we will coordinate our activities with your caregivers outside the hospital. You can also expect to receive information and, where possible, training about the self-care you will need when you go home.

Help with Your Bill and Filing Insurance Claims
Our staff will file claims for you with health care insurers or other programs such as Medicare and Medicaid. They also will help your doctor with needed documentation. Hospital bills and insurance coverage are often confusing. If you have questions about your bill, contact our business office. If you need help understanding your insurance coverage or health plan, start with your insurance company or health benefits manager. If you do not have health coverage, we will try to help you and your family find financial help or make other arrangements. We need your help with collecting needed information and other requirements to obtain coverage or assistance.

While you are here, you will receive more detailed notices about some of the rights you have as a hospital patient and how to exercise them. We are always interested in improving. If you have questions, comments or concerns, please contact: (relevant department here)

REVIEW FOR CERTIFICATION

The phlebotomist has a legal responsibility to follow standards of care in delivering health care services. Violation of public laws may lead to criminal prosecution, and violation of private laws may lead to civil suits. Injuries to patients that result from failure to follow the standard of care may result in a malpractice judgment or criminal prosecution. Medical malpractice is the most common civil action brought against health care professionals. Proof of malpractice requires findings of duty, dereliction, injury, and direct cause. The phlebotomist is usually covered by malpractice insurance carried by the institution. HIPAA establishes the legal right of the patient to have the privacy of his or her health information protected. Protection of patient confidentiality is not only a legal obligation under HIPAA, but also an ethical duty to the patient. The phlebotomist should not discuss a patient's case with anyone who is not authorized to know and should never conduct discussions in public. Test results must not be released to anyone who is not authorized to receive them.

BIBLIOGRAPHY

Department of Health and Human Services: National Standards to Protect the Privacy of Personal Health Information. Accessed June 8, 2006: http://www.hhs.gov/ocr/hipaa/

Ernst DJ: Four Indefensible Phlebotomy Errors and How to Prevent Them. Journal of Healthcare Risk Management. Spring 1998.

Ernst DJ: Phlebotomy on Trial. Medical Laboratory Observer. April 1999.

Faber V: Understanding Medicolegal Issues: Key to Avoid Phlebotomy Malpractice Suits. Advance for Medical Laboratory Professionals. March 13, 1995.

Judson K, Hicks S: Law and Ethics for Medical Careers, ed 2. New York, Glencoe, 1999.

STUDY QUESTIONS

1. List four reasons why health care costs have increased.
2. Explain the type of laws OSHA creates.
3. Define plaintiff.
4. Give three scenarios in which a phlebotomist may be held liable.
5. Define negligence.
6. Define malpractice.
7. What does it mean to breach confidentiality?
8. What measures can phlebotomists take to protect themselves against malpractice suits?
9. Patient communication is an important aspect of malpractice claims. Give three examples of effective communication that may help to avoid a lawsuit.
10. Explain the difference between criminal actions and civil actions, and how each can pertain to phlebotomy.
11. Explain professional liability. Give at least three examples of duties that the phlebotomist can perform and patient care duties that the phlebotomist cannot perform.
12. Name three elements that a plaintiff must prove in a malpractice suit.
13. Describe the meaning of the following statement: "A phlebotomist who does so is derelict in his or her duty."
14. In defense against malpractice, what is the key in defending oneself?
15. What is liability insurance? Why would a phlebotomist have the need to carry liability insurance?
16. How does the phlebotomist maintain doctor–patient integrity?
17. Most judgments are settled in out-of-court settlements. Describe what happens when cases are not settled as easily.
18. Give at least one example of how a phlebotomist may commit a negligent act.

CERTIFICATION EXAM PREPARATION

1. Administrative agencies such as OSHA create which type of law?
   a. statutory
   b. case
   c. administrative
   d. federal

2. The failure to perform an action consistent with the accepted standard of care is:
   a. negligence
   b. assault
   c. malpractice
   d. dereliction

3. The four elements of negligence are:
   a. malpractice, tort, liability, negligence
   b. confidentiality, litigation, contract, felony
   c. duty, dereliction, injury, direct cause
   d. injury, direct cause, privacy, tort

4. The phlebotomist's duties and performance level should be outlined in the:
   a. floor book
   b. safety manual
   c. OSHA guidelines
   d. policies and procedure manual

5. When a phlebotomist breaches the duty of care to a patient, this is known as:
   a. direct cause
   b. civil action
   c. dereliction
   d. assault

6. A tort comes from a(n):
   a. out-of-court settlement
   b. civil action
   c. public law
   d. criminal action

7. _____ are the basis for most medical malpractice suits.
   a. Unintentional torts
   b. Criminal actions
   c. Felonies
   d. Misdemeanors

8. The principal defense against a malpractice suit is:
   a. to show burden of proof
   b. to reach an out-of-court settlement
   c. to deny liability
   d. to show that the standard of care was followed

9. The phlebotomist has a legal responsibility to do which of the following?
   a. maintain the integrity of the doctor–patient relationship
   b. maintain patient confidentiality
   c. follow the standard of care
   d. all of the above

10. Medical information that is linked to a specific patient is called
    a. confidentially protected information
    b. protected health information
    c. private health information
    d. protected confidential information

11. Which of the following is not found in The Patient Care Partnership?
    a. The patient can expect protection of his or her privacy.
    b. The patient can expect high quality hospital care.
    c. The patient can expect involvement in his or her care.
    d. The patient can expect the cheapest care possible.

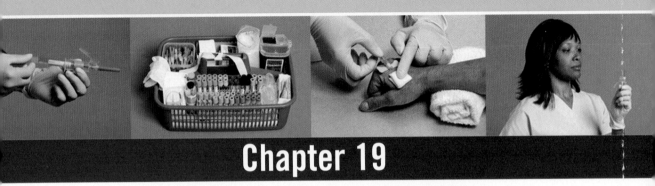

Chapter 19

Point-of-Care Testing

OBJECTIVES

After completing this chapter, you should be able to:

1. Define point-of-care testing and explain its
   advantages and disadvantages.
2. Discuss the importance of quality-assurance
   activities in point-of-care testing.
3. Describe the testing principle and clinical
   usefulness of:
   a. hematocrit
   b. hemoglobin
   c. prothrombin time

   d. activated coagulation time
   e. glucose
   f. cardiac troponin T
   g. cholesterol
   h. blood gases and electrolytes
   i. occult blood
   j. "dipstick" urinalysis
   k. pregnancy testing
4. Describe the major features of an electrocardiogram,
   and outline important points of patient preparation.

KEY TERMS

alternate site testing
cardiac cycle
cardiac troponin T
conduction system
depolarization
electrocardiogram
electrocardiography

human chorionic gonadotropin
leads
point-of-care testing
P-R interval
P wave
QRS complex
Q-T interval

rapid group A streptococcus
repolarization
sinoatrial node
ST segment
stylus
T wave

ABBREVIATIONS

ACT: activated coagulation time
APTT: activated partial thromboplastin time
AST: alternate site testing
CLIA: Clinical Laboratory Improvement Amendments of 1988
ECG, EKG: electrocardiogram

g/dL: grams per deciliter
HCG: human chorionic gonadotropin
PCV: packed cell volume
POCT: point-of-care testing
PT: prothrombin time
TnT: troponin T

Point-of-care testing is the performance of analytical tests at the "point of care," which may be at the bedside, in the clinic, or even in the patient's home. Tests are done with small portable instruments that offer significant time and cost savings in many situations. Blood tests typically performed as point-of-care test include many in chemistry and hematology. Additionally, the multiskilled phlebotomist may perform electrocardiography, occult blood analysis, urinalysis, pregnancy testing, and rapid group A streptococcus ("strep") testing.

ADVANTAGES OF POINT-OF-CARE TESTING

Point-of-care testing (POCT) refers to the performance of analytical tests immediately after obtaining a sample, often in the same room that the patient is seen in (the "point of care"). POCT is also known as **alternate site testing** (AST). POCT may be performed at the bedside, in the intensive care unit or emergency room, or in outpatient settings such as a clinic, physician's office, nursing home, assisted living center, or the patient's own home. Box 19-1 lists special

considerations to keep in mind when drawing blood at a patient's home.

The advantages of POCT are considerable. By "bringing the lab to the patient," the turn-around time for obtaining test results is shortened, allowing more prompt medical attention, faster diagnosis and treatment, and potentially decreased recovery time. Most tests performed as POCT are Clinical Laboratory Improvement Amendments (CLIA)–waived tests. The FDA decides which tests are CLIA-waived based on the ease of performing and interpreting the test. A CLIA-waived test is not subject to regulatory oversight by government authorities. The FDA web site maintains a complete list of waived tests.

An essential feature of a CLIA-waived test is that the testing equipment and procedure is so simple and accurate that erroneous results are very unlikely. Results are read directly from digital displays or monitors on the instrument. Although the direct cost per test is often more with these instruments, the total cost to the laboratory is often less when the time and cost for sample delivery or after-hours staffing of the lab are considered.

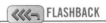 **FLASHBACK**

You learned about CLIA in Chapter 2.

Tests such as bleeding times have always been done at the bedside. The significant expansion of POCT in recent years has been possible because of the development of miniaturized analytical equipment, and microcomputers. Instruments used in POCT are small, portable, and often hand-held, with some tests requiring no instruments at all, only a card or reagent strip or "dipstick." In general, POCT instruments are easy to use, the required training is simple, and they can be used by a variety of medical professionals, including phlebotomists, nurses, nurse assistants, and physicians.

Although these instruments are easy to use, the importance of carefully following the manufacturer's instructions cannot be overemphasized. For

> **BOX 19-1**   Reminders for Performing Phlebotomy in a Patient's Home
>
> 1. When obtaining the specimen, always have the patient sitting or reclining in a safe, comfortable chair or bed.
> 2. Be aware of the nearest bathroom or sink. Carry antiseptic towelettes for hand washing.
> 3. Carry a cell phone for emergencies.
> 4. Always bring biohazard containers for specimen transport and removal of sharps.
> 5. Make sure that the patient has completely stopped bleeding before leaving.
> 6. Recheck the phlebotomy area to ensure that all the materials used during the procedure have been properly removed and disposed of.
> 7. Preserve the specimen for transport at the proper temperature.

example, some manufacturers follow the traditional method of wiping away the first drop of blood from a dermal puncture and using subsequent drops for testing. However, a few instrument makers use the first drop of blood for their procedures. Using the second drop with such instruments would give false readings.

Of course, quality assurance and controls are still essential for the use of POCT instruments, just as they are with lab-based instrumentation. The laboratory is usually responsible for documentation and maintenance of POCT instruments. Finally, proper and adequate training for all personnel performing these procedures is critical in order to implement POCT successfully. Strict adherence to guidelines regarding calibrating equipment, running controls, performing maintenance, and keeping records is a must for a POCT program. Failure in any one of these areas can lead to erroneous test results and negative consequences for patients.

COMMON TESTS PERFORMED AT THE POINT OF CARE

Here we discuss some of the most common point-of-care tests likely to be performed by the phlebotomist. A more complete list is given in Box 19-2.

> **BOX 19-2** Point-of-Care Tests
>
> B-type natriuretic peptide
> Complete blood count (hemoglobin and hematocrit)
> Coagulation testing (ACT, PT, APTT)
> Glucose
> Cardiac troponin T
> Cholesterol
> Multiple chemistry panels (arterial blood gases, electrolytes, blood urea nitrogen)
> Electrocardiography

Hematology

Anemia and Polycythemia Evaluation

The level of red blood cells in the blood can be determined by a hematocrit, in which a sample of blood in a capillary tube is sealed and spun in a centrifuge to pack the red blood cells at the bottom. The packed cell volume (PCV) is determined by placing the tube against a readout scale and is reported as a percentage of the total blood volume (Figure 19-1). Mylar-wrapped hematocrit tubes minimize the danger of broken glass and provide an extra level of safety.

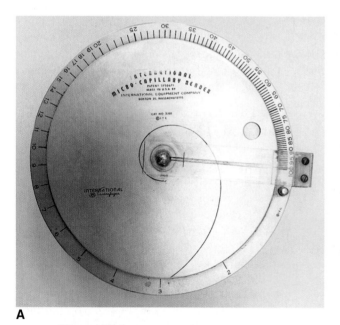

A

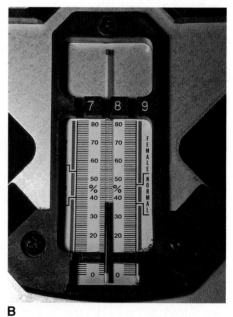

B

Figure 19-1
Examples of microhematocrit tube readers. **A,** Stand-alone readout device. **B,** Built-in reader in a microhematocrit centrifuge. (*A* from Stepp CA, Woods MA: Laboratory Procedures for Medical Office Personnel. Philadelphia, WB Saunders, 1998; *B* from Chester GA: Modern Medical Assisting. Philadelphia, WB Saunders, 1998.)

FLASHBACK

You learned about collecting a sample for hematocrit testing in Chapter 10.

A simpler, faster method of anemia testing uses a hand-held hemoglobin analyzer (Figure 19-2). Such instruments can use arterial, venous, or dermal blood specimens and typically give readouts in less than a minute. A blood sample is placed into a microcuvette, which is then inserted into the machine for a reading. Rather than determining PCV, the instrument determines the hemoglobin value in grams per deciliter (g/dL), which can be tracked over the disease course or be used to determine the response to therapy.

Coagulation Monitoring

Coagulation monitoring is used to monitor patients with clotting disorders who are receiving therapy. There are several hand-held instruments used for bedside measurement. Some use only a single drop of whole blood obtained from a dermal puncture; others use citrated blood obtained by venipuncture. Most give results in 5 minutes or less.

Heparin therapy may be monitored by determining the activated coagulation time (ACT). A small volume of blood is collected in a prewarmed tube that contains a coagulation activator. The tube is incubated at 37°C for 1 minute and then inspected by tilting the tube to determine whether a clot is present. If not, the tube is inspected every 5 seconds thereafter, with incubation continuing between observations. An automated ACT tester is available as well. The activated partial thromboplastin time (APTT) can also be used to monitor heparin therapy. With recent advances in POCT instrumentation, physicians now have a choice of tests for monitoring heparin therapy (Figure 19-3). Oral anticoagulant therapy using warfarin (Coumadin) is monitored by the prothrombin time (PT) test. CLIA-waived PT testing instruments are frequently used in physicians' offices and clinics (Figure 19-4).

Chemistry

Glucose

Bedside glucose monitoring is the most common chemistry test done by POCT. Glucose is determined with dermal puncture and reagent strips.

FLASHBACK

You learned about bedside glucose testing in Chapter 10.

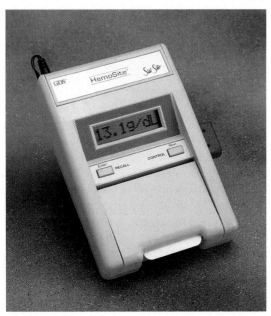

Figure 19-2
Hand-held instruments such as the Stat-Site system can analyze hemoglobin quickly and accurately. This system can also analyze blood cholesterol levels. (Courtesy GDS Technology, Inc., Elkhart, IN.)

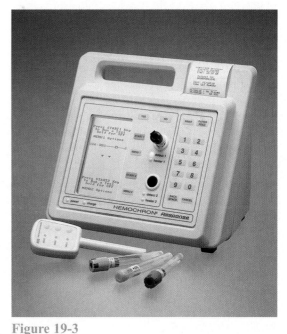

Figure 19-3
The Hemochron system is designed to manage the effects of anticoagulation drugs such as heparin. (Courtesy ITC, Edison, NJ.)

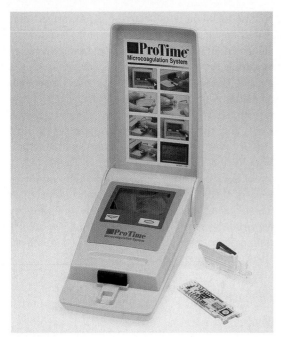

Figure 19-4
The ProTime Microcoagulation System for prothrombin time testing is designed to safely manage warfarin (Coumadin) therapy. (Courtesy ITC, Edison, NJ.)

Cardiac Troponin T

Cardiac troponin T (cardiac TnT) is part of a protein complex in cardiac muscle that aids the interaction of actin and myosin. Damaged cardiac muscle releases cardiac TnT, and the serum level of cardiac TnT rises within 4 hours after an acute myocardial infarction (heart attack). It may stay elevated for up to 2 weeks, and its level may help determine the extent of damage and the patient's prognosis. Therefore, monitoring of cardiac TnT can provide valuable information for a patient with a possible myocardial infarction. Bedside determination is performed using anticoagulated whole blood, and results are available within 15 minutes (Figure 19-5).

Cholesterol

Cholesterol levels may be determined as part of a routine examination or to monitor therapy with cholesterol-lowering drugs. Some POCT determinations use a one-step, disposable color card test rather than a machine. These use whole blood from either a dermal puncture or a heparinized venous sample. Blood is applied to a card, and a color determination is made after the reaction takes place. Other cholesterol POCT methods use instrumentation (see Fig. 19-2).

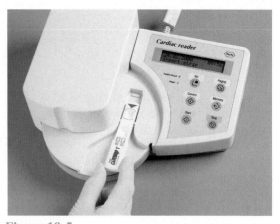

Figure 19-5
The Cardiac Reader system allows rapid determination of the cardiac markers troponin T and myoglobin from a single whole blood sample. (Courtesy Roche Diagnostics, Indianapolis, IN.)

Blood Gases and Electrolytes

Several instruments are available that can analyze arterial blood gases (Po_2, Pco_2, and pH) and common electrolytes (sodium, potassium, calcium, chloride, and bicarbonate). Some systems are small enough to be hand-held; others require a cart. They are particularly useful when frequent or rapid chemistry determinations must be made, such as in the emergency room or intensive care unit. Because of their complexity, all these instruments require careful calibration and more training than do simpler instruments such as hemoglobin analyzers.

B-Type Natriuretic Peptide

B-type natriuretic peptide (BNP), also known as brain natriuretic peptide, is a hormone made by the heart in response to expansion of ventricular volume and pressure overload. Its production increases in patients with congestive heart disease (CHD). The measurement of BNP at the bedside allows the practitioner to quickly differentiate between chronic obstructive pulmonary disease (COPD) and CHD, which may have similar symptoms. BNP can also be monitored to determine the effectiveness of CHD therapy. The BNP test requires a whole blood sample collected in EDTA.

ELECTROCARDIOGRAPHY

Electrocardiography is a method for recording the electrical activity of the heart. The output of the electrocardiograph is a tracing, called an

electrocardiogram (ECG or EKG). The ECG is used to diagnose heart disease such as ischemia, myocardial infarction, or fibrillation.

With the increasing demand for multiskilled personnel, developing the ability to perform electrocardiography is a natural progression for phlebotomists. It is beyond the scope of this chapter to give a complete introduction to this topic. Here we give the broad outlines needed to understand electrocardiography and present the basics of patient preparation and ECG recording.

The Cardiac Cycle

As you learned in Chapter 7, each heartbeat cycle includes a contraction and relaxation of each of the four chambers of the heart. This contraction is triggered and coordinated by electrical impulses from the heart's pacemaker, called the **sinoatrial node,** located in the upper wall of the right atrium. Electrical impulses spread out from there through the heart's **conduction system,** triggering the coordinated contraction of the heart muscle. The **cardiac cycle** refers to one complete heartbeat, consisting of **depolarization** (contraction) and **repolarization** (recovery and relaxation) of both the atria and the ventricles. The electrical activity occurring during this cycle is recorded on the ECG.

The normal ECG consists of a tracing with five prominent points where the graph changes direction. These are arbitrarily known as P, Q, R, S, and T (Figure 19-6). The regions immediately surrounding each point are known as the **P wave**, Q wave, and so on. As shown in the figure, the sections joining these points are known variously as segments, complexes, or intervals. Each part of the graph corresponds to a particular portion of the cardiac cycle and can be analyzed to determine how the heart is functioning (Table 19-1).

Important parameters that can be determined from the ECG include the time intervals between different phases of the cardiac cycle, which indicate conduction efficiency, and the size of the electrical signals, which may be correlated with an increase or decrease of heart muscle mass. For instance, ischemia may be associated with elongation of the Q-T interval, and myocardial injury may cause elevation of the ST segment above its normal position. The duration of the cardiac cycle can be read directly from the ECG, because each small square represents a known unit of time (Figure. 19-7).

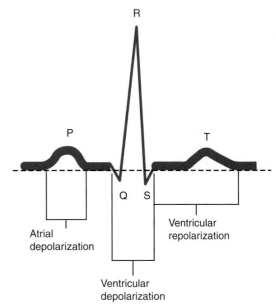

Figure 19-6

ECG tracing depicting P, Q, R, S, and T cycle. (Modified from Flynn JC Jr: Procedures in Phlebotomy, ed 3. Philadelphia, Saunders, 2005.)

Electrocardiogram Equipment

The electrical activity of the heart is recorded with 12 numbered electrodes that are placed in defined locations on the patient's chest, arms, and legs (Figure 19-8). The electrodes may be applied with an electrolyte solution to increase conductivity. A wire, or **lead**, is attached to each electrode (note that many practitioners use "lead" to refer to both wire and electrode, and "12-lead EKG" is a common phrase meaning the use of 12 electrodes). The leads pass to the ECG machine through a cable. The tracing is made on heat- and pressure-sensitive paper by a **stylus**.

TABLE 19-1 Electrocardiogram Measurements

ECG Section	Heart Activity
P wave	Atrial depolarization
P–R interval	Time between atrial contraction and ventricular contraction
QRS complex	Ventricular depolarization
ST segment	Time between ventricular depolarization and the beginning of repolarization
T wave	Ventricular repolarization
Q–T interval	Time between ventricular depolarization and completion of repolarization

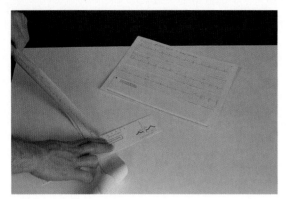

Figure 19-7
Analyzing an ECG tracing.

Performing an Electrocardiogram

The machine and the patient should be positioned away from electrical equipment, including televisions, air conditioners, and other functioning appliances. The patient must be disrobed from the waist up, and the lower legs must be exposed. The patient should be lying down and must remain still during the ECG (Figure 19-9). Electrode locations are cleaned with alcohol and shaved of hair, if necessary. Disposable adhesive electrodes are available, or electrolyte cream or gel is applied if reusable electrodes are being used. Electrodes are applied to the proper locations (as outlined in Box 19-3) and secured in place. The machine is turned on, and the recording is made. Many ECG machines automatically cycle through the 12 electrodes; alternatively, the technician switches the machine by hand to record from each electrode for a short time. After successfully recording from each electrode, the electrodes are removed, the skin is cleaned, and the patient can get dressed.

OTHER CLIA-WAIVED TESTS

The number of CLIA-waived tests is growing, owing to both advances in bioanalytical chemistry and the recognition that such tests allow more flexible delivery of care by a wider range of staff. The following tests are commonly performed as CLIA-waived tests, though not necessarily at the bedside or with hand-held instruments.

Occult Blood

This test uses a card kit. The stool specimen is placed on the card, and the reagent is added to the test area (Figure 19-10). Detection of occult blood

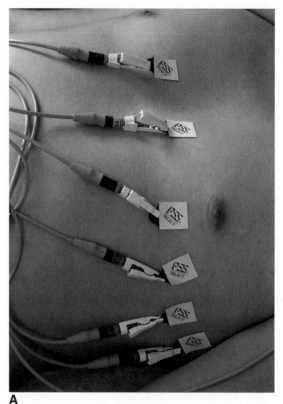

A

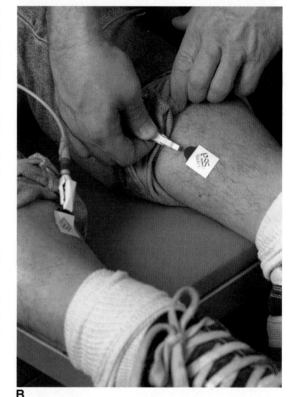

B

Figure 19-8
ECG electrodes are attached to the chest (**A**) and to the right and left legs (**B**), as well as to the arms.

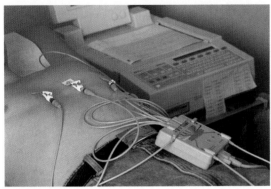

Figure 19-9
Patient and equipment position during an ECG.

BOX 19-3 Placement of Chest Electrodes

V_1, fourth intercostal space to right of sternum
V_2 fourth intercostal space to left of sternum
V_3 midway between position 2 and position 4
V_4 fifth intercostal space at the left midclavicular line
V_5 fifth intercostal space at the left anterior axillary line
V_6 fifth intercostal space at the left midaxillary line

---

in feces is used in the diagnosis of digestive tract diseases such as gastric ulcers or colon cancer. The patient must be informed of dietary restrictions that need to be followed before the test.

Urinalysis

Many commonly requested urine tests can be performed using a "dipstick," a plastic strip with reagents embedded in it. Tests may include pH, protein, glucose, ketones, bilirubin, urobilinogen, blood, leukocyte esterase, nitrite, and specific gravity. Before testing begins, the urine specimen must be at room temperature and thoroughly mixed. The urine strip is briefly and completely immersed in a well-mixed fresh urine specimen (Figure 19-11). After removal, excess urine is blotted from the side of the strip (Figure 19-12). The color change on the strip is compared with the reference color chart on the bottle at the appropriate time (Figure 19-13).

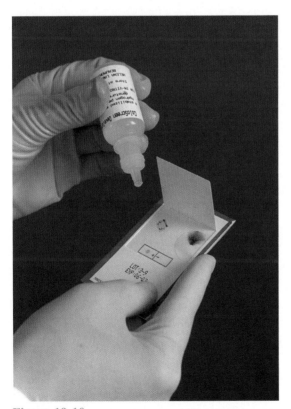

Figure 19-10
Applying developer to the occult blood card.

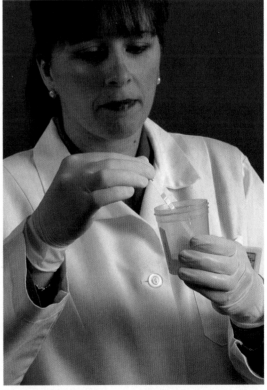

Figure 19-11
In a routine urinalysis procedure, the strip is completely immersed in the urine and then evaluated against the control, usually found in the bottle.

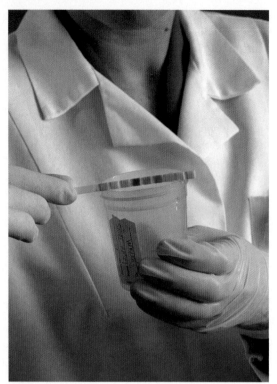

Figure 19-12
Remove excess urine by withdrawing the strip along the side of the container.

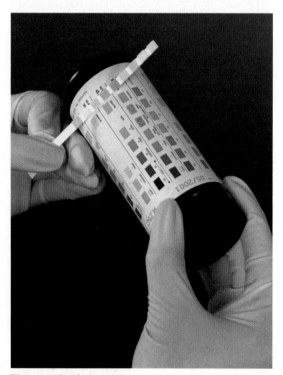

Figure 19-13
Compare the color change on the strip with the chart on the bottle.

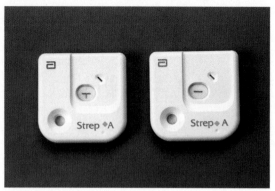

Figure 19-14
Rapid strep test results.

Pregnancy

A pregnancy test detects the presence of **human chorionic gonadotropin** (HCG), a hormone produced by the placenta after implantation of a fertilized egg. This hormone is present in both urine and serum, and test kits are available for each.

Rapid Group A Streptococcus

This test detects group A streptococcus (*Streptococcus pyogenes*) from a throat culture. The procedure usually requires extracting the sample to isolate bacterial carbohy rates, followed by the addition of reagents and the development of a color change. Test results are generally available within 3 to 5 minutes (Figure 19-14).

REVIEW FOR CERTIFICATION

Point-of-care testing refers to the performance of analytical tests immediately after obtaining a sample, often in the same room in which the patient is seen. Most tests performed as POCT are CLIA-waived tests, and the results are read directly from digital displays or monitors on the instrument. POCT instruments are easy to use, training is simple, and they can be used by a variety of medical professionals, including phlebotomists, nurses, nurse assistants, and physicians. Carefully following the manufacturer's instructions is important for obtaining accurate results. Hematology tests commonly performed as POCT include anemia and polycythemia evaluation by hematocrit or a hand-held hemoglobin analyzer; coagulation monitoring; heparin therapy monitoring using the ACT or APTT; and oral anticoagulant therapy via the PT. Chemistry tests include glucose; cardiac troponin T; cholesterol, using either a machine or a card test; arterial blood gases; and electrolytes. Electrocardiography provides an ECG tracing that can be used to diagnose heart disease. The ECG includes waves and other features corresponding to particular portions of the cardiac cycle, which can be analyzed to determine how the heart is functioning. Numbered electrodes, called leads, are placed in defined locations on the patient's chest, arms, and legs. The machine and the patient should be positioned away from electrical equipment, and the patient should be lying down and must remain still during the ECG. Other tests performed as POCT include occult blood testing using a card kit, urinalysis with a dipstick reagent stick, pregnancy testing for the presence of HCG, and rapid group A strep from a throat culture.

BIBLIOGRAPHY

Kost GJ, et al: Point-of-Care Testing: Principles, Management, and Clinical Practice. Philadelphia, McGraw-Hill, 1999.
Price CO, Hicks JM (eds): Point-of-Care Testing. Washington, DC, AACC Press, 1999.

STUDY QUESTIONS

1. Define point-of-care testing, and state four locales in which it may occur.
2. State an advantage and a disadvantage of point-of-care testing.
3. Describe the use of and the need for adherence to quality-assurance and quality-control procedures when performing POCT.
4. State two hematology tests that can be performed as POCT, and indicate how the test is done.
5. State four chemistry tests that can be performed as POCT, and indicate how the test is done.
6. Name the five waves that make up an ECG.
7. Name the heart activity that corresponds to the following:
   a. P wave
   b. QRS complex
   c. ST segment
8. Describe how to perform a "dipstick" urinalysis test.
9. Explain why it is important to follow the manufacturer's instructions when performing POCT.
10. Describe the POCT that can be used to evaluate:
   a. anemia
   b. Coumadin therapy
   c. cholesterol
   d. arterial blood gases
11. List the common electrolytes that can be measured by POCT.
12. Describe the normal ECG pattern.
13. Relate the ECG tracing to cardiac activity.
14. List the dipstick tests that are routinely performed on random urine specimens.
15. What types of specimens are used to determine pregnancy?
16. List the adherence guidelines for a POCT program. List the detrimental outcomes of failing to adhere to these guidelines.
17. The microcuvette tests and measures _____ and is essential in _____.
18. List the process used in ACT and the timed intervals if a clot does not form.
19. List the three analytes obtained in an arterial blood gas sample and the common electrolytes.
20. List the proper electrode placement for the precordial leads of an ECG.

CERTIFICATION EXAM PREPARATION

1. The percentage of packed red blood cells in a volume of blood is known as the:
   a. hemoglobin
   b. red blood cell count
   c. packed cell volume
   d. erythrocyte sedimentation rate

2. A hand-held hemoglobin analyzer gives a readout whose units are:
   a. g/mL
   b. g/dL
   c. kg/L
   d. g/mL

3. What point-of-care test can be used to monitor heparin therapy?
   a. PT or APTT
   b. ACT or APTT
   c. ACT or PT
   d. PT or TT

4. What test can provide valuable information regarding whether a patient has experienced a myocardial infarction?
   a. hemoglobin
   b. cholesterol
   c. cardiac troponin T
   d. glucose

5. What test can be used to screen for colon cancer?
   a. hemoglobin
   b. glucose
   c. cholesterol
   d. occult blood

6. Determination of HCG is used to evaluate:
   a. liver disease
   b. anemia
   c. urinary tract infection
   d. pregnancy

7. What type of specimen is used for the occult blood test?
   a. blood
   b. urine
   c. feces
   d. saliva

8. What streptococcus group is detected when performing a rapid strep test on a throat culture?
   a. group A
   b. group B
   c. group C
   d. group D

9. Before performing the dipstick test for a routine urinalysis, what two pretesting conditions must be met?
   a. Specimen must be at room temperature and well mixed.
   b. Specimen must be refrigerated and centrifuged.
   c. Specimen must be warmed to body temperature and well mixed.
   d. Specimen must be at room temperature and centrifuged.

10. For a POCT program to be successful, which of the following must be incorporated?
    a. adherence to the manufacturer's instructions
    b. use of quality-assurance and quality-control procedures
    c. proper and adequate training of all personnel
    d. all of the above

Appendix A

Metric System Measurements

Prefix	Meaning	Decimal	Exponent
deci-	tenth	0.1	10^{-1}
centi-	hundredth	0.01	10^{-2}
milli-	thousandth	0.001	10^{-3}
micro-	millionth	0.000001	10^{-6}
nano-	billionth	0.000000001	10^{-9}
deca-	ten	10	10^{1}
kilo-	thousand	1,000	10^{3}
mega-	million	1,000,000	10^{6}

Volume Units

liter (L)
deciliter (dL)
milliliter (mL)
microliter (μL)
cubic centimeter (cc or cm³)

Volume Conversions

1 L = 1,000 mL
1 L = 10 dL
1 dL = 100 mL
1 mL = 1,000 μL
1 mL = 1 cc

Mass Units

gram (g)
kilogram (kg)
milligram (mg)
microgram (μg)

Mass Conversions

1 kg = 1000 g
1 g = 1000 mg
1 mg = 1000 μg

Volume-to-Mass Conversions

Water has a density of 1 g/mL. Thus, the volume of water in milliliters is equivalent to its weight in grams.

Temperature Units

	Degrees Fahrenheit	Degrees Centigrade
Freezing point of water	32	0
Room temperature	72	22
Normal body temperature	98.6	37
Boiling point of water	212	100

Temperature Conversions

To convert from Centigrade to Fahrenheit:

$$(°C + 40) \times 9/5 - 40 = °F$$

Example:

$$(20°C + 40) \times 9/5 - 40 = 68°F$$

To convert from Fahrenheit to Centigrade:

$$(°F + 40) \times 5/9 - 40 = °C$$

Example:

$$(110°F + 40) \times 5/9 - 40 = 43.3°C$$

Appendix B

Common English-Spanish Phrases for Phlebotomy

General Rules of Spanish Pronunciation

Vowels: Pronunciation of vowels in Spanish is straightforward, since each vowel has one and only one sound:

a = ah
e = eh
i = ee
o = oh
u = oo

Emphasis: Emphasis goes on the last syllable unless the last letter is n, s, or a vowel. In those cases, it goes on the next-to-last syllable. Accent marks also indicate stressed syllables.

English
Spanish
Phonetic pronunciation

1. **Greeting the patient:**

   Please
   Por favor
   Por fah-VOR

   Thank you
   Gracias
   GRAH-see-as

   Good morning
   Buenos dias
   Bway-nos DEE-as

   Good afternoon
   Buenas tardes
   Bway-nas TAR-des

   Good evening
   Buenas noches
   Bway-nas NO-ches

2. **Checking patient identification:**

   What is your name?
   ¿Cómo se llama usted?
   CO-mo seh YA-ma oo-STED?

May I see your identification bracelet?
¿Puedo ver su brazalete de identificación?
Poo-EH-do vair soo BRA-sa-LET-eh de ee-dent-ih-fi-cah-see-ON

3. **Informing the patient that you need to take a blood sample:**

   Your doctor has ordered some laboratory tests.
   Su médico ha ordenado un análisis de laboratorio.
   Soo MEH-dee-co ah OR-den-AH-doe oon ah-NAH-lee-sees de lah-BOR-ih-TOR-ee-o

   I have to take some blood for testing.
   Tengo que sacarle sangre para un análisis.
   TENG-go keh sah-CAR-leh SANG-gray PAH-rah oon ah-NAH-lee-sees

   I am going to take a blood sample for testing.
   Voy a tomarle una muestra de sangre para análisis.
   VOY ah to-MAR-lay OON-ah moo-ES-tra de SANG-gray PAH-rah ah-NAH-lee-sees

   Have you had anything to eat or drink in the last 12 hours?
   ¿Ha comido o bebido algo en las últimas doce horas?
   Hah co-MEE-doh oh beh-BEE-doh AL-go en las UL-tee-mas DOH-seh OR-as?

4. **Collecting the blood sample:**

   Please make a fist.
   Por favor haga un puño.
   Por fah-VOR HAH-ga oon POON-yo

   Is the tourniquet too tight?
   ¿Está demasiado apretado el torniquete?
   Eh-STAH deh-MAH-see-AH-doh AH-preh-TAH-doh el TOR-nih-KET-eh?

   You are going to feel a small prick.
   Usted va a sentir un pequeño piquete.
   oo-STED vah ah sen-TEER oon peh-KEN-yo pih-KET-eh

Please keep your arm straight.
Por favor, mantenga su brazo firme.
Por fah-VOR, man-TENG-ah soo BRA-so
   FEER-meh

You can now relax your arm and fist.
Usted puede relajar su brazo y puño.
oo-STED PWED-eh REH-la-HAR soo BRA-zo
   ee POON-yo

5. **Asking the patient to give you a urine sample:**

You need to give us a urine sample for testing.
Usted tiene que darnos una muestra de orina para
   análisis.
oo-STED tee-EN-eh keh DARN-ohs OON-ah
   moo-ES-tra de oh-REEN-ah PAH-rah ah-
   NAH-lee-sees

6. **Useful phlebotomy terms:**

tourniquet
torniquete
TOR-nih-KET-eh

blood
sangre
SANG-gray

arm
brazo
BRA-so

right arm
brazo derecho
BRA-so de-RESH-oh

left arm
brazo izquierdo
BRA-so IS-kee-AIR-doh

needle
aguja
ah-GOO-ha

test, analysis
análisis
ah-NAH-lee-sees

urine
orína
oh-REEN-ah

urinalysis
análisis de la orína
ah-NAH-lee-sees de la oh-REEN-ah

sample
muestra
moo-ES-tra

finger stick
piquete del dedo
pih-KET-eh del DEH-doh

prick, stick
piquete
pih-KET-eh

finger
dedo
DEH-doh

7. **Names of laboratory tests:**

blood test
análisis de la sangre
ah-NAH-lee-sees de la SANG-gray

glucose level
nivel de glucosa
nee-VEL de glu-CO-sa

blood count
recuento sanguíneo
reh-KWEN-toh san-GEEN-ee-o

electrolytes
electrólitos
eh-lec-TRO-lee-toes

cholesterol
colesterol
co-LES-teh-ROL

triglycerides
triglicéridos
tree-glee-SEH-ree-dos

pregnancy test
análisis de embarazo
ah-NAH-lee-sees de EM-bar-AH-so

liver enzymes
enzimas del higado
en-SEE-mas del EE-gah-do

hepatitis C
hepatitis tipo C
heh-pa-TEE-tis TEE-po say

Appendix C
Competency Checklists

COMPETENCY CHECKLIST
Handwashing

Name _____ Date _____

Instructions

1. Properly demonstrate aseptic handwashing technique.
2. Demonstrate competency by: Performing the procedure of handwashing satisfactorily for the instructor. All steps must be completed as listed on the Competency Checklist.

Performance Standard

Properly wash hands using aseptic technique. Maximum time to complete assignment: 5 minutes.

Materials and Equipment

- Sink with running water
- Soap dispenser
- Paper towels

Procedure Record in the comments section any problems encountered while performing the procedure.			S = Satisfactory U = Unsatisfactory
You Must:	**S**	**U**	**Comments**
1. Remove all hand and wrist jewelry.			
2. Wet your hands with warm water.			
3. Apply soap to your hands.			
4. Scrub your hands together vigorously, working up a lather.			
5. Scrub palms, between fingers, under nails, and back of hands for at least 15 seconds.			
6. Rinse in a downward position.			
7. Dry your hands thoroughly with paper towels.			
8. Turn off the faucet with paper towels.			
9. Discard paper towels.			
Performance Standard Met _____ Yes _____ No Evaluator _____			***Comments*** Date _____

COMPETENCY CHECKLIST

Donning and Removing Personal Protective Equipment

Name _____ Date _____

Instructions

1. Properly demonstrate how to put on and take off personal protective equipment.
2. Demonstrate competency by: Demonstrating the correct order of putting personal protective equipment on and the appropriate order of removing and discarding it. All steps must be completed as listed on the Competency Checklist.

Performance Standard

Properly apply and remove personal protective equipment in the correct order. Maximum time to complete assignment: 8 minutes.

Materials and Equipment

- Gloves
- Gown or lab coat
- Goggles, mask, or face shield
- Biohazard waste container

Procedure			S = Satisfactory U = Unsatisfactory
Record in the comments section any problems encountered while performing the procedure.			
You Must:	**S**	**U**	**Comments**
Applying Personal Protective Equipment:			
1. Wash your hands.			
2. Put on lab coat or gown and fasten buttons or ties appropriately.			
3. Apply goggles, face mask, or face shield. If applying a mask, tie the mask on top, then on the bottom.			
4. Apply gloves over the cuffs of the lab coat or gown.			
Removing Personal Protective Equipment:			
5. Remove the first glove.			
6. Remove the second glove with the ungloved hand.			
7. Dispose of the gloves in a biohazard waste container.			
8. Remove the face mask, goggles, or face shield. If wearing a mask, untie the top ties, then the bottom ties, and discard in a biohazard waste container.			
9. Remove the gown or lab coat. If wearing a gown, turn it inside out as it is removed and discard in a biohazard waste container.			
10. Wash your hands.			
Performance Standard Met _____ Yes _____ No			*Comments*
Evaluator _____			Date _____

COMPETENCY CHECKLIST
Venipuncture (Evacuated Tube Method)

Name _____ Date _____

Instructions

1. Perform a venipuncture using the evacuated tube method.
2. Demonstrate competency by: Demonstrating the procedure for performing a venipuncture satisfactorily for the instructor. All steps must be completed as listed on the Competency Checklist.

Performance Standard

Successfully and properly perform a venipuncture using the evacuated tube method. Maximum time to complete assignment: 10 minutes.

Materials and Equipment

- Personal protective equipment
- Tourniquet
- Alcohol wipe
- Safety needle
- Disposable adapter
- Collection tubes
- 2×2 gauze
- Bandage
- Sharps container
- Biohazard waste container

Procedure			S = Satisfactory
Record in the comments section any problems encountered while performing the procedure.			U = Unsatisfactory

You Must:	S	U	Comments
1. Greet and identify the patient.			
2. Introduce yourself.			
3. Verify the lab tests ordered against the requisition.			
4. Position and prepare the patient.			
5. Explain the procedure to the patient.			
6. Wash your hands and don personal protective equipment.			
7. Assemble the equipment.			
8. Apply the tourniquet.			
9. Palpate the vein.			
10. Cleanse the site with an alcohol wipe and allow to air dry.			
11. Reapply the tourniquet (if necessary).			
12. Examine the safety needle.			
13. Anchor the vein.			
14. Insert the needle into the vein at the appropriate angle.			
15. Advance and change tubes in the appropriate order of draw.			
16. Remove the tourniquet.			

17. Mix anticoagulated tubes as they are removed from the adapter.		
18. Remove the last tube from the adapter before removing the needle. Activate the safety device.		
19. Remove the needle and discard in the sharps container.		
20. Apply pressure to the site with gauze.		
21. Label tubes with appropriate information.		
22. Check the site and apply a bandage.		
23. Thank the patient.		
24. Dispose of used supplies and materials.		
25. Remove personal protective equipment and wash your hands.		
26. Deliver specimens to appropriate departments.		
Performance Standard Met _____ Yes _____ No Evaluator _____		*Comments* Date _____

COMPETENCY CHECKLIST
Venipuncture (Syringe Method)

Name _____ Date _____

Instructions

1. Perform a venipuncture using the syringe method.
2. Demonstrate competency by: Demonstrating the procedure for performing a venipuncture satisfactorily for the instructor. All steps must be completed as listed on the Competency Checklist.

Performance Standard

Successfully and properly perform a venipuncture using the syringe method. Maximum time to complete assignment: 10 minutes.

Materials and Equipment

- Personal protective equipment
- Tourniquet
- Alcohol wipe
- Safety needle
- Syringe
- Syringe transfer device
- Collection tubes
- 2×2 gauze
- Bandage
- Sharps container
- Biohazard waste container

Procedure Record in the comments section any problems encountered while performing the procedure.			S = Satisfactory U = Unsatisfactory
You Must:	**S**	**U**	**Comments**
1. Greet and identify the patient.			
2. Introduce yourself.			
3. Verify the lab tests ordered against the requisition.			
4. Position and prepare the patient.			
5. Explain the procedure to the patient.			
6. Wash your hands and don personal protective equipment.			
7. Assemble the equipment.			
8. Apply the tourniquet.			
9. Palpate the vein.			
10. Cleanse the site with an alcohol wipe and allow to air dry.			
11. Reapply the tourniquet.			
12. Check the syringe plunger to verify free movement.			
13. Examine the needle.			
14. Anchor the vein.			
15. Insert the needle into the vein at the appropriate angle.			
16. Pull back the plunger evenly to withdraw blood.			
17. Remove the tourniquet.			
18. Remove the needle and activate the safety device.			

19. Apply pressure to the site with gauze.		
20. Transfer blood to evacuated tubes in the correct order of draw using the syringe transfer device.		
21. Mix any anticoagulated tubes as needed.		
22. Discard the syringe and needle into sharps container.		
23. Label tubes with appropriate information.		
24. Check the site and apply a bandage.		
25. Thank the patient.		
26. Dispose of used supplies and materials.		
27. Remove personal protective equipment and wash your hands.		
28. Deliver specimens to the appropriate departments.		
Performance Standard Met _____ Yes _____ No Evaluator _____		*Comments* Date _____

COMPETENCY CHECKLIST
Dermal Puncture (Finger Stick)

Name _____ Date _____

Instructions

1. Perform a dermal puncture.
2. Demonstrate competency by: Demonstrating the procedure for performing a dermal puncture satisfactorily for the instructor. All steps must be completed as listed on the Competency Checklist.

Performance Standard

Successfully and properly perform a dermal puncture. Maximum time to complete assignment: 10 minutes.

Materials and Equipment

- Personal protective equipment
- Alcohol wipe
- Skin puncture device
- Collection tubes (microtainers/capillary pipettes)
- Sealing caps or clay
- 2×2 gauze
- Bandage
- Sharps container
- Biohazard waste container

Procedure Record in the comments section any problems encountered while performing the procedure.			S = Satisfactory U = Unsatisfactory
You Must:	**S**	**U**	**Comments**
1. Greet and identify the patient.			
2. Introduce yourself and explain the procedure.			
3. Verify the lab tests ordered against the requisition.			
4. Wash your hands and don personal protective equipment.			
5. Assemble the equipment.			
6. Select the puncture site (and warm if necessary). Cleanse with alcohol and allow to air dry.			
7. Position and hold the finger and make the puncture in the appropriate area and position.			
8. Wipe away the first drop of blood.			
9. Collect the specimen in the appropriate containers, without air bubbles.			
10. Seal the specimen containers.			
11. Mix specimens with anticoagulant to prevent clot formation.			
12. Apply pressure to the puncture site with gauze.			
13. Bandage the puncture site appropriately based on patient's age.			
14. Label the specimens.			
15. Thank the patient.			

16. Dispose of used supplies and materials appropriately.			
17. Remove personal protective equipment and wash your hands.			
Performance Standard Met _____ Yes _____ No Evaluator _____			**Comments** Date _____

COMPETENCY CHECKLIST
Bleeding Time

Name _____ Date _____

Instructions

1. Successfully perform the bleeding time test.
2. Demonstrate competency by: Demonstrating the procedure for bleeding time satisfactorily for the instructor. All steps must be completed as listed on the Competency Checklist.

Performance Standard

Determine platelet function, as well as the significance of the test result. Maximum time to complete assignment: 15 minutes.

Materials and Equipment

- Personal protective equipment
- Blood pressure cuff
- Alcohol wipe
- Automated bleeding time puncture device
- Filter paper
- Stopwatch or timer with second hand
- Butterfly bandage
- Sharps container
- Biohazard waste container

Procedure Record in the comments section any problems encountered while performing the procedure.	S = Satisfactory U = Unsatisfactory		
You Must:	**S**	**U**	**Comments**
1. Greet and identify the patient.			
2. Identify yourself and explain the procedure.			
3. Verify the lab tests ordered against the requisition.			
4. Wash your hands and don personal protective equipment.			
5. Assemble the equipment.			
6. Position the patient's arm on a flat, steady surface.			
7. Select and cleanse the incision site with alcohol and allow to air dry.			
8. Apply the blood pressure cuff on the arm and inflate to 40 mm Hg.			
9. Position the incision device.			
10. Make the incision and start the timer.			
11. Wick blood onto the filter paper every 30 seconds after timer starts.			
12. Stop the timer when blood is no longer absorbed by the filter paper and record the time.			
13. Deflate and remove the blood pressure cuff.			
14. Cleanse the puncture site and apply a butterfly bandage.			
15. Instruct the patient on puncture site and bandage care.			

16. Correctly dispose of used supplies and materials.			
17. Thank the patient.			
18. Remove personal protective equipment and wash your hands.			
Performance Standard Met _____ Yes _____ No Evaluator _____			***Comments*** Date _____

COMPETENCY CHECKLIST
Venipuncture (Winged Infusion Method)

Name _____ Date _____

Instructions

1. Perform a venipuncture using the winged infusion method.
2. Demonstrate competency by: Demonstrating the procedure for performing a venipuncture satisfactorily for the instructor. All steps must be completed as listed on the Competency Checklist.

Performance Standard

Successfully and properly perform a venipuncture using the winged infusion method. Maximum time to complete assignment: 10 minutes.

Materials and Equipment

- Personal protective equipment
- Tourniquet
- Alcohol wipe
- Winged infusion set
- 2×2 gauze
- Evacuated tubes or syringe
- Bandage
- Sharps container
- Biohazard waste container

Procedure Record in the comments section any problems encountered while performing the procedure.			S = Satisfactory U = Unsatisfactory
You Must:	**S**	**U**	**Comments**
1. Greet and identify the patient.			
2. Introduce yourself.			
3. Verify the lab tests ordered against the requisition.			
4. Explain the procedure to the patient.			
5. Wash your hands and don personal protective equipment.			
6. Assemble the equipment.			
7. Apply the tourniquet around the wrist.			
8. Choose the puncture site.			
9. Cleanse the site with an alcohol wipe and allow to air dry.			
10. Reapply the tourniquet (if necessary).			
11. Anchor the vein.			
12. Holding the butterfly wings, insert the needle into the vein at the appropriate angle.			
13. Advance the needle and hold in place by one wing with the thumb of the opposite hand.			
14. Collect the sample in accordance with the method being used (evacuated tubes or syringe).			
15. Release the tourniquet, remove the needle, and activate the safety device.			

16. Apply pressure to the site with gauze.			
17. Mix anticoagulated tubes if applicable.			
18. Discard the needle and tubing in sharps container.			
19. If using a syringe, transfer blood to evacuated tubes. Use a syringe transfer device.			
20. Label tubes with appropriate information.			
21. Check the site and apply a bandage.			
22. Thank the patient.			
23. Dispose of used supplies and materials.			
24. Remove personal protective equipment and wash your hands.			
25. Deliver specimens to appropriate departments.			

Performance Standard Met

_____ Yes

_____ No

Evaluator _____

Comments

Date _____

COMPETENCY CHECKLIST
Modified Allen Test

Name _____ Date _____

Instructions

1. Properly perform the modified Allen test.
2. Demonstrate competency by: Demonstrating the procedure for determining collateral circulation satisfactorily for the instructor. All steps must be completed as listed on the Competency Checklist.

Performance Standard

Determine the presence of collateral circulation, as well as the significance of the test result. Maximum time to complete assignment: 5 minutes.

Materials and Equipment

- Towel

Procedure	S = Satisfactory
Record in the comments section any problems encountered while performing the procedure.	U = Unsatisfactory

You Must:	S	U	Comments
1. Extend the patient's wrist over a towel and position the hand palm up.			
2. Locate the radial and ulnar pulse sites by palpating with the appropriate fingers.			
3. Ask the patient to make a fist.			
4. Compress both arteries.			
5. Ask the patient to open and close the fist until the palm blanches.			
6. Release pressure on the ulnar artery and observe the color of the patient's palm.			
7. State and record a positive or negative result.			
8. Explain the significance and appropriate action to take for the test result.			
Performance Standard Met _____ Yes _____ No			*Comments*
Evaluator _____			Date _____

COMPETENCY CHECKLIST
Radial Artery Puncture

Name _____ Date _____

Instructions

1. Properly perform a radial artery puncture following the step-by-step procedure.
2. Demonstrate competency by: Demonstrating the procedure for performing a radial artery puncture for the instructor. All steps must be completed as listed on the Competency Checklist.

Performance Standard

Perform a radial artery puncture with accuracy and minimal discomfort. Maximum time to complete assignment: 12 minutes.

Materials and Equipment

- Personal protective equipment
- Alcohol wipe
- Povidone-iodine tincture
- 2×2 gauze
- Blood gas syringe (heparinized)
- Safety needle, needle block, Luer cap
- Cup of ice chips
- Bandage
- Sharps container
- Biohazard waste container

Procedure Record in the comments section any problems encountered while performing the procedure.			**S = Satisfactory** **U = Unsatisfactory**
You Must:	**S**	**U**	**Comments**
1. Assemble the equipment.			
2. Greet and identify the patient, introduce yourself, and explain the procedure.			
3. Verify that the patient is in a respiratory steady state.			
4. Wash your hands and don personal protective equipment.			
5. Verify the lab tests ordered against the requisition.			
6. Perform the modified Allen test to assess collateral circulation in the hand.			
7. Locate the radial artery.			
8. Cleanse the puncture site with 70% isopropyl alcohol and allow to air dry.			
9. Cleanse the puncture site with povidone-iodine tincture and allow to air dry.			
10. Administer local anesthetic and wait 1 to 2 minutes.			
11. Cleanse your index finger with alcohol and place it over the area where the needle should enter the artery.			

12. Hold the syringe like a dart, bevel up, and insert the needle at a 45- to 60-degree angle distal to your finger until blood appears in the needle hub.			
13. Allow arterial pressure to fill the syringe.			
14. Remove the needle and apply direct pressure to the puncture site with folded gauze for at least 5 minutes.			
15. While applying pressure, expel air from the syringe, activate safety device, and plant the needle into the rubber block.			
16. Mix the specimen with heparin.			
17. Place specimen in ice chips.			
18. Check the site and remove the povidone-iodine with an alcohol wipe.			
19. Apply a pressure bandage of gauze.			
20. Check for a pulse distal to the puncture site.			
21. Remove and discard the needle into a sharps container.			
22. Place the Luer cap on the syringe, label the specimen, and return to ice chips.			
23. Dispose of used supplies and materials; remove personal protective equipment and wash your hands.			
24. Thank the patient.			
25. Deliver the specimen immediately to the lab.			
Performance Standard Met _____ Yes _____ No Evaluator _____			*Comments* Date _____

COMPETENCY CHECKLIST
Blood Culture

Name _____ Date _____

Instructions

1. Properly perform a blood culture collection.
2. Demonstrate competency by: Demonstrating the procedure for collecting a blood culture satisfactorily for the instructor while adhering to aseptic technique. All steps must be completed as listed on the Competency Checklist.

Performance Standard

Collect a blood culture with accuracy. Maximum time to complete assignment: 10 minutes.

Materials and Equipment

- Personal protective equipment
- Alcohol wipe
- Povidone-iodine tincture
- 2×2 gauze
- Tourniquet
- Bandages
- Aerobic blood culture bottle
- Anaerobic blood culture bottle
- Safety needle
- Disposable adapter
- Sharps container
- Biohazard waste container

Procedure Record in the comments section any problems encountered while performing the procedure.			S = Satisfactory U = Unsatisfactory
You Must:	**S**	**U**	**Comments**
1. Greet and identify the patient.			
2. Identify yourself and explain the procedure.			
3. Verify the lab tests ordered against the requisition.			
4. Wash your hands and don personal protective equipment.			
5. Assemble the equipment.			
6. Apply the tourniquet, identify the puncture site, and remove the tourniquet.			
7. Vigorously scrub the site with alcohol.			
8. Vigorously scrub the site with povidone-iodine and allow to air dry.			
9. Cleanse the tops of the blood culture bottles.			
10. Reapply the tourniquet without contaminating the site.			
11. Perform the venipuncture.			
12. Inoculate each bottle in the correct order and mix the samples.			
13. Release the tourniquet, remove the needle, activate the safety device, and apply pressure.			
14. Label the blood culture bottles correctly.			

15. Remove povidone-iodine from the patient's arm and apply a bandage.		
16. Discard used materials and supplies appropriately.		
17. Thank the patient.		
18. Remove personal protective equipment and wash your hands.		
Performance Standard Met _____ Yes _____ No Evaluator _____		***Comments*** Date _____

COMPETENCY CHECKLIST
Blood Smear Preparation

Name _____ Date _____

Instructions

1. Successfully prepare a blood smear.
2. Demonstrate competency by: Demonstrating the procedure for preparing a blood smear satisfactorily for the instructor. All steps must be completed as listed on the Competency Checklist.

Performance Standard

Accurately prepare a peripheral blood smear. Maximum time to complete assignment: 5 minutes.

Materials and Equipment

• Gloves
• Clean glass slides

Procedure Record in the comments section any problems encountered while performing the procedure.	**S = Satisfactory** **U = Unsatisfactory**		
You Must:	**S**	**U**	**Comments**
1. Wash your hands and put on gloves.			
2. Apply a small drop of blood to the correct area of the slide.			
3. Place the spreader at the correct angle in front of the blood drop.			
4. Pull the spreader back to contact the blood drop.			
5. Move the spreader forward in continuous motion.			
6. Repeat steps 2 through 5 to prepare a second slide.			
7. Allow the smears to dry.			
8. Properly label the smears.			
9. Examine the blood smears for quality and acceptability.			
10. Remove gloves and wash your hands.			
Performance Standard Met _____ Yes _____ No			***Comments***
Evaluator _____			Date _____

COMPETENCY CHECKLIST
Throat Swab

Name _____ Date _____

Instructions

1. Properly perform a throat swab.
2. Demonstrate competency by: Demonstrating the procedure for performing a throat swab satisfactorily for the instructor. All steps must be completed as listed on the Competency Checklist.

Performance Standard

Successfully and properly perform a throat swab. Maximum time to complete assignment: 5 minutes.

Materials and Equipment

- Personal protective equipment
- Tongue depressor
- Flashlight
- Collection swab
- Transport tube with transport media
- Biohazard waste container

Procedure Record in the comments section any problems encountered while performing the procedure.			**S = Satisfactory** **U = Unsatisfactory**
You Must:	**S**	**U**	**Comments**
1. Greet and identify the patient.			
2. Introduce yourself.			
3. Verify the lab tests ordered against the requisition.			
4. Explain the procedure to the patient.			
5. Wash your hands and don personal protective equipment.			
6. Assemble the equipment.			
7. Position the patient.			
8. Depress the patient's tongue with a tongue depressor and inspect the back of the throat with the flashlight to locate inflamed areas.			
9. Quickly touch the tip of the swab to the tonsils and any other inflamed areas.			
10. Return the swab to the holder.			
11. Crush the ampule at the bottom of the holder containing the transport media.			
13. Thank the patient.			
14. Dispose of used supplies and materials.			
15. Remove personal protective equipment and wash your hands.			
16. Deliver the specimen to the appropriate department.			

Performance Standard Met			*Comments*
_____ Yes			
_____ No			
Evaluator _____			Date _____

Appendix D
Common Abbreviations

AAAHP	American Association of Allied Health Professionals
ABG	arterial blood gases
ACT	activated coagulation time
ACTH	adrenocorticotropic hormone
ADH	antidiuretic hormone
AIDS	acquired immunodeficiency syndrome
ALP	alkaline phosphatase
ALT	alanine aminotransferase
AMT	American Medical Technologists
APTT	activated partial thromboplastin time
ASCLS	American Society of Clinical Laboratory Science
ASCP	American Society for Clinical Pathology
ASPT	American Society for Phlebotomy Technicians
AST	aspartate aminotransferase
AV	atrioventricular, arteriovascular
BBP	blood-borne pathogen
BC	blood culture
BNP	brain natriuretic peptide
BT	bleeding time
BUN	blood urea nitrogen
BURPP	bilirubin, uric acid, phosphorus, and potassium
CAP	College of American Pathologists
CBC	complete blood count
CCU	cardiac care unit
CK	creatine kinase
CLIA	Clinical Laboratory Improvement Amendments of 1988
CLS	clinical laboratory scientist
CLSI	Clinical Laboratory Standards Institute
CLT	clinical laboratory technician
CNA	certified nursing assistant
COC	chain of custody
COPD	chronic obstructive pulmonary disease

CPT	certified phlebotomy technician
CQI	continuous quality improvement
C&S	culture and sensitivity
CSF	cerebrospinal fluid
CT	computed tomography
CVC	central venous catheter
DIC	disseminated intravascular coagulation
Diff	differential
DOB	date of birth
DOT	Department of Transportation
ECG, EKG	electrocardiogram
EDTA	ethylenediaminetetraacetic acid
EIA	enzyme immunoassay
EP	expanded precautions
ER	emergency room
ESR	erythrocyte sedimentation rate
FBS	fasting blood glucose
FDA	Food and Drug Administration
FDP	fibrin degradation product
FSH	follicle stimulating hormone
FUO	fever of unknown origin
g/dL	grams/deciliter
GGT	gamma glutamyl transferase
GH	growth hormone
GTT	glucose tolerance test
HCG	human chorionic gonadotropin
Hct	hematocrit
HDL	high-density lipoprotein
HEPA	high efficiency particulate air filtration
Hgb	hemoglobin
HIPAA	Health Insurance Portability and Accountability Act
HLA	human leukocyte antigen
HMO	health maintenance organization
ICU	intensive care unit
INR	international normalized ratio
IRS	Internal Revenue Service

IV	intravenous	PHI	protected health information
		PICC	peripherally inserted central catheter
JCAHO	Joint Commission on Accreditation of Healthcare Organizations	PKU	phenylketonuria
		PMN	polymorphonuclear
LD	lactate dehydrogenase	Po_2	partial pressure of oxygen
LDL	low-density lipoprotein	POCT	point-of-care testing
LH	luteinizing hormone	POL	physician office lab
LIS	Laboratory Information Services	PPE	personal protective equipment
LPN	licensed practical nurse	PPO	preferred provider organization
		PT	prothrombin time
MCH	mean corpuscular hemoglobin	PTT	partial thromboplastin time
MCHC	mean corpuscular hemoglobin concentration	QA	quality assurance
MCV	mean corpuscular volume	QC	quality control
MHC	major histocompatibility complex	QNS	quantity not sufficient
MIS	manager of information services		
MLT	medical laboratory technician	RBC	red blood cell (or count)
MRI	magnetic resonance imaging	RDW	red cell distribution width
MSDS	materials safety data sheet	RIA	radioimmunoassay
MSH	melanocyte-stimulating hormone	RN	registered nurse
MT	medical technologist	RPT	registered phlebotomy technician
		RT	respiratory therapist
NAACLS	National Accrediting Agency for Clinical Laboratory Sciences	SCID	severe combined immune deficiency
NCCLS	National Committee for Clinical Laboratory Standards	SE	sweat electrolytes
NFPA	National Fire Protection Association	Seg	segmented neutrophils
NIDA	National Institute on Drug Abuse	SPS	sodium polyanetholesulfonate
NK	natural killer	SST	serum separator tube
NP	nasopharyngeal		
NPA	National Phlebotomy Association	T_3	triiodothyronine
		T_4	thyroxine
OGTT	oral glucose tolerance test	TBP	transmission-based precautions
O&P	ova and parasites	TLC	tender loving care
OR	operating room	TnT	troponin T
OSHA	Occupational Safety and Health Administration	t-PA	tissue plasminogen activator
		TQM	total quality management
		TSH	thyroid stimulating hormone
PBT	phlebotomy technician		
PCA	patient care assistant	VAD	vascular access device
Pco_2	partial pressure of carbon dioxide		
PCT	patient care technician	WBC	white blood cell (or count)
PCV	packed cell volume	WIS	winged infusion set
PET	positron emission tomography		

Appendix E
Mock Certification Exam

1. What is phlebotomy?
   A. A trained professional in blood drawing
   B. The legal standards for a person who performs blood-drawing skills
   C. The process of drawing blood
   D. All of the above are correct

2. What is a phlebotomist?
   A. A trained professional in blood drawing
   B. The legal standards for a person who performs blood-drawing skills
   C. The process of drawing blood
   D. All of the above are correct

3. Which of the following is not part of a phlebotomist's point-of-care job-related duties?
   A. Taking blood pressure
   B. Instructing patients on urine specimen collection
   C. Performing a tracheostomy
   D. Performing basic laboratory tests

4. All of the following are considered hazards, except:
   A. Bending your knees when lifting heavy objects
   B. Airborne viruses and bacteria
   C. Handling broken glass when wearing gloves
   D. All of the above are hazards

5. All of the following are true about laboratory safety, except:
   A. You may store food in the laboratory refrigerator
   B. Protect your feet from spills
   C. Always wear required personal protection equipment
   D. All of the above are correct

6. As written in the Patient's Bill of Rights, the patient has the right to:
   A. Refuse treatment
   B. Not participate in experimental procedures
   C. Know the name of the phlebotomist
   D. All of the above are correct

7. Certification is evidence that:
   A. The phlebotomist is working in the field
   B. The phlebotomist has demonstrated proficiency in the area of blood drawing
   C. The phlebotomist is licensed in the field
   D. The phlebotomist is accredited in the field

8. Which of the following is not an OSHA-required personal protection equipment?
   A. Steel-toe shoes
   B. Goggles
   C. Chin-length face shield
   D. Full-length lab coat

9. The Clinical Laboratory Improvement Amendment of 1988 follows guidelines and standards set by the:
   A. CLIA '88
   B. CLSI
   C. JCAHO
   D. CDC

10. Samples collected from a patient in a nursing home are sent to:
    A. POL
    B. CDC
    C. Reference laboratory
    D. An urgent care center

11. Quality assurance for laboratory personnel includes all of the following, except:
    A. Specimen collection procedures
    B. Specimen transport processes
    C. Specimen-processing policies
    D. The laboratory supervisor's home telephone number

12. Personal protection equipment must be provided by the:
    A. Centers for Disease Control and Prevention
    B. OSHA
    C. Employee
    D. Employer

13. Which of the following personal protection equipment must a phlebotomist use when performing a skin puncture or venipuncture?
    A. Goggles
    B. Gloves
    C. Masks
    D. Caps and booties

14. Under HIPAA, protected health information is defined as:
    A. Information that the patient refuses to disclose to the doctor
    B. Any test result
    C. Any part of a patient's health information that is linked to information that identifies the patient
    D. Information that summarizes the patient's insurance coverage

15. Employers must provide vaccination against _____ free of charge.
    A. Hepatitis A virus
    B. Hepatitis B virus
    C. Hepatitis C virus
    D. Hepatitis delta virus

16. Which of the following would be a reason for rejection of a specimen by the lab?
    A. Patient's name, date of birth, and the date and time are written on the label and requisition slip
    B. Specimen containing an additive has been inverted
    C. An ESR has been collected in a red-topped tube
    D. All of the above are reasons for rejections

17. The quality of the test result depends on:
    A. The type of specimen
    B. The source of the specimen
    C. The time lapsed between collection of the specimen and analyzing the specimen
    D. Whether the sample is going to be analyzed for glucose or phosphate

18. The purpose of quality control is to:
    A. Check machinery with automated procedures
    B. Ensure that proper laboratory procedures are being followed
    C. Ensure that adequate patient care is being provided
    D. All of the above are correct

19. A specimen may be rejected by the lab if:
    A. The tube was not initialed
    B. The blood is hemolyzed
    C. The tube was not transported properly
    D. All of the above are correct

20. Transport bags have a separate compartment (pouch) for requisitions in order to:
    A. Safeguard the requisition
    B. Keep the specimen from getting lost
    C. Prevent contamination if the specimen leaks
    D. Ensure the requisition goes to central receiving and the specimen to the processing lab

21. _____ is the most important step in phlebotomy and other testing procedures.
    A. Proper patient identification
    B. Proper hand washing
    C. Proper specimen handling
    D. Collecting sufficient blood

22. When identifying a patient, the phlebotomist must:
    A. Ask the patient to give his or her name and DOB
    B. Check the patient's ID band
    C. Ask the patient to present a photo ID
    D. All of the above are correct

23. When an admitted patient is not wearing an ID band, the phlebotomist must:
    A. Ask the patient for a picture ID
    B. Not draw blood from this patient
    C. Simply question the patient and confirm the date of birth
    D. Contact the nursing station and request an ID band be placed on the patient

24. What is the proper procedure for a phlebotomist to follow if a physician or clergy is in the patient's room at the time of draw?
    A. Ask the physician or clergy to step outside
    B. Draw the blood with the physician or clergy present
    C. Return at another time if the specimen is not a STAT
    D. Both A and C are correct

25. What should the phlebotomist do if he or she cannot communicate with the patient?
    A. Communicate with the hands
    B. Leave the room; let the doctor draw
    C. Draw the blood without consent
    D. All of the above are correct

26. Most tubes containing additives should be inverted:
    A. Once
    B. 3 times
    C. 5–8 times
    D. Tubes containing additives should not be inverted

27. The additive within the lavender-topped tube is:
    A. No additive
    B. Heparin
    C. SPS or ACD
    D. EDTA

28. The green-topped tube contains:
    A. No additive
    B. Heparin
    C. SPS or ACD
    D. EDTA

29. The yellow-topped tube contains:
    A. No additive
    B. Heparin
    C. SPS or ACD
    D. EDTA

30. The glass red-topped tube contains:
    A. No additive
    B. Heparin
    C. SPS or ACD
    D. EDTA

31. Which of the following tubes contain(s) sodium fluoride and potassium oxalate?
    A. Red-topped tube
    B. Lavender-topped tube
    C. Gray-topped tube
    D. All tubes with splash guards

32. Which of the following tubes would hold a glucose specimen for 24 hours?
    A. Red-topped tube
    B. Lavender-topped tube
    C. Gray-topped tube
    D. All tubes with splash guards

33. In which tube would a phlebotomist collect an erythrocyte sedimentation rate?
    A. Red-topped tube
    B. Lavender-topped tube
    C. Gray-topped tube
    D. All tubes with splash guards

34. Cardiac enzymes are drawn in:
    A. Red-topped tube
    B. Lavender-topped tube
    C. Gray-topped tube
    D. All tubes with splash guards

35. Which of the following tubes yield(s) a serum specimen?
    A. Red-topped tube
    B. Lavender-topped tube
    C. Gray-topped tube
    D. All of the above yield a serum specimen

36. Coagulation studies include all of the following, except:
    A. Prothrombin time
    B. Complete blood count
    C. Partial thromboplastin time
    D. Platelet function

37. A blood donation given by a patient for use during his or her surgical procedure is called:
    A. An autologous donation
    B. A cryoprecipitated donation
    C. A Willebrand's collection
    D. None of the above

38. Why should a glass red-topped tube be drawn before a green-topped tube?
    A. Additives in the red-topped tube will not interfere with the tests performed on the green-topped tube
    B. Red-topped tubes are always the very first tube drawn
    C. Since there are no additives in the red-topped tube, it cannot contaminate the green-topped tube
    D. Green-topped tubes are always the very last tube drawn

39. Which of the following is false for blood culture collection?
    A. Must be collected in the red- and marbled-topped tube
    B. Area must be prepped with iodine or other antibacterial agent before draw
    C. Tourniquet is not used for blood culture collection
    D. Both A and C are false for blood culture collection

40. Which of the following is correct for arterial blood gas collection?
    A. Must be collected in a red- and marbled-topped tube
    B. Area must be prepped with iodine before draw
    C. A tourniquet is used in the collection
    D. Both B and C are correct

41. A heparinized needle and syringe are necessary in the collection of:
    A. Blood culture
    B. ESR
    C. ABG
    D. Heparin levels

42. A Hemogard top:
    A. Is a plastic top that fits over the stopper
    B. Is only used on the lavender top tube
    C. Is used to reduce aerosol and splattering of blood
    D. Both A and C are correct

43. Cold agglutinin test must be maintained at a temperature of:
    A. 37°F
    B. 32°C
    C. 32°F
    D. 37°C

44. Chilling a specimen will:
    A. Speed up the metabolic process
    B. Maintain the stability of the specimen during transport
    C. Prevent problems in tubes containing EDTA
    D. Facilitate the processing process

45. Specimens for which of the following tests must be kept chilled?
    A. Ammonia
    B. Pyruvate
    C. Lactic acid
    D. All of the above

46. When labeling tubes, all of the following information must be placed on them, except:
    A. Patient's name
    B. Date
    C. Time of draw
    D. Patient's diagnosis
    E. Phlebotomist's initials

47. Which of the following is not needed for a routine phlebotomy procedure?
    A. Gloves
    B. Tourniquet
    C. Alcohol
    D. Iodine

48. What additional equipment may be needed when drawing blood from a patient in the premature nursery?
    A. Small butterfly needles
    B. Rewards, stickers, and toys
    C. Anesthesia
    D. Additional personal protection equipment

49. The depth of a heel puncture cannot exceed:
    A. 5.3 mm
    B. 2.4 cm
    C. 2.0 mm
    D. 1.3 mm

50. The tourniquet is placed _____ above the site of draw.
    A. 5–7 inches
    B. 3–4 inches
    C. 1–2 inches
    D. 4–6 inches

51. When a tourniquet is left on too tight, capillaries may rupture, causing:
    A. A rash
    B. Pain
    C. Urticaria
    D. Petechiae

52. Which of the following is true when using a tourniquet during a phlebotomy procedure?
    A. Never tie a tourniquet on open sores
    B. Tying a tourniquet too tightly can cause petechiae
    C. Leaving a tourniquet on too long can cause hemoconcentration
    D. All of the above are correct

53. A phlebotomist must inspect the needle for:
    A. Burrs
    B. Expiration date
    C. Bevel facing up
    D. All of the above are correct

54. Which of the following is the smallest needle?
    A. 18 gauge
    B. 19 gauge
    C. 20 gauge
    D. 21 gauge

55. A butterfly needle should be used:
    A. For patients with sclerosed veins and one tube being drawn
    B. On adults' dorsal and metacarpal veins
    C. On pediatric and geriatric patients
    D. All of the above are correct

56. A tube holder is used to connect needle and evacuated tube in order to:
    A. Prevent contact between the needle and tube
    B. Ensure a firm stable connection between them
    C. Keep blood from entering the adapter
    D. Allow a syringe to be used

57. The proper way to dispose of a needle is to:
    A. Recap it and put it into a sharps container
    B. Throw it recapped into a biohazard bag
    C. Put it into a sharps container, without recapping, immediately after withdrawing it from a patient
    D. Collect it in a cup and dispose of it later

58. Factors to consider in site selection prior to a venipuncture are:
    A. Scars or burns
    B. Edema
    C. Mastectomy
    D. All of the above are correct

59. Which of the following are correct for ending the phlebotomy procedure?
    A. Remove the needle, remove the tube, remove the tourniquet
    B. Remove the tourniquet, apply pressure, remove the needle, discard the needle in sharps container
    C. Remove tourniquet, remove tube, place gauze, remove needle, apply pressure, discard needle in sharps container
    D. Remove needle, apply pressure, discard needle in biohazards bag

60. The most commonly occurring complication in phlebotomy is:
    A. Convulsions
    B. Short draw
    C. Hypovolemia
    D. Hematoma

61. A tourniquet that has been left on too long can cause:
    A. Petechiae
    B. Hemolysis
    C. Hemoconcentration
    D. All of the above

62. What should a phlebotomist do first if a patient has syncope during a phlebotomy procedure?
    A. Go quickly for help
    B. Apply a cold compress
    C. Remove the needle and tourniquet, and apply pressure
    D. Attempt to wake the patient by speaking loudly

63. Which of the following are signs and symptoms of syncope?
    A. Small red dots at the site of draw
    B. Black and blue discoloration at the site
    C. Cold, damp, clammy skin
    D. All of the above are correct

64. Blood that has seeped from a vein into tissue is called:
    A. Hemoconcentration
    B. Hematoma
    C. Petechiae
    D. Short draw

65. Which of the following may cause vein occlusion?
    A. Dermal puncture
    B. CABG
    C. Sphygmomanometer
    D. Chemotherapy

66. Which of the following complications may occur if the phlebotomist punctures a bone?
    A. Hematoma
    B. Hemoconcentration
    C. Arteriosclerosis
    D. Osteomyelitis

67. Veins that are hard and cord-like are called:
    A. Thrombosed
    B. Sclerosed
    C. Collapsed
    D. Tortuous

68. The term that means the rupturing of red blood cells is:
    A. Hemostasis
    B. Hemoglobin
    C. Hemolysis
    D. Hematoma

69. High bilirubin levels can lead to:
    A. Mismatched blood groups
    B. Breakdown of antibodies
    C. Jaundice, which can lead to brain damage
    D. All of the above are correct

70. Thrombosis is:
    A. An autoimmune reaction
    B. Blood pooled in the legs
    C. Clot formation within a blood vessel
    D. Inflammation of the thyroid gland

71. Which of the following will cause a shortened bleeding time in a bleeding time test?
    A. Aspirin
    B. Infection
    C. Hair at incision site
    D. Scratching of a capillary

72. A hematoma can be prevented if:
    A. Pressure is applied on the vein until bleeding stops completely
    B. A bandage is immediately placed on the vein
    C. The needle is removed before the tourniquet is released
    D. All of the above are correct

73. Aspirin may affect a patient's:
    A. HCG
    B. CBC
    C. Bleeding time
    D. Heparin time

74. In a CSF collection the phlebotomist will:
    A. Obtain the specimen from the patient
    B. Transport the specimen to the lab
    C. Process the microbiology specimen under the microscope
    D. All of the above are always done by a certified phlebotomist technician

75. Body fluid collections are:
    A. Always obtained/collected by a phlebotomist
    B. Always a STAT specimen
    C. Collected in a sterile container
    D. Both A and C are correct

76. The process for collecting amniotic fluid is known as:
    A. An amniocentesis
    B. An amnioectomy
    C. An amniotomy
    D. An amniology

77. The amniotic fluid must be:
    A. Transferred into a sterile container
    B. Protected from light
    C. Transported immediately to the lab for analysis
    D. All of the above are correct

78. Prompt delivery to the lab of semen samples is necessary to determine _____ in fertility testing.
    A. Viability
    B. Volume
    C. V_{max}
    D. All of the above are correct

79. Fecal specimens are collected for:
    A. Ova and parasite testing
    B. Testing for digestive abnormalities
    C. Occult blood analysis
    D. All of the above

80. What is the best sample to determine blood pH and blood gases?
    A. Capillary blood
    B. Venous blood
    C. Arterial blood
    D. Cerebrospinal fluid

81. An un-iced ABG must be delivered to the lab within:
    A. 1 hour
    B. 5–10 hours
    C. 5–10 minutes
    D. 2 hours

82. Arterial blood gas must be processed immediately in order to minimize:
    A. Blood loss into tissue
    B. Hematoma
    C. Petechiae
    D. Changes in the analyte

83. All of the following are safety equipment for arterial blood gas collection, except:
    A. Small rubber block
    B. Fluid retention gown
    C. Heparinized syringe and needle
    D. Face shield

84. If the Modified Allen test is negative,
    A. Another artery must be selected for blood collection
    B. The patient does not have hepatitis B
    C. Dermal puncture may proceed
    D. Sweat electrolytes are unlikely to be positive for cystic fibrosis

85. The NPC culture is used to diagnose:
    A. Whooping cough
    B. Croup
    C. Upper respiratory infections
    D. All of the above are correct

86. The SE test is used to diagnose:
    A. Whooping cough
    B. Elevated levels of salt
    C. Cystic fibrosis
    D. All of the above are correct

87. Which procedure is normally collected by a nurse or respiratory therapist?
    A. Glucose tolerance test
    B. Routine blood collection
    C. Arterial blood gas
    D. Capillary/dermal punctures

88. Dermal punctures can be used as an alternate for all of the following except:
    A. CBC
    B. Glucose tolerance test
    C. ESR
    D. Arterial blood gas

89. Which of the following would be a reason for performing a dermal puncture?
    A. Patients who require frequent blood draws
    B. Patients with burns on the arms
    C. Patients who are at risk for venous thrombosis
    D. All of the above are correct

90. Which of the following is the reason for cleansing the first drop of blood in a dermal puncture?
    A. To rid the sample of arterial blood
    B. To rid the specimen of fluid from tissue
    C. To rid the specimen of potassium
    D. All of the above are correct

91. When collecting blood from a child, the phlebotomist should:
    A. Consider the psychological aspect of the draw
    B. Log the amount of blood collected to avoid depletion
    C. Collect dermal punctures whenever possible
    D. All of the above are correct

92. Which of the following should a phlebotomist NOT do when drawing blood from a child?
    A. Use the patient identification process
    B. Explain the procedure
    C. Tell the child that the procedure will not hurt
    D. During the draw, tell the child "just a few more seconds"

93. What does the phlebotomist look for when identifying a newborn?
    A. The first and last name on the ID band
    B. The hospital identification number and the last name
    C. The date of birth
    D. The mother's ID bracelet

94. Improper cleansing of a venipuncture site can cause:
    A. Hematoma
    B. Septicemia
    C. Petechiae
    D. All of the above are correct

95. A pathogen is:
    A. The invasion and growth of a microorganism
    B. An infectious disease-causing microorganism
    C. Always a bacterium
    D. Never a virus

96. Which of the following components is needed in order to make what is known as the chain of infection?
    A. Causative agent
    B. Etiology
    C. Doppler
    D. All of the above are correct

97. A health care–related infection is:
    A. An infection contracted within a health care institution
    B. An infection that requires hospitalization
    C. An infection that is only significant when a patient is immunocompromised
    D. All of the above

98. When a patient has a highly contagious disease, he or she is placed in:
    A. Enteric isolation
    B. Reverse isolation
    C. Strict isolation
    D. Blood and body fluid precautions

99. A patient who is known to have a blood-transmissible disease is placed on:
    A. Enteric isolation
    B. Reverse isolation
    C. Strict isolation
    D. Blood and body fluid precautions

100. A patient who has diarrhea and bacterial gastroenteritis is placed on:
    A. Enteric isolation
    B. Reverse isolation
    C. Strict isolation
    D. Blood and body fluid precautions

101. Patients within a neonatal ICU/burn unit or the recovery room are in:
    A. Enteric isolation
    B. Reverse isolation
    C. Strict isolation, blood and body fluid precautions
    D. Wound and body fluid precautions

102. The most frequently occurring laboratory healthcare-related infection is:
    A. HIV
    B. HBV
    C. HCV
    D. HAV

103. An infection is:
    A. A disease-causing microorganism
    B. The invasion and growth of a pathogen
    C. Always caused by bacteria
    D. Never caused by a virus

104. Microorganisms that cause disease are:
    A. Pathogenic
    B. Normal flora
    C. Nonpathogenic
    D. None of the above

105. Which of the following are causative agents?
    A. Only bacteria
    B. Airborne vectors
    C. Bacteria, viruses, protozoa, fungi
    D. Direct, indirect vectors

106. Elevation of _____ is an indication of an infection.
    A. Erythrocytes
    B. Leukocytes
    C. Thrombocytes
    D. Megakaryocytes

107. Red blood cells are:
    A. Erythrocytes
    B. Leukocytes
    C. Thrombocytes
    D. Platelets

108. The primary function of a red blood cell is to:
    A. Fight infections
    B. Carry iron
    C. Carry iodine
    D. Carry hemoglobin

109. The most abundant white blood cell is:
    A. The lymphocyte
    B. The basophil
    C. The neutrophil
    D. The megakaryocyte

110. The liquid portion of blood is:
    A. Serum
    B. Hemoglobin
    C. The sediment
    D. Plasma

111. The average adult has approximately how much blood?
    A. 0.05 liter
    B. 5 liters
    C. 0.5 liter
    D. 15 liters

112. The vein most subject to venipuncture is:
    A. The antecubital
    B. The basilic
    C. The median cubital
    D. All of the above

113. Veins carry:
    A. Deoxygenated blood away from the heart
    B. Oxygenated blood away from the heart
    C. Blood back to the heart
    D. All of the above

114. Arteries carry:
    A. Deoxygenated blood away from the heart
    B. Oxygenated blood away from the heart
    C. Deoxygenated blood back to the heart
    D. Oxygenated blood back to the heart

115. The outermost layer of the heart is:
    A. The epicardium
    B. The myocardium
    C. The endocardium
    D. The mesocardium

116. The contractile layer of the heart is:
    A. The epicardium
    B. The myocardium
    C. The endocardium
    D. The mesocardium

117. The upper receiving chamber of the heart is:
    A. The atrium
    B. The ventricle
    C. The aorta
    D. The valves

118. Which of the following heart chambers has the thickest myocardium?
    A. The right atrium
    B. The right ventricle
    C. The left atrium
    D. The left ventricle

119. Which of the following are the semilunar valves?
    A. The mitral valve and the bicuspid valve
    B. The aortic valve and the pulmonary valve
    C. The tricuspid valve
    D. Both A and C are correct

120. Which of the following are atrioventricular valves?
    A. The mitral or bicuspid valve
    B. The aortic valve and the pulmonic valve
    C. The tricuspid valve
    D. Both A and C are correct

121. The aorta is:
    A. The major vein
    B. The major artery
    C. A peripheral artery
    D. A systemic vein

122. The pulmonary vein will carry blood:
    A. To the heart from the lung
    B. To the lung from the heart
    C. To the heart from the brain
    D. To the lung from the brain

123. The exchange of oxygen and carbon dioxide occurs in:
    A. The capillaries
    B. The loops of Henle
    C. The bronchi
    D. All of the above are correct

124. Anatomy is:
    A. The structure of the human body
    B. The function of the human body
    C. Homeostasis
    D. Hemostasis

125. Physiology is:
    A. The structure of the human body
    B. The function of the human body
    C. Homeostasis
    D. Hemostasis

126. The main function of the kidneys is:
    A. The retention of urine
    B. The filtering of waste from blood
    C. The concentration of water
    D. Removal of solid waste products
127. Blood in the urine is called:
    A. Hemostasis
    B. Hemoconcentration
    C. Hematuria
    D. Hemoccult
128. A loss of pituitary gland function:
    A. Is likely to be very serious, since this gland regulates many others
    B. Is likely to be very serious, since this gland produces digestive enzymes
    C. Is unlikely to be very serious, since this gland only affects fertility
    D. Is unlikely to be very serious, since this gland only affects hair growth
129. Homeostasis is:
    A. The ability of the body to return to normal conditions under stress
    B. The ability of the blood to clot whenever necessary
    C. When a person has had adequate sleep and has not eaten in 12 hours
    D. The ability of the body to recognize an invading organism
130. Hemostasis is:
    A. The ability of the body to return to normal conditions under stress
    B. The ability of the blood to clot whenever necessary
    C. When a person has had adequate sleep and has not eaten in 12 hours
    D. The ability of the body to recognize an invading organism
131. When a person has had adequate rest and has not eaten in 12 hours, it is called:
    A. Homeostasis
    B. Hemostasis
    C. Basal state
    D. Permanent immunity
132. The building blocks of all living things are:
    A. Cells
    B. Systems
    C. Nuclei
    D. Organs
133. The blood cells that carry oxygen are:
    A. White blood cells
    B. Platelets
    C. Red blood cells
    D. Tissue cells

134. Groups of cells working together to perform the same job are called:
    A. Organs
    B. Systems
    C. Ligaments
    D. Tissues
135. The location where bones come together is called:
    A. Pivot
    B. Joint
    C. Ligament
    D. Junction
136. The appendicular and the axial are two main divisions of the:
    A. Pelvic girdle
    B. Spinal column
    C. Skeleton
    D. Joints
137. The bones within the spinal column are called:
    A. Vertebrae
    B. Long bones
    C. Short bones
    D. Back bones
138. The three kinds of muscles in the body are:
    A. Skeletal, striated, voluntary
    B. Involuntary, smooth, striated
    C. Cardiac, involuntary, smooth
    D. Voluntary, involuntary, cardiac
139. The beginning of a muscle is attached to a bone that the muscle cannot move. This is called:
    A. Insertion
    B. Voluntary
    C. Involuntary
    D. Origin
140. Which kind of muscle straightens a part of the body?
    A. Flexor
    B. Extensor
    C. Striated
    D. Involuntary
141. The stomach passes food into the:
    A. Large intestines
    B. Gallbladder
    C. Esophagus
    D. Small intestines
142. Compared to arteries, veins:
    A. Have thinner walls
    B. Carry blood under lower pressure
    C. May be closer to the surface of the skin
    D. All of the above

143. Substances that speed up digestion are called:
    A. Chemicals
    B. Enzymes
    C. Compounds
    D. Elements

144. Tissue fluid is returned to the circulation through the:
    A. Lymphatic system
    B. Digestive system
    C. Nervous system
    D. Endocrine system

145. Which is the correct ratio of plasma to formed elements in the blood?
    A. 45% plasma, 55% formed elements
    B. 50% plasma, 50% formed elements
    C. 55% plasma, 45% formed elements
    D. 60% plasma, 40% formed elements

146. Digestion begins in the:
    A. Esophagus
    B. Stomach
    C. Small intestine
    D. Mouth

147. When you exhale you rid the body of:
    A. Oxygen
    B. Carbon dioxide
    C. Nitrogen
    D. Electrolytes

148. The organs of the excretory system are:
    A. Kidneys, ureter, bladder, urethra
    B. Kidneys, skin, lungs, large intestines
    C. Skin, lungs, small intestines, large intestines
    D. Liver, heart, kidneys, large intestines

149. Tiny microscopic hairs called _____ are found in all of the air passages of the body.
    A. Alveoli
    B. Mucus
    C. Flagella
    D. Cilia

150. The master gland in the endocrine system is (are):
    A. The ovaries or testes
    B. The thyroid
    C. The pituitary
    D. The thymus

Appendix F

Answers to Chapter Questions and Mock Certification Exam

Chapter 1

Study Questions

1. Phlebotomy is the practice of drawing blood samples for analysis.
2. Five personal characteristics that a professional phlebotomist should possess are interpersonal skills, organizational skills, the ability to handle stress, professionalism, and ability to be detail oriented.
3. A phlebotomist must adhere to safety regulations, interact with patients, keep accurate records, and operate computers.
4. Licensure is a documented permit issued by a government agency that grants the bearer permission to perform a service.
5. CEUs are required educational units to remain certified that provide updates on new regulations and techniques to help refresh skills.
6. Organizations that provide accreditation for phlebotomy programs are the American Medical Technologists (AMT), National Accrediting Agency for Clinical Laboratory Sciences (NAACLS), National Phlebotomy Association (NPA), and American Society of Phlebotomy Technicians (ASPT).
7. Organizations that provide certification for phlebotomists are the American Society of Clinical Pathologists (ASCP), NPA, American Certification Agency for Health Care Professionals (ACA), AMT, ASPT, and National Credentialing Agency (NCA).
8. Phlebotomists may wish to become members of a professional organization in order to follow changes in the field and learn new techniques.
9. A patient must be informed of intended treatments and their risks and must give consent before these treatments are performed; this is known as informed consent.
10. Confidentiality is the concept by which information regarding the patient should not be discussed with anyone not involved with the patient's treatment.
11. Ancient phlebotomy procedures ranged from leeches to cutdowns. These practices were used to bleed a person and thus rid that person of his or her ailment.
12. Modern-day phlebotomy has set protocols, procedures, and guidelines. Phlebotomy is used in the diagnosis and treatment of disease and as a therapeutic procedure.
13. Job-related duties in the phlebotomist's job description may include: correctly and positively identifying the patient; choosing the appropriate equipment for obtaining the sample; selecting and preparing the site for collection; collecting the sample; ensuring patient comfort and safety; and correctly labeling the sample.
14. Required personal characteristics a phlebotomist must have include dependability, honesty, integrity, positive attitude, professional detachment, professional appearance, interpersonal skills, telephone skills, and communication skills.
15. (This answer is up to the student's discretion and class discussion.)
16. Two of the most important legal aspects to a phlebotomist are obtaining informed consent and maintaining patient confidentiality.

Certification Exam Preparation

1. b	5. d
2. b	6. d
3. a	
4. c	

Chapter 2

Study Questions

1. The four branches of support personnel in the hospital organizational system are fiscal, support, nursing, and professional services.
2. The two main areas of the lab are the anatomic and clinical areas; the phlebotomist works in the clinical area.
3. A physician specializing in pathology oversees the lab.
4. Lab tests performed in the coagulation department:

Test	Therapy monitored
PT	Coumadin
INR	Coumadin
APTT	Heparin

5. The immunology department performs tests to monitor the immune response through the detection of antibodies.
6. Molecular diagnostics characterize genetic and biochemical techniques used to diagnose genetic disorders, analyze forensic evidence, and track diseases.
7. Liver function tests: ALT, AST, GGT, ALP, enzymes, and bilirubin.
8. The microbiology department performs culture and sensitivity testing.
9. CLIA '88 mandates that facilities that perform patient testing meet performance standards to ensure the quality of procedures.
10. JCAHO stands for the Joint Commission on Accreditation of Healthcare Organizations.
11. The Clinical Laboratory Standards Institute sets lab standards and guidelines.
12. A phlebotomist may also be employed in HMOs, PPOs, POLs, nursing homes, urgent care centers, or reference labs.
13. The Immunohematology/Blood Bank Department is the laboratory that has a special patient/specimen identification process. Mislabeling or mishandling these specimens may result in a patient's death.
14. The technologist looks for agglutination of specimens; if the specimen agglutinates, the blood type is not compatible and cannot be transfused to the patient. If the blood does not agglutinate, the blood type is compatible with that of the patient and can be transfused.
15. Professional services are services that are provided at the request of the physician to aid in the diagnosis and treatment of a patient. Examples of professional services are physical

therapy, occupational therapy, and respiratory therapy.

Certification Exam Preparation

1. d	8. c
2. c	9. b
3. c	10. c
4. a	11. b
5. b	12. a
6. d	13. c
7. c	

Chapter 3

Study Questions

1.
Safety hazard	Example
Biological	bacteria, viruses
Sharps	needles, lancets, broken glass
Electrical	high-voltage equipment
Chemical	lab reagents, preservatives
Latex sensitivity	gloves
Physical	wet floors, lifting heavy objects
Fire, explosive	oxygen, chemicals
Radioactive,	x-ray equipment, reagents

2. Safety precautions include wearing personal protective equipment; never storing food with biohazard substances; protecting feet from spills, slips, and falling; avoiding putting things in the mouth in the work area; avoiding eye-hand contact in the work area; not wearing loose clothing, hair, or jewelry that can get caught in equipment or contaminated.
3. Never recap after collection—needle sticks can occur.
4. Hazardous material labels must display a warning to alert you to the hazard, an explanation of the hazard, a list of precautions to reduce risk, and first aid measures to take in case of exposure.
5. A materials safety data sheet provides information on the chemical, its hazards, the procedure for its cleanup, and first aid in case of exposure.
6. A chemical hygiene plan describes all safety procedures, special precautions, and emergency procedures used when working with chemicals.
7. If a chemical spills on your arm, proceed to the safety shower, flush the area for 15 minutes, and go to emergency room for treatment.
8. In the event of electrical shock to someone, turn off the equipment or break contact between the

equipment and the victim using a nonconductive material; do not touch the victim until the risk of further shock is removed; call 911; start CPR if indicated; keep the victim warm.

9. **Extinguisher type**   **Contains**

Extinguisher type	Contains
A	Pressurized water or soda and acid
BC	Carbon dioxide or foam
ABC	Dry chemical
Halon	Chlorofluorocarbons

10. The protocol for assistive breathing: determine consciousness; if there is no response, call 911 and begin rescue breathing; the victim should be flat on a firm surface, and the airway should be checked; position the victim's head; if the victim is not breathing, pinch the nose shut, place your mouth over the victim's mouth, and exhale; check to see if the victim's chest rises (clear airway); give two full ventilations and check for breathing; continue until breathing occurs or until assistance arrives.

11. Skin conditions associated with latex use:

Irritant contact dermatitis: redness, swelling, itching

Allergic contact dermatitis: the body's immune system reacts to proteins absorbed through the skin

Anaphylaxis: rapid severe immune reaction, airway may swell shut, heart rate increases, blood pressure decreases

12. OSHA (Occupational Safety and Health Administration) regulates all work environments in order to prevent accidents. They provide guidelines for accident prevention.

13. To control a bleeding emergency, one MUST apply pressure to the area or wound, elevate the limb unless it is fractured, and maintain pressure until medical help arrives.

14. The early signs of shock include pale, cold, clammy skin; tachycardia (rapid pulse); shallow breathing; weakness; nausea and/or vomiting. In case of shock, keep the victim warm and lying down with the airway open, and call for professional assistance.

15. The plan to follow during a disaster emergency varies from institution to institution. It is important to learn and know your institution's disaster plan.

Certification Exam Preparation

1.	c	4.	d
2.	a	5.	c
3.	b	6.	d

7.	a	10.	c
8.	d	11.	d
9.	d	12.	c

Chapter 4

Study Questions

1. Infection is the invasion and growth of disease-causing microorganisms in the human body.
2. Four classifications of pathogens: viruses, bacteria, fungi, protists
3.

Disease	Infectious organism that it is caused by
AIDS	Human immunodeficiency virus (HIV)
Hepatitis	Hepatitis virus (A, B, C, D, E, and G)
Tuberculosis	Mycobacterium tuberculosis
Strep throat	Streptococcus
Syphilis	Treponema pallidum
Gonorrhea	Neisseria gonorrhoeae
Malaria	Plasmodium
Trichomoniasis	Trichomonas vaginalis
Oral/genital herpes	Herpes simplex

4. Health care–related infections are contracted by a patient during a hospital stay due to direct contact with other patients or by failure of hospital personnel to follow infection control protocols.
5. The chain of infection is made up of a source, means of transmission, and susceptible host.
6. The chain of infection is broken by preventing transmission, which can be achieved by hand washing, using personal protective equipment, isolating patients at risk of spreading or contracting infections, and using standard precautions.
7. Direct contact involves the transfer of microorganisms from an infected person to a susceptible host by body contact; indirect contact involves contact between a susceptible host and contaminated object.
8. Fomites are objects, whereas vectors are organisms.
9. Hand washing is the most effective way to prevent the spread of infection.
10. Personal protective equipment includes fluid-resistant gowns, masks, respirators, face shields, gloves, and shoe covers.
11. Standard precautions are an infection control method that uses barrier protection and work control practices to prevent direct skin contact with biohazardous materials.

12. Blood-borne pathogens: syphilis; HIV; hepatitis A, B, C, D, and E; HTLV types I and II; malaria; babesiosis; Colorado tick fever.

13. Hepatitis B may be stable in dried blood for at least 7 days.

14. Bleach should be in contact with a contaminated area for 20 minutes for complete disinfection.

15. In 1992 OSHA issued standard precautions, which dictated that employers must have a written blood-borne pathogen exposure control plan and provide personal protective equipment to all workers (health care and others) at no charge to the employee. The standard precautions also dictated that employers must provide hepatitis B vaccine, free follow-up care for accidental exposure, and yearly safety training, and ensure that needles are not being recapped.

Certification Exam Preparation

1. d	7. c
2. b	8. c
3. c	9. b
4. d	10. c
5. c	11. b
6. c	12. a

Chapter 5

Study Questions

1. The parts of a word always include a root and may include a suffix or prefix.

2. | *Prefix* | *Meaning* |
|---|---|
| ante- | before |
| anti- | against |
| brady- | slow |
| hyper- | above |
| hypo- | below |
| inter- | between |
| intra- | within |
| neo- | new |
| micro- | small |
| poly- | many |
| post- | after |
| tachy- | fast |
| cirrho- | yellow |
| cyan- | blue |
| erythro- | red |
| hemi- | half |
| nano- | billionth |
| epi- | on, over |
| rube- | red |

peri-	around
tetra-	four
lute-	yellow

3. | *Root* | *Meaning* |
|---|---|
| agglut- | clump together |
| angio- | vessel |
| bili- | bile |
| cardio- | heart |
| derm- | skin |
| heme- | blood |
| hepato- | liver |
| oste- | bone |
| phago- | eat |
| -pnea | breath |
| pulmon- | lung |
| ren- | kidney |
| thromb- | clot |
| tox- | poison |

4. | *Suffix* | *Meaning* |
|---|---|
| -emia | blood condition |
| -plasty | shape |
| -tomy | cut |
| -oma | tumor, growth |
| -penia | deficiency |
| -pathy | disease |
| -plegia | paralysis |
| -stasis | stopping |
| -itis | inflammation |
| -genous | originating from |

Abbr.	*Meaning*
SOB	shortness of breath
q	every
DOB	date of birth
ASAP	as soon as possible
IV	intravenously
NPO	nothing by mouth
OR	operating room
UTI	urinary tract infection
stat	immediately
qns	quantity not sufficient
FUO	fever of unknown origin
CVA	cerebrovascular accident
COLD	chronic obstructive lung disease
hypo	hypodermically
OB	obstetrics
MI	myocardial infarction
Rx	prescription
STD	sexually transmitted disease
O_2	oxygen
P	pulse
NB	newborn
TB	tuberculosis

AIDS	acquired immunodeficiency syndrome
Prep	prepare

5. | **Singular form** | **Plural form** |
|---|---|
| papilla | papillae |
| testis | testes |
| larynx | larynges |
| scapula | scapulae |
| vertebra | vertebrae |
| appendix | appendices |

Certification Exam Preparation

1. a	6. d
2. d	7. a
3. b	8. b
4. b	9. b
5. c	10. c

Chapter 6

Study Questions

1. Homeostasis is the steady state of good health.
2. | **Tissue** | **Example** |
|---|---|
| Epithelial | lining of gut, surface of the eye |
| Muscle | heart |
| Nerve | neurons, spinal cord |
| Connective | bone, blood |
3. C. The nucleus contains DNA.
4. A. The plasma membrane regulates the flow of materials in and out of the cell.
5. B. Mitochondria are "power plants" of the cell.
6. D. Cytoplasm contains cellular material.
7. The anatomic position is the body erect, facing forward, arms at the sides, and palms forward.
8. Body cavities are spaces within the body that contain major organs.
9. E. Ventral is the front surface of the body.
10. G. Posterior is the back surface of the body.
11. B. Lateral is toward the side.
12. C. Medial is toward the middle.
13. A. Prone is lying on the abdomen facing down.
14. H. Supine is lying on the back.
15. D. Extension is straightening the joint.
16. F. Inferior is below.
17. The three body planes:
    Frontal—vertical division (front and back)
    Sagittal—vertical division (left and right)
    Transverse—horizontal division (top and bottom)
18. Hematopoiesis is the formation of blood cells.

19. Lab tests used to assess for bone and joint disorders:

Lab test	**Tests for**
ALP	bone metabolism marker
UA	gout
RF	rheumatoid arthritis
Calcium	mineral calcium imbalance
Magnesium mineral	magnesium imbalance
ANA	systemic lupus erythematosus
ESR	general inflammation test
Synovial fluid analysis	arthritis
Uric acid	gout

20. *Osteomyelitis* is a bone infection that can be caused by improper phlebotomy technique.
21. Lab tests used to assess for muscle disorders: aldolase, AST, troponin, myoglobin, CK, CK-MM, CK-MB, lactate dehydrogenase.
22. The divisions of the central nervous system are the brain and spinal cord.
23. Lab tests used to assess for digestive disorders: CBC, amylase, lipase, ALP, ALT, AST, GGT, bilirubin, HBsAg, ammonia, hepatitis antibody, carotene, O&P, gastrin, occult blood, stool culture.
24. External respiration is the exchange of gases in the lungs, whereas internal respiration is the exchange of gases at the cellular level.
25. The endocrine system maintains homeostasis in conjunction with the nervous system by producing hormones.
26. | **Joint type** | **Examples** |
|---|---|
| Immovable | facial bones, cranium (synarthrosis) |
| Partially movable | vertebrae (amphiarthrosis) |
| Free moving | elbow, shoulder, knee (diarthrosis) |

Certification Exam Preparation

1. c	11. b
2. b	12. a
3. a	13. d
4. b	14. c
5. b	15. c
6. a	16. d
7. c	17. c
8. c	18. a
9. b	19. b
10. d	20. b

Chapter 7

Study Questions

1. The circulatory system transports blood containing oxygen and nutrients throughout the body and picks up metabolic waste products for disposal.
2. Pulmonary circulation carries blood between the heart and lungs for gas exchange, whereas systemic circulation carries blood between the heart and the rest of the body.
3. Veins carry blood toward the heart; arteries carry blood away from the heart.
4. The four valves of the heart are atrioventricular, pulmonary semilunar, bicuspid, aortic semilunar.
5. Contraction of the heart is known as systole, and relaxation is known as diastole.
6. The three layers surrounding the lumen of veins and arteries are tunica adventitia, media, and intima.
7. The yellow liquid portion of whole blood, containing fibrinogen, is known as plasma.
8. The formed elements constitute 45% of blood volume.
9. A phagocyte attacks and digests bacteria.
10. B cells produce antibodies.
11. The extrinsic pathway begins with the release of tissue factor by endothelial cells. The intrinsic pathway begins when the plasma coagulation factors contact materials exposed when blood vessels are damaged.
12. Autoimmunity is an attack by the immune system on the body's own tissues. Examples include rheumatoid arthritis, systemic lupus erythematosus, myasthenia gravis, and multiple sclerosis.
13. The lymph organs include lymphatic vessels, lymph nodes (the tonsils are the largest lymph nodes in the body), the spleen, the thymus, and the thoracic and right lymphatic ducts. Lymphedema is one lymphatic disorder; it constitutes an accumulation of fluid blocking a lymphatic vessel. Lymphoma is another disorder; it characterizes a tumor of a lymph gland. Hodgkin's disease is a type of lymphoma.
14. The types of immunity include nonspecific and specific immunity. Nonspecific immunity refers to the defense against infectious agents independent of the specific chemical markers on their surfaces. Nonspecific immunity encourages inflammation and phagocytosis. Specific immunity involves the molecular recognition of antigens on the surface of a foreign agent. Specific immunity involves the antigen/antibody response, also called *humoral immunity*.
15. In the coagulation process, enzymes enter the common pathway, reacting with Factors X and V to convert circulating inactive prothrombin to active thrombin.

Certification Exam Preparation

1. a	9. b
2. a	10. b
3. c	11. b
4. b	12. c
5. d	13. d
6. c	14. a
7. a	15. b
8. c	

Chapter 8

Study Questions

1. A tourniquet prevents venous flow out of the arm.
2. The gauge of a needle indicates the diameter of the needle's lumen.
3. If a large-gauge needle is used in venipuncture, collection is slower and blood cells may be hemolyzed (destroyed) as they pass through the narrower opening.
4. The rubber sleeve on the multisample needle keeps the needle from becoming contaminated or injuring you or the patient, and it keeps blood from leaking onto or into the adapter or tube holder, especially when changing tubes.
5. An advantage of the syringe method is that blood appears in the hub when the vein has been entered.
   A disadvantage of the syringe method is that there is the potential for needle stick when depositing blood into the collection tube.
6. When blood tubes are evacuated, a vacuum is created within the tube so a measured amount of blood will flow in easily.
7. Unused blood tubes must be discarded when they expire because out-of-date tubes may have decreased vacuum, preventing a proper fill, or they may have additives that degrade over time.
8. SPS is sodium polyanetholesulfonate. It is an additive that prevents blood from clotting.
9. Blood collected in a tube with an anticoagulant must be mixed thoroughly after collection by gently and repeatedly inverting the tube.

10. Thixotropic gel forms a barrier between blood cells and serum or plasma, thus preventing contamination and allowing easy separation.
11. Glycolysis is a cellular reaction used to harvest energy from glucose.
12. Blood specimens used for analysis are whole blood, serum, and plasma.
13. B. brown—lead analysis
14. A. red—blood bank
15. I. light blue—coagulation
16. G. lavender—CBC
17. C. gray—glucose tolerance test
18. E. black—sedimentation rate
19. D. gold Hemogard—chemistry testing
20. F. green—arterial blood gases
21. H. dark (royal) blue—trace metals
22. 3   light blue
    6   lavender
    5   green
    2   red
    1   yellow (sterile)
    7   gray
    4   gold Hemogard

Certification Exam Preparation

1. a	11. a
2. c	12. d
3. a	13. b
4. c	14. b
5. c	15. a
6. d	16. a
7. b	17. d
8. b	18. b
9. b	19. a
10. b	20. d

Chapter 9

Study Questions

1. It is extremely important to correctly and positively identify the patient in any phlebotomy procedure.
2. To properly identify a patient, match the information on the requisition with the information on the patient's identification band (for inpatients) or with information provided by the patient (for outpatients).
3. Information typically found on a requisition form is the patient's name, date of birth, the patient's hospital ID number (for inpatients), the patient's room number and bed (for inpatients), the patient's doctor's name or code, the type of test requested, and the test status.
4. When requisitions are received, you should examine them for the necessary information; check for duplicates or errors; group them together for the same patient; prioritize them; and gather all the equipment you will need to perform the collections.
5. Hemoconcentration is an increase in the ratio of formed elements to plasma caused by leaving the tourniquet on too long.
6. The three veins in the antecubital area suitable for venipuncture are: median cubital, cephalic, and basilic.
7. The median cubital vein is the first choice for venipuncture because it is large and well anchored and does not move when the needle is inserted.
8. Veins feel spongy, bouncy, and firm on palpation; arteries pulsate; tendons feel rigid.
9. To help locate a vein, tap the arm, have the patient make a fist, or warm the site with a warm towel or hot pack.
10. A hematoma is a reddened swollen area in which blood collects under the skin. It can form when the extra pressure from the tourniquet forces blood out through the puncture.
11. The correct position for the arm after venipuncture is straight or slightly bent, but not bent back over the puncture site.
12. To correctly label blood tubes, label them at the bedside using a pen or permanent marker. The label must have the patient's name and identification number, the date and time of collection, and the collector's initials or identification number. If labels are computer generated, make sure all the information is present, and then add the collector's initials or identification number.
13. To correctly transfer blood to collection tubes with a syringe, place the tube in a tube holder and pierce the stopper with the needle. Never hold the tube in your hand during the transfer. Allow the vacuum to pull the blood into the tube, without applying any pressure to the plunger.
14. The requisition slip must contain the patient's identification/chart number, the patient's last name/first name, the patient's date of birth, the physician's name, and the test(s) ordered.
15. Phlebotomists must set up their equipment and wash their hands in order to prevent self-contamination, as the equipment being handled may have pathogenic contamination. If phlebotomists wash their hands, put on gloves, and

then handle their equipment, they may inadvertently pick up debris from the equipment and acquire the properties for an infectious growth.

Certification Exam Preparation

1. a	9. b
2. b	10. a
3. c	11. c
4. c	12. b
5. b	13. b
6. c	14. b
7. c	15. c
8. c	

Chapter 10

Study Questions

1. Sites commonly used for adult capillary collection are the palmar surface of the distal segments of the third and fourth fingers or the big toe.

2. Dermal puncture is preferred for children because the young child's smaller veins and lower blood volume make standard venipuncture difficult and potentially dangerous.

3. Dermal puncture may be advisable for patients undergoing frequent glucose monitoring or frequent blood tests, obese patients, patients with IVs in place, geriatric patients, patients with burns or scars, patients at risk for venous thrombosis, restrained patients, and patients at risk for anemia, hemorrhage, infection, organ or tissue damage, arteriospasm, or cardiac arrest.

4. The first drop of blood in a dermal puncture is wiped away with clean gauze to prevent contaminating the sample with tissue fluid.

5. Micropipets are typically used for the collection of samples for arterial blood gas determinations.

6. The Unopette system allows you to collect a very small blood sample, which is diluted to the correct volume for analysis in the Unopette reservoir. The system includes a capillary pipet in a holder, a pipet shield, and a sealed reservoir containing diluent. This system is useful for CBC tests when a large sample is not needed for other tests.

7. Warm washcloths or heel warmers can be used to stimulate blood flow to the capillaries.

8. Specific areas of the skin to avoid when performing a capillary stick include areas with scars, cuts, bruises, rashes, or edema, and callused, burned, bluish, and infected areas, as well as previous puncture sites.

9. Heel sticks are preferred to finger sticks in children under the age of 1 year.

10. Unless alcohol air dries before a capillary stick, stinging, hemolysis, and contamination can occur. Alcohol also can interfere with the formation of rounded drops of blood on the skin surface.

11. Povidone-iodine may elevate test results for bilirubin, uric acid, phosphorus, and potassium, and therefore is not recommended for use with dermal puncture.

12. The third and fourth fingers are acceptable to use for dermal puncture.

13. The order of collection for a dermal puncture is: (1) blood smears; (2) platelet counts, CBCs, and other hematology tests; (3) other tests.

14. The bleeding time test measures the length of time required for bleeding to stop after an incision is made. It helps assess the overall integrity of primary hemostasis, involving the vascular system and platelet function.

15. Small children may remove bandages and choke on them; therefore, it is not recommended that bandages be used on children younger than 2 years.

Certification Exam Preparation

1. a	9. b
2. d	10. b
3. c	11. b
4. c	12. d
5. d	13. d
6. b	14. b
7. c	15. c
8. b	

Chapter 11

Study Questions

1. If a patient is not in the room when you come to collect a specimen, every effort must be made to locate that patient by checking with the nursing station.

2. If a patient is not wearing an ID bracelet, contact the nursing station so that one can be attached by the nurse on duty. Unless an ID band is on the patient, you must not draw blood. Specific policies regarding the resolution of patient identification problems may vary from institution to institution, so be sure to follow the policy of your institution.

3. Unconscious patients should be treated just as you would conscious ones: identify yourself

and describe the procedure. They may be able to hear you, even if they cannot respond.

4. Potential barriers to communicating with a patient: sleeping or unconscious patients; presence of physicians, clergy, or visitors; apprehensive patients; language problems; patient refusal.

5. Hemolysis is the destruction of red blood cells, resulting in the release of hemoglobin and cellular contents into the plasma.

6. Veins that are occluded are blocked. Occluded veins feel hard or cordlike and lack resiliency.

7. When performing a dorsal hand stick, the tourniquet is applied around the wrist below the antecubital fossa.

8. Povidone iodine must be used when collecting for a blood alcohol test. Alcohol can adversely affect test results.

9. Hemoconcentration can be caused by a tourniquet that is on longer than 1 minute, pumping of the fist, sclerosed or occluded veins, long-term IV therapy, or dehydration.

10. Before syncope, a patient's skin often feels cool, damp, and clammy.

11. If a needle's bevel has stuck to the vein wall, slightly rotate the needle to correct its position.

12. Too much vacuum on a small vein can cause it to collapse during a blood draw. During the syringe method, it may occur when the plunger is pulled too quickly.

13. The policy at most institutions is that a second try is acceptable. After a second unsuccessful try, another phlebotomist should be found to draw blood from the patient.

14. Reflux of an additive during collection can be prevented by keeping the patient's arm angled downward, so that the tube is always below the site, allowing it to fill from the bottom up. Also, remove the last tube from the needle before removing the tourniquet or needle.

15. Reasons why specimens may be rejected include: no requisition form; unlabeled or mislabeled specimens; incompletely filled tubes; defective tubes; collection in the wrong tube; hemolysis, clotted blood in an anticoagulated specimen; contaminated specimens and containers; improper special handling.

Certification Exam Preparation

1. c	5. a		
2. d	6. c		
3. d	7. a		
4. a	8. d		

9. c	13. c
10. b	14. b
11. d	15. b
12. b	

Chapter 12

Study Questions

1. To reduce a child's anxiety before a draw, prepare your material ahead of time; perform the procedure in a room that is not the child's hospital room; be friendly, cheerful, and empathetic; explain the procedure in child's terms; do not say that the procedure won't hurt, and say that it's okay to say "ouch"; give children choices whenever possible, such as which arm or finger they want to use or the type of bandage they prefer.

2. When performing venipuncture on patients younger than 2 years, use shorter needles, if possible, and use the smallest gauge consistent with the requirements of the tests. Butterflies and smaller tube sizes should be used. If the patient is younger than 1 year, a heel stick should be performed, rather than venipuncture.

3. EMLA is a topical anesthetic cream used in pediatric patients to numb the venipuncture site.

4. Children can be immobilized during a draw by wrapping newborns or infants in receiving blankets. Older children need to be restrained. They may be seated in the lap of a parent or assistant who hugs the child's body and holds the arm not being used in the draw, or they may be lying down with the parent or assistant leaning over the child, holding the unused arm securely.

5. Bilirubin is light sensitive. Bili lights should be turned off during collection, and the specimen should be shielded from light.

6. A PKU sample is collected via capillary stick onto a special filter paper supplied in a kit provided by the state agency responsible for PKU tests.

7. Physical changes the elderly undergo include skin that is less elastic and thinner; a tendency to bruise more easily; longer healing times; more fragile, less elastic, and narrower blood vessels; loss of supporting connective tissue, leading to "loose skin"; loss of muscle tissue, allowing veins to move from their usual locations; arteries that are closer to the surface.

8. To perform a draw on an elderly patient, be especially careful with patient identification; be aware of the frequency of blood draws; be especially gentle; do not apply the tourniquet as

tightly; place the arm on a pillow and have the patient grip a washcloth while the arm is supported by rolled towels; do not "slap" the arm to find a vein; anchor the vein firmly; apply pressure longer to ensure bleeding has stopped.

9. VAD is an acronym for "vascular access device." It is a tube that is inserted into either a vein or an artery and is used to administer fluids or medications, monitor blood pressure, or draw blood.

10. To draw blood from a patient who has an IV line, have the nurse turn off the IV drip before the draw (less than 2 minutes); apply the tourniquet distal to the IV insertion site; select a vein distal to the IV insertion site and in a different vein; discard the first 5 mL of blood drawn, since it will be contaminated with IV fluid; note on the requisition that the specimen was drawn from an arm with an IV, and identify the IV solution.

11. Types of VADs: CVC (Broviac, Groshong, Hickman, triple lumen); implanted port; PICC; arterial line; heparin or saline lock; AV shunt (external, internal).

12. In a phlebotomy procedure, a child may experience a fear of the unknown and a fear of pain. As a phlebotomist, you must explain the procedure in detail to the child, using words the child understands. The phlebotomist should speak to the child during the entire procedure, letting the child know how much longer the procedure will last.

13. Since a newborn is under reverse isolation, additional protection equipment is needed. Blood should be drawn from the infant's heel. The amount collected, tests, and their frequency must be recorded in order to prevent blood depletion.

14. Besides the PKU test, neonates are also screened for hypothyroidism, galactosemia, homocystinuria, maple syrup disease, biotinidase deficiency, and sickle cell anemia.

15. Common disorders affecting the elderly population include hearing loss, Parkinson's disease, stroke, arthritis, and tremors, all of which can make blood collection difficult.

Certification Exam Preparation

1. c	9. d
2. c	10. a
3. c	11. c
4. a	12. c
5. c	13. d
6. b	14. c
7. c	15. b
8. b	

Chapter 13
Study Questions

1. Arterial collection is most often used for testing ABGs.

2. Abnormal ABG values can be produced by: COPD, lung cancer, diabetic coma, shock, cardiac or respiratory failure, neuromuscular disease.

3. Normal blood pH is 7.35.

4. Acidosis is indicated by a lower pH, whereas alkalosis is indicated by a higher pH.

5. A syringe used for venipuncture is not heparinized, whereas a syringe used for arterial puncture is pretreated with heparin (glass or gas-impermeable plastic) to prevent coagulation.

6. Povidone iodine must be used in addition to alcohol for arterial puncture.

7. Lidocaine may be used to numb an arterial puncture site.

8. Safety precautions to take when collecting arterial blood: wear a fluid-resistant gown, face protection, and gloves; use a puncture-resistant container for sharps and a small rubber or latex block for the needle.

9. For blood gas collection, 21- or 22-gauge needles are most often used.

10. Collateral circulation is the accessory supply of blood to a region by more than one artery. Collateral circulation is tested using the modified Allen test.

11. The needle should be inserted at an angle 45 to 60 degrees above the plane of the skin for an arterial collection.

12. Pressure should be applied to the puncture site for 5 minutes after an arterial collection.

13. An arteriospasm is the spontaneous constriction of an artery in response to pain.

14. ABG sampling errors include: using too much or too little heparin; insufficient mixing; allowing air bubbles to enter the syringe; using an improper plastic syringe; using an improper anticoagulant; puncturing a vein instead of an artery; exposing the specimen to the atmosphere after collection.

15. ABG specimens may be rejected due to: inadequate volume of specimen for the test; clotting; improper or absent labeling; using the wrong syringe; air bubbles in the specimen; failure to ice the specimen; too long a delay in delivering the specimen to the lab.

16. Capillary blood gas testing is most commonly performed on pediatric patients, as they generally

should not be subjected to the deep punctures required for ABG testing. This procedure is usually performed on the heel.

17. Capillary blood is not as desirable as arterial blood for testing blood gases because capillary blood is a mixture of blood from the capillaries, venules, and arterioles, and it is mixed with tissue fluid. In addition, this method of collection is open to the air, and the specimen may exchange gases with room air before it is sealed.

Certification Exam Preparation

1. b	7. c
2. a	8. b
3. d	9. a
4. c	10. c
5. d	11. a
6. d	

Chapter 14

Study Questions

1. Basal state is the body's state after 12 hours of fasting and abstinence from strenuous exercise.
2. Blood composition is influenced by: age; altitude; dehydration; environment; gender; pregnancy; stress; diet; diurnal variation; drugs; exercise; body position; smoking.
3. Timed specimens are most often used to monitor medication levels, changes in a patient's condition, and normal diurnal variation in blood levels at different times of the day.
4. OGTT is an acronym for "oral glucose tolerance test." It is a test used to screen for diabetes mellitus and other disorders of carbohydrate metabolism.
5. TDM means "therapeutic drug monitoring." It is often used to adjust drug dosing in patients.
6. Blood cultures are ordered to test for the presence of microorganisms in the blood.
7. Aseptic collection technique and drawing the correct volume are critical for meaningful BC results.
8. A potential blood donor must: (1) register by providing identifying information and written consent; (2) interview with a trained interviewer and provide a medical history; (3) submit to a physical exam, which includes hemoglobin testing.
9. Cold agglutinins must be kept warm until the serum is separated from the cells. They can be wrapped in an activated heel-warmer pack or placed in the incubator.

10. Tests that require transport on ice include: ABGs; ammonia; lactic acid; pyruvate; glucagon; gastrin; adrenocorticotropic hormone; parathyroid hormone.
11. Chain of custody is a protocol that ensures that a sample is always in the custody of a person legally entrusted to be in control of it. The chain begins with patient identification and continues through every step of the collection and testing process. Chain of custody documentation includes special containers, seals, and forms, as well as the date, time, and identification of the handler.
12. For blood alcohol testing: the site must not be cleaned with alcohol, as this will falsely elevate the result (use soap, water, and gauze or another nonalcoholic antiseptic solution instead); tubes must be filled as full as the vacuum allows to minimize the escape of alcohol from the specimen into the space above; the specimen should not be uncapped because that also allows alcohol to escape and compromises the integrity of the sample before testing.
13. To prepare a blood smear: Place a drop of blood on a clean slide 1/2 to 1 inch from the end, centered between the two slides; place the spreader onto the first slide at a 25- to 30-degree angle and draw it back to just contact the blood drop; move the spreader forward in one continuous movement to the end of the slide. The blood will be drawn along over the slide; dry and label the slides, using a pencil on the frosted end.
14. To prepare a thick malaria smear: place a large drop of blood on a slide and spread it out to about the size of a dime; let the sample dry for at least 2 hours.
15. Therapeutic phlebotomy is often used in the treatment of polycythemia. The prefix poly- means "excessive" or "a lot"; the root word cyte means "cell"; the suffix -emia means "blood." Polycythemia is excessive red blood cell production.

Certification Exam Preparation

1. b	8. d
2. d	9. a
3. c	10. c
4. c	11. b
5. a	12. c
6. a	13. d
7. b	14. b

Chapter 15

Study Questions

1. Random urine specimens can be collected at any time. They are used to screen for obvious abnormalities in the concentration of proteins, glucose, and other significant constituents of urine.
2. A first morning specimen is collected after the patient wakes up. It is a very concentrated specimen. A timed specimen is collected over a 24-hour period to provide a single large specimen. Typically, the first morning sample is discarded in a timed specimen.
3. To collect a midstream clean-catch specimen, the patient should cleanse the area surrounding the urethra; next, the patient should begin voiding into the toilet; then the container should be brought into the urine stream until sufficient urine has been collected; the remainder of the urine should be voided into the toilet.
4. Fecal specimens are collected to look for intestinal infection and screen for colorectal cancer.
5. Semen specimens are collected to determine whether viable sperm are present, either for fertility testing or to assess the success of a vasectomy. Semen may also be collected as a forensic specimen from a rape victim.
6. Nasopharyngeal specimens are collected to diagnose whooping cough, croup, pneumonia, and other upper respiratory tract infections.
7. The SE test is used to help diagnose cystic fibrosis.
8. In CSF collections, three tubes are collected. Tube 1 is delivered to the chemistry lab; tubes 2 and 3 are delivered to the microbiology and hematology labs. Which department receives which tube is set by the policies of the institution.
9. Amniotic fluid is collected to analyze the presence of certain genetic disorders, such as Down syndrome. It can be analyzed for lipids (to indicate lung development), bilirubin (associated with hemolytic disease), and proteins (associated with other abnormalities such as spina bifida).
10. A throat culture is collected from the back of the mouth around the tonsils and uvula with a swab. A nasopharyngeal culture is collected through the nose.
11. Pleural fluid is found in the lungs and thoracic cavity. Synovial fluid is found in the knee joint. Cerebrospinal fluid is found in the brain and spinal cord. All of these specimens are collected by a physician only.
12. A 24-hour collection may detect low levels of certain proteins and hormones. This specimen needs to be preserved with an added preservative or by refrigeration.
13. The methods used to induce sweat in an SE test are by iontophoresis and the drug pilocarpine. Sweat is collected on a sterile filter paper, which must be covered with paraffin and handled with forceps or sterile gloves. The chloride level is obtained via weight and coulometrical analysis.

Certification Exam Preparation

1. a	6. a
2. c	7. a
3. c	8. a
4. b	9. b
5. d	10. b

Chapter 16

Study Questions

1. Tubes with anticoagulant should be inverted gently and completely 5 to 10 times immediately after the sample is drawn.
2. Tests affected by glycolysis include glucose, calcitonin, phosphorus, aldosterone, and a number of enzymes.
3. No more than 2 hours should pass between collection of the sample and separation of cells from plasma or serum.
4. Specimens that must be maintained at 37°C during transport and handling should be warmed in a heel warmer before and after collection. Some tests require warming of the sample in a 37°C incubator before testing.
5. Chilling a specimen slows down metabolic processes and keeps analytes stable during transport and handling.
6. Minimum documentation to be included with each specimen delivered to the lab should include the patient's name, hospital number and room number, specimen type, date and time of delivery to the drop-off area, and the name of the person depositing the specimen.
7. Disadvantages of pneumatic tube systems include unreliability of the system, speed of delivery, potential for specimen damage during transport, and cost of the alternative.
8. An accession number is a unique identifying number used for cataloging a sample in the lab.

9. A centrifuge must carry a balanced load, or the rotor of the centrifuge may spin out of center, which can damage the centrifuge and cause samples to break.
10. Aliquots are small portions of a specimen transferred into separate containers for distribution to a variety of lab departments. All tubes into which aliquots are placed should be labeled before filling and then capped before delivery to the appropriate department. Aliquots are removed with any one of several types of disposable pipetting systems.
11. To remove a stopper from a tube, place a 4×4-inch piece of gauze over the top and pull the stopper straight up, twisting it if necessary. Do not rock it from side to side or "pop" it off.
12. Stat specimens should be transported to the lab immediately after being drawn, whereas routine specimens should be delivered to the lab within 45 minutes of being drawn.
13. Tubes must be transported in an upright position to allow complete clot formation, prevent sample contamination due to prolonged contact with the stopper, and reduce the formation of aerosol during uncapping.
14. Delivery of specimens in a timely manner will ensure the quality of test results.
15. One light-sensitive analyte is bilirubin. To transport, the specimen must be protected from light—the tube must be wrapped in aluminum foil, or an amber-colored tube must be used. Other light-sensitive analytes include vitamin B_{12}, carotene, folate, and urine porphyrin.

Certification Exam Preparation

1. c	6. d
2. c	7. c
3. b	8. c
4. b	9. b
5. d	

Chapter 17

Study Questions

1. Quality assurance is a set of methods used to guarantee quality patient care, including the methods used for patient preparation and collection and transportation protocols. These methods ensure better care, help reduce errors and improve the quality of test results, and save money. Quality assurance programs are mandated by the Joint Commission on Accreditation of Healthcare Organizations (JCAHO).
2. Quality control refers to the quantitative methods used to monitor the quality of procedures to ensure accurate test results. Quality control is part of quality assurance, which is a larger set of methods that guarantees quality patient care through a specific program, including both technical and nontechnical procedures.
3. JCAHO's role is to mandate quality assurance programs, requiring that a systemic process be in place to monitor and evaluate the quality of patient care.
4. Documentation processes include a procedure manual for lab procedures, a floor book detailing schedules and other information, the identification of variables that may affect patient care and test results, and continuing education for all members of the lab staff.
5. A procedure manual contains protocols and other information about all the tests performed in the lab, including the principle behind the test, the purpose of performing it, the specimen type the test requires, the collection method, and the equipment and supplies required.
6. A delta check helps to identify patient identification errors. This check compares previous patient results with current results and alerts lab personnel to the possibility of error if the difference ("delta") between the two sets of results is outside the limit of expected variation.
7. The patient's physical condition at the time of the collection has a significant effect on the sample quality. If a phlebotomist must draw from a patient who smokes, the phlebotomist must document this factor. Since smoking can affect the variables of many tests, the phlebotomist's documentation of this factor will aid in the interpretation of test results.
8. Each aliquot must be properly labeled as to the source and the additives present.
9. The purpose of quality phlebotomy is to ensure that a systemic process is in place to monitor and evaluate the quality of patient care, as mandated by JCAHO.
10. The philosophy and purpose of total quality management (TQM) are to focus on continuous improvements in the quality of services provided by the lab. The role of this program is to set guidelines and to evaluate and change its due process and standards as needed to reflect its philosophy.

11. The procedure manual contains protocols and other information about tests performed in the lab.

12. The procedure manual lists all of the procedures, processes, protocols, and handling and transport guidelines for each phlebotomy procedure. The floor log book lists patients, their room numbers, specimens collected, phlebotomists' initials, the dates and times of collection, and their outcomes.

13. Analytical variables exist in requisition handling, equipment, identification, preparation and specimen collection, transport, and processing. Variables are problems and errors that can arise in any of these areas. Variables for each area vary.

14. One negative outcome of improper patient identification is a patient's death. The wrong medication can be administered based on erroneous tests results. To ensure proper patient identification, the phlebotomist MUST ask the patient his or her name and date of birth, and then compare such information with the requisition slip. If the patient is an inpatient, the same is done, but the patient's identification number is also matched with the requisition slip.

15. Variables of which phlebotomists must be aware vary based on the procedure they are performing. Such variables may include patient identification, delta check, patient preparation for specimen collection, specimen collection, transport, time constraints, processing, and separation time.

Certification Exam Preparation

1. d	6. b
2. d	7. c
3. c	8. a
4. b	9. d
5. c	

Chapter 18

Study Questions

1. Health care costs have increased due to the gradual inflation in the price of all goods and services; the growing sophistication of medical technology; the need for highly trained operators of health care delivery; the fast pace of drug discovery and development; an increase in the number of tests ordered by doctors.

2. OSHA creates administrative laws; these laws are given the force of law by the statutory laws that created OSHA.

3. A plaintiff is a person claiming to have been harmed by a defendant in a court of law.

4. To be liable for an action means that you are legally responsible for it and can be held accountable for its consequences. Scenarios include reusing a needle, thereby infecting a patient with a disease; probing for a vein and damaging a nerve; failing to perform a physician-ordered test, and having the patient suffer harm as a result. There are many more ways in which a phlebotomist could be held liable for his or her actions.

5. Negligence is the failure to perform an action consistent with the accepted standard of care.

6. Malpractice is the delivery of substandard care that results in harm to a patient.

7. To breach confidentiality means to reveal test results or any information about the patient to anyone not directly involved in that patient's care; to discuss a patient's care in a public place; to release medical information concerning a patient to anyone not specifically authorized to acquire it; to leave patient records out where anyone can glance at them.

8. Phlebotomists can adopt several measures to protect them from malpractice suits, such as precise and detailed documentation, clear patient communication, and following procedures and protocols accurately. Some phlebotomists opt to purchase their own liability insurance.

9. Effective communication includes giving clear information to the patient in order to obtain consent, explaining the procedure in order for the patient to fully understand what will happen, and always getting a clear "Yes" or "I understand" response from the patient.

10. A criminal action is taken when a public law is violated. There is a jury trial in the presence of a district attorney. A phlebotomist can be prosecuted under criminal action for assault or battery, using dirty needles, or patient misidentification. If a patient dies as a consequence of a wrongful action by the phlebotomist, the charge against the phlebotomist can be manslaughter.
A civil action is the violation of private law. A civil action is taken when the accused injures the plaintiff. A civil action suit for a phlebotomist can result from reusing needles, careless probing, or an accidental stick.

11. Professional liability is being legally responsible for your actions, and failure to act. Phlebotomists are bound to act within the realm of

their training; they are professionally liable if they do not. Phlebotomists can perform venipunctures and assist the physician and nurse in specimen collection. Phlebotomists cannot perform a tracheostomy or amniocentesis, collect a CSF, or perform other procedures for which they have not been trained.

12. The plaintiff MUST prove duty, dereliction, injury, and direct cause in a malpractice suit.

13. The statement "a phlebotomist who does so is derelict in his or her duty" means that the phlebotomist has not followed the set standards of care. For example, if a phlebotomist has trouble with a venipuncture procedure and fails to call for help as he or she was trained to do, he or she is being derelict in duty.

14. The key defense against a malpractice suit is to show that the standards of care were followed. Clear, precise documentation is vital in proving such.

15. Liability insurance covers monetary damage that must be paid if the defendant loses a liability suit. Phlebotomists should carry liability insurance in case they are accused in a civil action and the health care institution will not cover such charges.

16. The phlebotomist maintains doctor-patient integrity by allowing test results to be given to the patient by the physician.

17. When a case cannot be settled easily, the case will go to a jury trial and judgment.

18. A phlebotomist may commit a negligent act if he or she does not follow the standards of care for the procedure being performed.

Certification Exam Preparation

1.	c	6.	b
2.	a	7.	a
3.	c	8.	d
4.	d	9.	d
5.	c	10.	d
		11.	d

Chapter 19

Study Questions

1. Point-of-care testing (POCT) is the performance of analytical tests immediately after obtaining a sample at the "point of care," such as the bedside, clinic, intensive care unit or emergency department, physician's office, nursing home, assisted living center, or patient's home.

2. Advantages to point-of-care testing include shorter turnaround times for obtaining test results, allowing more prompt medical attention, faster diagnosis and treatment, potentially decreased recovery time, and decreased costs to the lab. Disadvantages include misleading test results due to improperly following manufacturer's directions, inadequate training of personnel, improper maintenance, and poor record keeping.

3. Quality assurance and controls are essential for use of POCT instruments. The lab is usually responsible for documentation and maintenance of POCT instruments, and proper and adequate training for all personnel performing these procedures is critical in order to successfully implement POCT. Strict adherence to guidelines regarding calibration, running controls, performing maintenance, and record keeping is a must for a POCT program. Failure in any one of these areas can lead to misleading test results and negative consequences for the patient.

4. Hematology tests that can be performed as POCT include anemia and polycythemia evaluation and coagulation monitoring. (See the chapter discussion on specific tests and how to perform them.)

5. Chemistry tests that can be performed as POCT include glucose, cardiac troponin T, cholesterol, blood gases, and electrolytes. (See the chapter discussion on specific tests and how to perform them.)

6. The five waves that make up an ECG are P, Q, R, S, and T.

7. The heart activity corresponding to the P wave is atrial depolarization.
The heart activity corresponding to the QRS complex is ventricular depolarization.
The heart activity corresponding to the ST segment is ventricular repolarization.

8. To perform a dipstick urinalysis test, make sure the fresh urine specimen is at room temperature and thoroughly mixed; completely and briefly immerse the urine strip into the urine specimen; remove excess urine from the strip by tapping the side of the strip on the container; the color change on the strip is then compared to the reference color chart on the bottle at the appropriate time.

9. It is extremely important to follow the manufacturer's directions when performing POCT because manufacturers tend to vary in their methods of testing. If their specific method of

testing is not followed, inaccurate test results can occur.

10. Anemia may be evaluated using a hand-held hemoglobin analyzer or a hematocrit reading.
    Coumadin therapy may be monitored by using the prothrombin time test.
    Cholesterol may be evaluated by using color card testing or instrumentation.
    Arterial blood gases may be evaluated by using hand-held analyzers.

11. The common electrolytes that can be measured by POCT include sodium, potassium, calcium, chloride, and bicarbonate.

12. The normal ECG pattern consists of a tracing with five prominent points where the graph changes direction. These are known as P, Q, R, S, and T. The sections joining these points are known as segments, complexes, or intervals. Each part of the graph corresponds to a particular portion of the cardiac cycle and can be analyzed to determine how the heart is functioning.

13. Important parameters that can be determined from the ECG include the time intervals between different phases of the cardiac cycle, which indicate conduction efficiency, and the size of the electrical signals, which may be correlated with increase or decrease of heart muscle mass. The duration of the cardiac cycle can be read directly from the ECG, because each small square represents a known unit of time.

14. The dipstick tests most commonly performed on random urine specimens include protein, pH, glucose, ketones, bilirubin, urobilinogen, blood, leukocyte esterase, nitrite, and specific gravity.

15. A dipstick urine test is commonly used to determine pregnancy, measuring the presence of HCG. This hormone, produced by the placenta after implantation of a fertilized egg, is present in urine.

16. The adherence guidelines in order for a POCT program to be successful are calibration, running controls, performing maintenance, and record keeping. Not adhering to the guidelines can result in inaccurate test results and negative consequences for the patient.

17. The microcuvette tests and measures the hemoglobin value and is essential in determining the response to therapy.

18. ACT is the activated coagulation time. Blood collected in a prewarmed tube is incubated at 37°C for 1 minute and then inspected by tilting the tube to determine whether a clot has formed. If a clot does not form at 1 minute, the tube is examined every 5 seconds, until a clot forms.

19. The analytes obtained in the ABG are Po_2, Pco_2, pH, and the common electrolytes tested are sodium, potassium, calcium, chloride, and bicarbonate.

20. The electrode placements for the precordial leads of an ECG are:
    V1—fourth intercostal space, right margin of the sternum
    V2—fourth intercostal space, left margin of the sternum
    V3—between position 2 and 4
    V4—fifth intercostal space, junction of midclavicular line
    V5—fifth intercostal space, anterior axillary line
    V6—fifth intercostal space, midaxillary line

Certification Exam Preparation

1.	c	6.	d
2.	b	7.	c
3.	b	8.	a
4.	c	9.	a
5.	d	10.	d

MOCK EXAM ANSWERS

1. C
2. A
3. C
4. A
5. A
6. D
7. B
8. A
9. B
10. C
11. D
12. D
13. B
14. C
15. B
16. C
17. C
18. D
19. D
20. C
21. A
22. D

23. D	76. A
24. D	77. D
25. A	78. A
26. C	79. D
27. D	80. C
28. B	81. C
29. C	82. D
30. A	83. C
31. C	84. A
32. C	85. D
33. B	86. C
34. A	87. C
35. A	88. C
36. B	89. D
37. A	90. B
38. C	91. D
39. A	92. C
40. B	93. B
41. C	94. B
42. D	95. B
43. D	96. A
44. B	97. A
45. D	98. C
46. D	99. D
47. D	100. A
48. D	101. B
49. C	102. B
50. B	103. B
51. D	104. A
52. D	105. C
53. D	106. B
54. D	107. A
55. D	108. D
56. B	109. C
57. C	110. D
58. D	111. B
59. C	112. C
60. D	113. C
61. D	114. B
62. C	115. A
63. C	116. B
64. B	117. A
65. D	118. D
66. D	119. B
67. B	120. D
68. C	121. B
69. C	122. A
70. C	123. A
71. C	124. A
72. A	125. B
73. C	126. B
74. B	127. C
75. B	128. A

129. A	140. B
130. B	141. D
131. C	142. D
132. A	143. B
133. C	144. A
134. D	145. C
135. D	146. D
136. C	147. B
137. A	148. B
138. D	149. D
139. D	150. C

Glossary

accepted standard of care the consensus of medical opinion on what is adequate patient care in a particular situation

accession number unique identifying number used for cataloging a sample in the lab

accreditation official approval of a program from a professional organization

aerobic bacteria bacteria that need oxygen

aerosol mist of droplets

agglutination sticking together

AIDS acquired immunodeficiency syndrome due to human immunodeficiency virus (HIV) infection

airborne infection isolation precautions precautions that are used with patients known or suspected to have serious illnesses transmitted by airborne droplet nuclei

airborne transmission spread of infection either by airborne droplet nuclei or dust particles that contain microorganisms

aliquot portion of sample

allergic contact dermatitis allergic reaction following skin contact with an allergen

allergy inappropriately severe immune reaction to an otherwise harmless substance

amniocentesis collection of amniotic fluid for detection of inherited diseases and other abnormalities

anaerobic bacteria bacteria that live without oxygen

analyte substance being analyzed

anaphylaxis severe immune reaction in which the airways may swell and blood pressure may fall

anatomic/surgical pathology area one of the two main branches of the clinical laboratory, responsible for analyzing cells and tissues

ancillary blood glucose test bedside test to determine blood glucose level, performed by dermal puncture

anticoagulants additives that prevent blood clotting

arterial blood gases (ABG) tests to determine the concentrations of oxygen and carbon dioxide in arterial blood and the pH of the blood

arterial line a vascular access device that is placed in an artery

arteriospasm rapid contraction of the arterial wall

arteriovenous (AV) shunt an artificial connection between an artery and a vein

autoimmunity a condition in which the immune system attacks the body's own tissues

autologous donation donation of a patient's own blood for use at a later time

B cell antibody-producing cell

basilic vein a prominent vein in the antecubital fossa

bacteriostatic an agent that prevents growth of bacteria

biotinidase deficiency inherited metabolic disorder

bleeding time (BT) test a test that measures the length of time required for bleeding to stop after an incision is made

blood bank the department that deals with blood for transfusions; also called *immunohematology department*

blood-borne pathogens infectious agents carried in the blood

blood type the presence and type of antigens on the surface of red blood cells

brachial artery large artery in the antecubital fossa

Broviac a type of central venous catheter; see *central venous catheter*

bulbourethral gland gland supplying fluid for semen

BURPP bilirubin, uric acid, phosphorus, and potassium

butterfly see *winged infusion set*

calcaneus heel bone

capillary blood gas testing alternative to arterial blood gas testing

capillary tube (microhematocrit tube) small plastic tubes used primarily for hematocrit tests

cardiac cycle set of events in one complete heartbeat

cardiopulmonary resuscitation (CPR) emergency manual means to maintain breathing and circulation

catheterized urine sample urine sample collected via a catheter inserted into the bladder

CD4 + cells see *helper T cell*

cellular immunity T-cell mediated immunity

central venous catheter most common vascular access device, inserted into one of the large veins emptying into the heart

central venous line see *central venous catheter*

centrifuge separating components of a sample based on density by using machine that spins a sample at a very high speed

certification verification that an individual has demonstrated proficiency in a particular area of practice

cervix narrow opening between vagina and uterus

chain of custody (COC) protocol that ensures the sample is always in the custody of a person legally entrusted to be in control of it

chain of infection a continuous link between the infection source, means of transmission, and susceptible host

chemical hygiene plan plan that describes all safety procedures, special precautions, and emergency procedures used when working with chemicals

chemistry panel a group of chemistry tests

Clinical Lab Improvement Amendments of 1988 federal law that mandated regulation of all facilities that performed patient testing

clinical laboratory the hospital branch that analyzes samples from a patient at the request of the physician or other health care personnel

Clinical Laboratory Standards Institute nonprofit organization that sets standards and guidelines under the Clinical Lab Improvement Amendments of 1988 (formerly National Committee for Clinical Laboratory Standards)

clinical pathology area one of the two main branches of the clinical laboratory, responsible for analyzing blood and other body fluids

clot activators additives that stimulate clotting

coagulation clotting

cold agglutinins antibodies often formed in response to infection with *Mycoplasma pneumoniae*

collateral circulation accessory supply of blood to a region by more than one artery

College of American Pathologists (CAP) accrediting agency; accreditation by CAP is required for Medicare/Medicaid reimbursement

combining form combination of the word root and the combining vowel

combining vowel a vowel added to a word root to make pronunciation easier

common vehicle transmission transmission by means of contaminated items such as food, water, medications, devices, and equipment

complete blood count an automated test used to test for conditions that affect the number and ratio of cell types in the blood

conduction system system of conductive cells in the heart that trigger contraction

contact precautions precautions used for patients known or suspected to have serious illnesses that are easily transmitted by direct patient contact or by contact with items in the patient's environment

contact transmission transfer of microorganisms from an infected or colonized person to a susceptible host by body surface–to–body surface contact or through contact with a contaminated object

continuing education units credits for participation in a continuing education program

continuous quality improvement major goal of total quality management

cryofibrinogen abnormal type of fibrinogen that precipitates when cold

cryoglobulin abnormal serum protein that precipitates when cold

culture and sensitivity tests to detect and identify microorganisms and to determine the most effective antibiotic therapy

cytokines chemical messengers that include interferons and interleukins

cytotoxic T cells lymphocytes that recognize antigens and directly destroy both foreign cells and infected host cells

damages monetary compensation

delta check quality assurance procedure that helps identify identification errors by comparing previous patient results with current results

depolarization contraction of the heart

dereliction a breach of the duty of care

differential a test to assess the ratio of the different types of white blood cells, and to look for changes in morphology (shape) of red blood cells and platelets

differential count determination of the proportions of the various blood cell types

diluent liquid for dilution

disinfectant an agent used to clean a surface other than living tissue

dorsalis pedis artery artery in the foot

DOT label Department of Transportation label, indicating the type of hazard, the United Nations hazard class number, and a specific identifying number

droplet nuclei particles smaller than 5 micrometers that remain suspended in the air for long periods of time

droplet precautions precautions used for patients known or suspected to have serious illnesses transmitted by large particle droplets

droplet transmission spread of infection through airborne droplets

8-hour specimen see *first morning specimen*

emesis nausea and vomiting

epididymis coiled tube in which sperm mature and are stored

essentials established standards and competencies used in an accredited program

estrogens hormones controlling the female reproductive cycle

expanded precautions precautions targeted at patients known or suspected to be infected with a highly transmissible pathogen

Exposure Control Plan a comprehensive document outlining all procedures and policies for preventing the spread of infection

external arteriovenous (AV) shunt AV shunt consisting of a cannula with a rubber septum, through which a needle may be inserted for drawing blood

fallopian tube tube through which an egg reaches the uterus

feathered edge a blood smear characteristic in which cells farther from the original drop appear to thin out

femoral artery artery in the groin area above the thigh

first morning specimen urine sample collected immediately after a patient wakens; also called *8-hour specimen*

fistula permanent internal connection between an artery and a vein

"flea" metal filing used to mix blood with additives in small tubes

floor book book that contains a variety of information pertinent to the smooth coordination of nursing staff and lab personnel, including laboratory schedules, sweep times, and written notification of any watch changes, plus information on patient preparation, specimen types and handling, and normal values

flow cytometry analytical technique used to identify cellular markers on the surface of white blood cells

fomite contaminated object

forensic related to legal proceedings

gauge a number describing the diameter of a needle's lumen

gonads testes and ovaries

glycolysis metabolic sugar breakdown within cells

Groshong a type of central venous catheter; see *central venous catheter*

health maintenance organization health care delivery system that functions as full-service outpatient clinics, providing all or almost all medical specialties under one roof

health care–associated infections infections contracted by a patient during a hospital stay

helper T cells regulators of the immune response

hematocrit test to determine the percentage of the blood volume that is red blood cells

hematoma a reddened, swollen area in which blood collects under the skin

hemochromatosis excess of iron in the blood

hemoconcentration an increase in the ratio of formed elements to plasma, usually caused by leaving the tourniquet on too long

hemolysis destruction of red blood cells

hemostasis the process by which the body stops blood from leaking out of a wound

heparin or saline lock a tube temporarily placed in a peripheral vein; used to administer medicine and draw blood

Hickman a type of central venous catheter; see *central venous catheter*

human chorionic gonadotropin (HCG) a hormone produced by the placenta after implantation of a fertilized egg

human leukocyte antigen (HLA) see major histocompatibility complex

humoral immunity antibody-based immunity

hyperventilation rapid shallow breathing

icteric related to jaundice

immunization deliberate provocation of an immune response to stimulate immune memory

immunohematology see *blood bank*

implanted port a chamber located under the skin and connected to an indwelling line

incident report prompt and complete documentation of the circumstances of an incident

infection an invasion by and growth of a microorganism in the human body that causes disease

informed consent consent to a procedure with full understanding of the risks and the right to refuse to undergo the procedure

interferon a type of cytokine

interleukin a type of cytokine

internal arteriovenous (AV) shunt AV shunt consisting of a fistula that uses the patient's tissue, a piece of bovine tissue, or a synthetic tube

iontophoresis induction of sweat by application of a weak electric current

iontophoretic pilocarpine test detection of salt levels in sweat; used as part of the diagnosis for cystic fibrosis

irritant contact dermatitis direct irritation of the skin by contact with a chemical irritant

isolation to separate an infection source from susceptible hosts, thereby breaking the chain of infection

Joint Commission on Accreditation of Healthcare Organizations organization that sets standards regarding systems to monitor and evaluate the quality of patient care

latex sensitivity response to latex proteins in gloves and other medical equipment; usually leads to contact dermatitis

leads ECG electrodes

liability insurance insurance that covers monetary damages that must be paid if the defendant loses a liability suit

liable to be legally responsible for an action or inaction

licensure a documented permit issued by a government agency, either municipal or state, that grants the bearer permission to perform a particular service or procedure

lipemic related to increased fats in the serum

Luer adapter a device for adapting a butterfly needle to an evacuated tube

lumen the hollow tube within a needle

lymphostasis lack of movement of lymph fluid

major histocompatibility complex set of surface proteins detected by the immune system that are used to distinguish self tissue from nonself

malpractice delivery of substandard care that results in harm to a patient

maple syrup disease inherited metabolic disorder

materials safety data sheet sheet that provides information on the chemical, its hazards, and procedures for cleanup and first aid

median antecubital vein a prominent vein in the antecubital fossa

memory cells B cells specialized to respond quickly upon the second encounter with an antigen

memory T cells T cells that are primed to respond rapidly if an antigen is encountered again later in life

microcollection tube small tube used to collect dermal puncture samples; "bullet"

micropipet (Caraway pipet or Natelson pipet) large glass capillary tube

midstream clean catch most common procedure for collecting any type of urine specimen

modified Allen test test for collateral circulation

molecular diagnostics department that analyzes DNA within a variety of tissues

multisample needle a double-ended needle designed to be used with an evacuated tube system

nasopharyngeal culture used to diagnose whooping cough, croup, pneumonia, and other upper respiratory tract infections

National Committee for Clinical Laboratory Standards see *Clinical Laboratory Standards Institute*

needle adapter translucent plastic cylinder connecting a multisample needle to an evacuated tube

negligence failure to perform an action consistent with the accepted standard of care

NFPA label National Fire Protection Association label that serves to warn fire fighters of the location of hazardous materials in the event of a fire

occluded blocked

occult blood specimen fecal specimen for detection of blood in the stool

order of draw the prescribed sequence in which tubes with different additives should be filled during a multitube collection

OSHA Occupational Safety and Health Administration; responsible for regulations governing workplace safety

osteochondritis painful inflammation of the bone or cartilage

osteomyelitis bone infection

out-of-court settlement a settlement in which the two parties reach an agreement without the intervention of a judge or jury

ovaries site of egg production

ovulation release of an egg

P wave part of the normal ECG tracing

palpation probing or feeling

partial pressure of carbon dioxide amount of carbon dioxide dissolved in the blood

partial pressure of oxygen amount of oxygen dissolved in the blood

pathogens infectious organisms

penis the male copulation organ

peripherally inserted central catheter a vascular access device threaded into a central vein after insertion into a peripheral (noncentral) vein

personal protective equipment fluid-resistant gowns, masks, respirators, face shields, shoe covers, and gloves

petechiae small red spots appearing on the skin that are caused by a tourniquet that is too tight

phlebotomy the practice of drawing blood

physician office lab physicians in a group practice that may employ a phlebotomist to collect patient samples

plaintiff person claiming to have been harmed by the defendant

plasma cells B cells specialized for producing antibodies

pneumatic tube system sample transport system in which samples are carried in a sealed container within a network of tubes

polycythemia excessive production of red blood cells

PR interval part of the normal ECG tracing

preanalytical variables variables that occur prior to performing the analysis of the specimen

preferred provider organization a group of doctors and hospitals who offer their services to large employers to provide health care to employees

prefix a word part preceding the root

procedure manual book that contains protocols and other information about all the tests performed in the lab, including the principle behind the test, purpose of performing it, specimen type the test requires, collection method, and equipment and supplies required

professional services hospital branch that, at the request of the physician, provides services that aid in the diagnosis and treatment of the patient; includes the clinical laboratory

progesterone hormone controlling the reproductive cycle

prostate gland supplying fluid for semen

protected health information any part of a patient's health information that is linked to information that identifies the patient

protective environment isolation of immunocompromised patients to prevent exposing them to infection

QRS complex part of the normal ECG tracing

QT interval part of the normal ECG tracing

quality assurance set of methods used to guarantee quality patient care

quality control quantitative methods used to monitor the quality of procedures

quality phlebotomy a set of policies and procedures designed to ensure the delivery of consistently high-quality patient care and specimen analysis

radial artery artery supplying the hand

radioactive hazard symbol symbol used to mark areas where radioactivity is used

random specimen a specimen that may be collected at any time

rapid Group A Strep test for the rapid detection of Group A *Streptococcus* bacteria

reagent test chemical

reference laboratory an independent laboratory that analyzes samples from other health care facilities

reflux flow of blood from the collection tube back into the needle and then into the patient's vein

repolarization relaxation and recovery of the heart after contraction

requisition form specifying which tests must be run or which samples to collect

reservoir a person carrying an infectious agent without being sick

respiratory steady state state required for ABG collection, in which blood gas concentrations are steady

reverse isolation see protective isolation

root the main part of a word

scalp artery artery used for arterial blood collection in infants

sclerosed hardened

scrotum sac containing the testes

seminal vesicles glands supplying fluid for semen

sepsis bacterial infection

serum plasma without its clotting factors

72-hour stool specimen specimen used for quantitative fecal fat determination

severe combined immune deficiency (SCID) inherited disorder marked by almost total lack of B and T cells

sharps needles, lancets, broken glass, and other sharp items

sickle-cell anemia inherited disorder of the hemoglobin molecule

ST segment part of the normal ECG tracing

standard precautions an infection control method that uses barrier protection and work control practices to prevent direct skin contact with blood, other body fluids, and tissues from all persons

standards established requirements used in an accredited program

STAT a requisition requiring immediate attention and processing

stylus recording pen of the ECG machine

suffix a word part following the root

suprapubic aspiration sample collected via a needle inserted through the abdominal wall into the bladder

sweat electrolytes salt present in normal sweat; used as part of the diagnosis for cystic fibrosis

syncope fainting

T wave part of the normal ECG tracing

testosterone principal male sex hormone

therapeutic phlebotomy removal of blood from a patient's system as part of the treatment for a disorder

thixotropic gel an inert additive used to separate cells from plasma during centrifugation

thrombosis clot formation within a blood vessel

timed specimens a series of samples often collected over 24 hours and combined to provide a single, large specimen

tort an injury to one person for which another person who caused the injury is legally responsible

total quality management entire set of approaches used by an institution to provide customer satisfaction

triple lumen see *central venous catheter*

tube advancement mark mark on a needle adapter indicating how far the tube can be pushed in without losing vacuum

tube holder see *needle adapter*

umbilical artery artery used for arterial collection in infants

unintentional torts unintentional injury; the basis for most medical malpractice claims

urethra tube carrying urine from the bladder

urgent care center an outpatient clinic that provides walk-in services to patients who cannot wait for a scheduled appointment with their primary health care provider

uterus site of egg implantation and fetal development

vagina passage in a female in which sperm and semen are deposited during intercourse

vas deferens tube in a male through which sperm reach the urethra

vascular access device a tube that is inserted into either a vein or artery; used to administer fluids or medications, monitor blood pressure, or draw blood

vector transmission transmission of infectious agents by organisms that are not harmed by their presence

venous thrombosis formation of a blood clot within a vein

winged infusion set small needle and flexible tube for delicate veins; "butterfly"

Index

Page numbers followed by b indicate
boxes; f, figures; and t, tables.